Mechanisms of Clinical Exercise Prescription

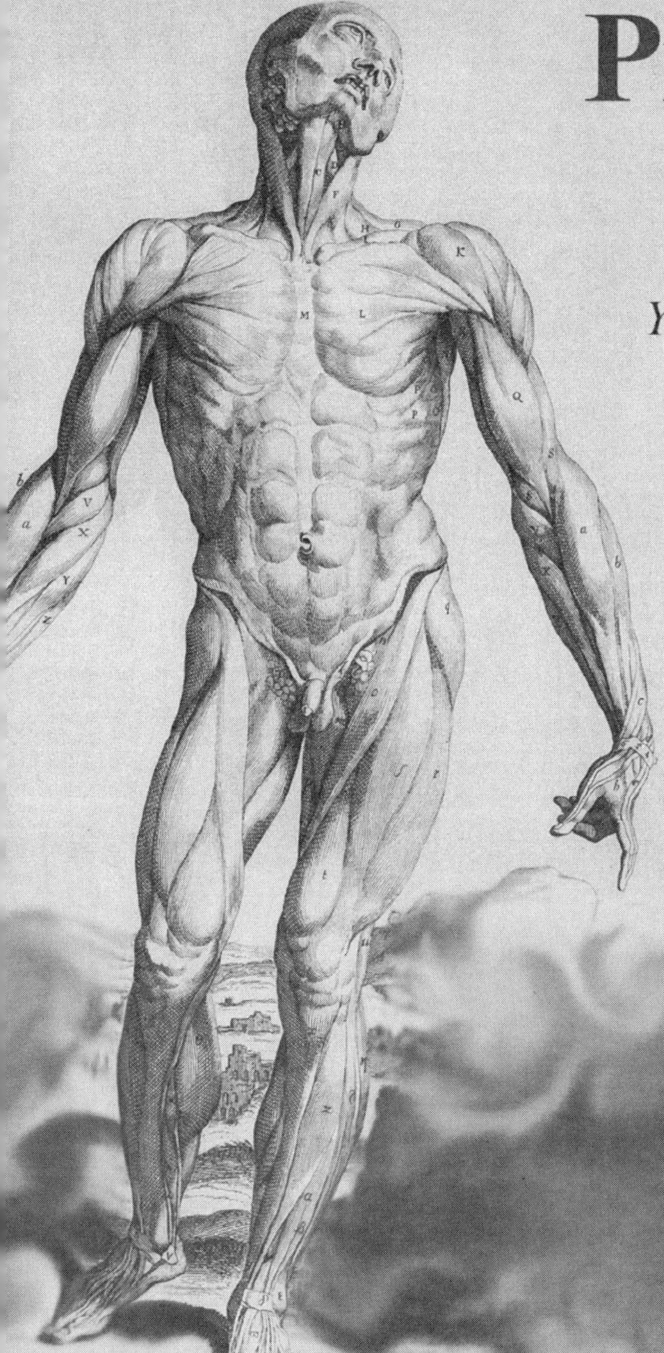

Yong-Seok Jee · Kang-Ho Kim

21st publishing

Preface

We are living in a modern age and are exposed to many lifestyle diseases (adult diseases), and many patients are already suffering from diseases. These adult diseases, along with a healthy lifestyle and regular exercise habits can be improved, prevented, and treatment can be expected. Unfortunately, many books related to this context are emerging, but in fact, it is not easy to understand how to manage patients by disease in the clinic. The purpose of this textbook is to compare the theories and the theories that have been published up to the present, based on the clinical experience up to now, in order to improve the understanding of mechanisms of exercise prescription based on human physiology and kinesiology in the training of health provider and exercise instructor.

In Chapter 1, Exercise and Health, we have described the reasons for exercise and the physiological changes during or after physical activity. In Chapter 2, Exercise and Nutrition, we have dealt with the right diet and the ratio of nutrients. In Chapter 3, Clinical Exercise Prescription, we have newly refurbished the principle and basis for practically managing the patient in the clinic, and prepared the interpretation of the electrocardiogram (ECG) more easily. In Chapter 4, Clinical Kinesiology discusses exercise methods that must be performed directly at the clinical hospital. Of course, considering clinical conditions, we have to emphasize flexibility exercise, cardiopulmonary endurance exercise, muscle strength and endurance exercise aiming at development of health related fitness. On the other hand, through Chapter 5, Clinical Sports Medicine, information and programs to be provided to various patients in the clinic were presented, and the characteristics of the drugs applied to each disease were discussed in detail.

This book features the latest information provided by American College of Sports Medicine (ACSM) and incorporates the contents provided by American Heart Association (AHA) and various official institutions in accordance with the Korean situation. We would also like to express our heartfelt gratitude to the disciples who helped to keep us close and to the 21st century company.

Yong-Seok Jee · Kang-Ho Kim

Contents

Chapter 4 Clinical Kinesiology 169

Chapter 5 Clinical Sports Medicine 209

Chapter 1

Exercise and Health

Goals

- To understand the meaning of the 2 QoL gotten through working out.
- To understand the changes of exercise metabolism in human physiology.
- To understand the mechanism of carbohydrate and fat during exercise.
- To understand the changes of physiological variables through physical training.

Why Should We Exercise?

In modern times, many of us live prosperous lives and reap great benefits from our sophisticated culture. However, can one truly say that we as a species are healthier than ever before? In fact, our ancestors had many physical ailments such as growth disorders, postural malformations, arthritis and neuralgia. This was due to the intense manual labor and physical activity that was required for them to survive. However, these ailments do not have the same characteristics of the adult disease, or lifestyle-related diseases, we suffer from today. In other words, we, living in modern times, have a whole new category of health problems to deal with known as hypokinetic disorders. Hypokinetic disorders are a result of a lack of physical activity in our daily lives, most likely due to scientific advancements in today's society. This lack of physical activity is often accompanied by irreverent and erroneous eating habits, leading to premature death from disorders such as obesity, diabetes mellitus, hypertension, heart disease, cancer, and cerebral stroke.

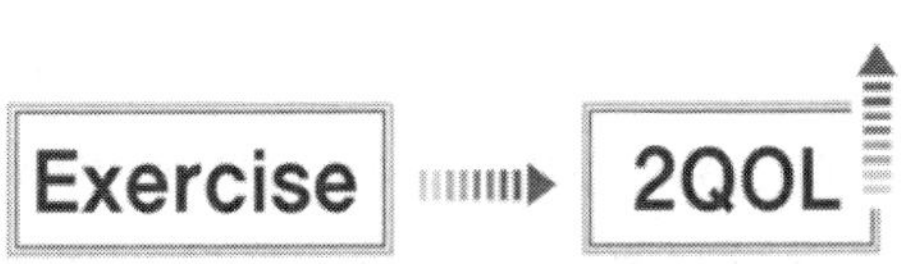

Hypokinetic disorders progress extremely slowly in the body without us knowing it, so once subjective symptoms begin to surface, the disorder has already progressed considerably. For this reason, prevention should be given priority over treatment. Proper eating habits and healthy lifestyles are important for prevention and treatment of these disorders, but frequent exercise is more important than anything else. This fact is highlighted further by the result of the recently published study, "Exercise can prevent cancer".[15,16] Ultimately, the reason we should exercise is to increase not only the quantity of life (QoL), but also the quality of life (QoL) through treatment as well as prevention of modern illnesses.

Mechanisms of Exercise Physiology in Human

Energy Production

A human body without the proper energy source simply cannot function - much like a car engine. In other words, the human body cannot move without energy. In this way, energy becomes the most important part of our life, and we cannot evaluate physical work without considering our energy source.

There are many different types of energy used by the human body, such as electrical, chemical, mechanical, and thermal energy, and they all have different characteristics. These types of energy can be converted to and from each other. For example, when we try to contract the biceps brachii while holding a 1.5 ㎏ dumbbell, the brain sends commands to the muscles via electrical energy through motor nerves in only raising that 1.5 ㎏ weight. When this command reaches the final part of the nerve and muscle (at the motor end plate), it sends chemical energy to the muscle to cause mechanical contraction. However, this example is only possible when there is enough energy in the muscle, therefore we must consume nutrients to maintain sufficient energy levels.

Carbohydrate and fat are the main nutrients that are used as energy in our body during exercise.[1] Fat produces about 9 ㎉ per gram, while carbohydrate produces around 4 ㎉ per gram. In this way, fat seems to be a much more efficient energy source, however, this is only the case if you have enough oxygen or if you are performing extremely low intensity exercise. Because the human body cannot inhale oxygen indefinitely, carbohydrate produces a lot more energy in less time when compared to fat. Thus, most of the energy used during exercise is supplied by carbohydrate. Nutrients and energy used during exercise are discussed in detail in Chapter 2, "Exercise and Nutrition".

Energy Source

All nutrients taken from food should be converted to adenosine triphosphate (ATP), a direct energy source in the body. Specifically, the absorbed nutrients are broken down and degraded by enzymes, resulting in a conversion to ATP, an energy source for physical activity. There are two ways in which ATP can be supplied to muscle cells. One way is through the anaerobic system which supplies ATP in the absence of oxygen, whereas the other way is through the aerobic system which produces and supplies ATP only when oxygen is present.

Anaerobic System

The process of energy release in the absence of sufficient oxygen levels, which includes the adenosine triphosphate and phosphocreatine (ATP-PC) system and the anaerobic glycolysis processes.

ATP-PC System

The ATP-PC system is the main source for short-term, high-intensity activities (e.g., leaps and short sprints), and it is the first fuel source for all forms of exercise, regardless of intensity. For example, during the first few seconds of a lightweight 5 ㎞ jog or moderate intensity indoor cycling, energy for muscle activity comes primarily from the ATP-PC system. This energy process depends on the chemical reaction of ATP, phosphocreatine (or creatine phosphate) and two different phosphagens, which involve myosin ATP enzyme (ATPase) and creatine enzyme (creatine kinase). ATPase catalyzes the decomposition of ATP to form adenosine diphosphate (ADP) and inorganic phosphate (Pi), which releases energy. Creatine enzyme catalyzes the synthesis of ATP from ADP and PC, and PC allows one phosphate group to bind to ADP to form ATP. These reactions supply energy at a rapid rate, but since ATP and PC are only stored in the muscle, the ATP-PC system does not supply enough energy for persistent or long-term activities. In general, Type II (fast-twitch) muscle fibers have more phosphagens than Type I (slow-twitch) muscle fibers.

The activity of the creatine enzyme mainly regulates the decomposition of PC. Increased ADP concentration in muscle cells promotes the activity of creatine enzyme, while the increase of ATP concentration inhibits the activity of creatine enzyme. At the beginning of exercise, ATP breaks down into ADP and releases energy for muscle contraction. This increase in ADP concentration activates the creatinine enzyme and promotes ATP formation through decomposition of PC. The activity of the creatine enzyme is maintained in an elevated state when the exercise continues at high intensity. On the other hand, if the exercise is stopped, or if low-intensity exercise is maintained to sustain a sufficient amount of ATP for the energy requirement of the muscle cells, the ATP concentration within the muscle cells is increased, which finally reduces enzyme activity. In fact, ATP and PC are separate substances that produce energy. In other words, ATP releases energy as it is decomposed into ADP and Pi, and PC releases energy as it is decomposed into Pi and C (creatine) [Fig. 1.1].

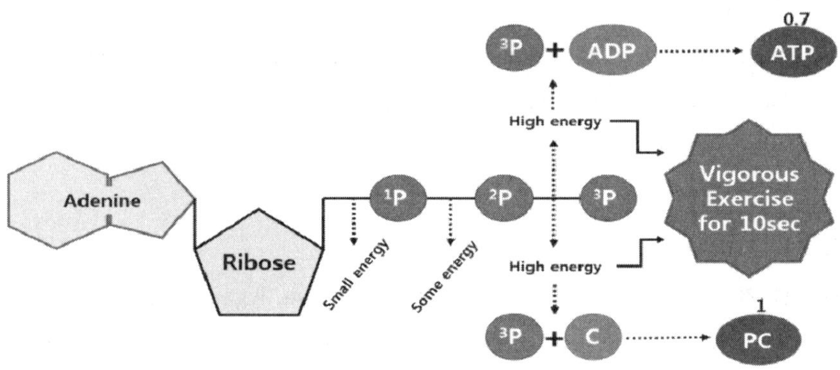

Fig. 1.1 ***Energy releasing process of ATP and PC***

Both substances work during exercise that require strong and vigorous power. However, the amount stored in muscles is limited, so it acts during movements that takes about 10 to 15 seconds, such as a 100 m sprint or a javelin throw.[3] Characteristically, when two substances are decomposed by enzymatic action to release energy, some energy is used to refill each other.

Glycolysis

Glycolysis refers to the decomposition process of carbohydrates in the state of insufficient oxygen, as shown in [Fig. 1.2]. It refers to the process in which either glycogen stored in muscle, or glucose present in blood, supply ATP. ATP supplied by glycolysis initially replenishes the ATP-PC system. After that, it becomes the main source of ATP for high-intensity muscle activity which can last about 2 minutes. An example of this system in use could be from a tennis game during a continuous volley. Glycolysis contains many enzymes that catalyze a series of chemical reactions. Enzymes for glycolysis are found in the protoplasm of the cell (myogenic for muscle cells).

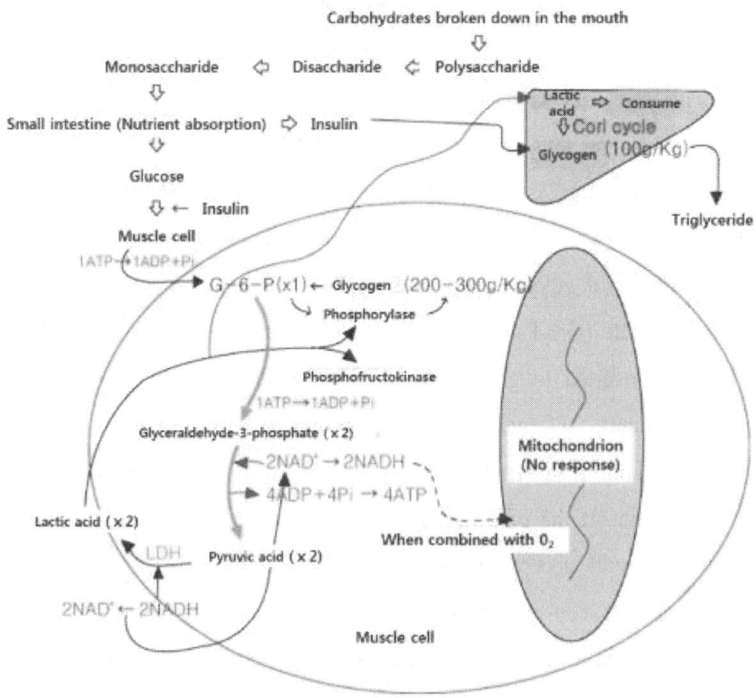

Fig. 1.2 ***Carbohydrate storage of muscles and liver and glycolitic processes in muscle cells***

Glycolysis occurs in one of two ways: fast glycolysis, or slow glycolysis. Pyruvic acid, the final product of fast glycolysis, provides ATP at a faster rate than slow glycolysis. Pyruvic acid can also be converted to lactic acid, leading to acidosis, which can cause muscle fatigue. However, pyruvic acid is also transported to mitochondria for energy production during the aerobic oxidation process. Fast glycolysis is often called anaerobic glycolysis, and slow glycolysis is called aerobic glycolysis. However, since glycolysis itself is not dependent on oxygen, these terms may be somewhat inappropriate for describing the process. The fate of the final product (pyruvic acid) is regulated by the energy requirements of the cell. If energy is to be supplied at a high rate (during resistance training for example), fast glycolysis is mainly used. On the other hand, at the beginning of a low intensity aerobic dance, slow glycolysis is activated because the energy requirement is low and oxygen is already present in the cells in sufficient quantities. Another interesting byproduct is the reduced form of nicotinamide-adenine dinucleotide (NADH), a substance that enters the electron transport chain (ETC) system for more advanced ATP production. The oxidized form of NAD can be expressed as NAD^+. The reduced form means that hydrogen is added. The final reaction of fast glycolysis and slow glycolysis can be summarized as shown in [Fig. 1.4].

As shown in [Fig. 1.2], the glucose absorbed in the small intestine is transported to the liver (100 g/kg) and muscles (200 to 300 g/kg) by the hormone insulin produced in the pancreas and the rest is transported to adipose tissue and stored in the form of triglyceride (TG).

During the process of glucose entry into muscle cells, ATP is consumed and converted to glucose-6-phosphate (G-6-P). G6P is converted to glycogen when it is stable, but once it is used, it is converted to glyceraldehyde-3-phosphate, which consumes another ATP molecule. Subsequently, D-glyceraldehyde-3-phosphate is oxidized by the NADH, an electron acceptor and a substitute for oxygen, to form 3 ATP molecules and to be converted to pyruvate. If the mitochondria do not accept hydrogen in an oxygen-deficient situation, pyruvate will accept hydrogen and form lactic acid.[2] In particular, lactate dehydrogenase (LDH) converts pyruvate to lactic acid more rapidly in this process. Ultimately, the formation of lactic acid can be said to be the recycling process of NAD, that is, the conversion of NADH to NAD [Fig. 1.3].

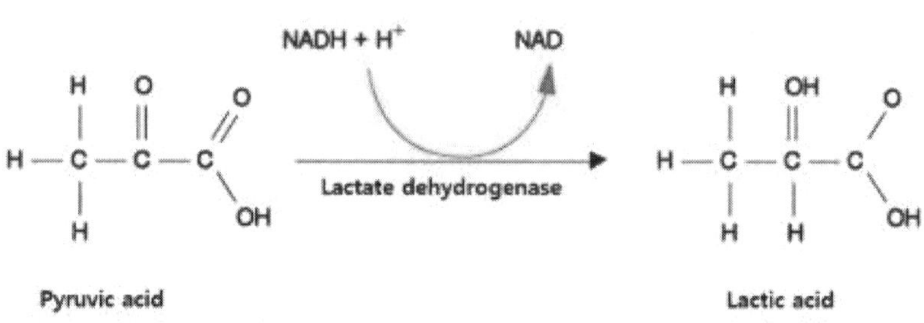

Fig. 1.3 ***Formation of lactic acid and NAD***[12]

When the supernatant adds two hydrogen atoms, lactic acid and NAD form, which can then be used in the process. This reaction is catalyzed by LDH.

Lactic acid produced in glycolysis reduces the activity of phosphorylase and phosphofructokinase (PFK), thereby inhibiting glycolysis and preventing prolonged exercise.[4] However, small amounts of lactic acid are delivered to the liver, some are consumed, and some are converted to carbohydrates. This process is called gluconeogenesis, or the Cori cycle. Glycolysis, like the ATP-PC system, is used when energy supply is needed quickly, but it works when exercising between 1 and 3 minutes, such as an 800-m run. Glycolysis is summarized in [Fig. 1.4].

Fast glycolysis

Glucose + $2P_i$ + 2ADP → 2 Lactic acid + 2 ATP + H_2O

↓

Energy → Moderate exercise for 1~3min

Slow glycolysis

Glucose + $2P_i$ + 2ADP + NAD^+ → 2 Pyruvic acid + 2 ATP + 2NADH + $2H_2O$

↓

Energy → Moderate exercise for 1~3min

Fig. 1.4 ***Energy release process in glycolysis***

Aerobic System

Exercises of moderate intensity, supplied with sufficient oxygen in muscle cells, do not accumulate lactate. In other words, if oxygen is sufficient during the glycolysis process in [Fig. 1.2], pyruvate is not converted to lactic acid, but instead enters the mitochondria. Pyruvate in mitochondria produces ATP via the TCA (tricarboxylic acid) cycle, the Krebs cycle, or the ETC. Once ATP is produced, the remaining chemical components of pyruvate are decomposed into carbon dioxide (CO_2) and water (H_2O). For reference, when oxygen supply is sufficient, mitochondria in muscle cells produce energy from carbohydrates, fats, and proteins [Fig. 1.5].

The Process of Using Carbohydrates

In aerobic systems, one molecule of carbohydrate is completely decomposed into CO_2 and H_2O to produce 38 ATP molecules. However, two of these molecules are produced by anaerobic glycolysis [Fig. 1.6]. When oxygen is sufficient, the pyruvate produced in the process of [Fig. 1.5] is decomposed by a chain reaction called the TCA cycle. The main purpose of the TCA cycle is to remove hydrogen from the reactants contained in the cycle.

Specifically, pyruvate from the aerobic process enters the TCA cycle after a slight change in chemistry. Once inside this cycle, two more advanced chemical reactions take place. That is, the release of CO_2 from the lungs, and the oxidation1) of hydrogen ions (H^+) and electrons (e^-), which go into the ETC system for further chemical conversion.[14]

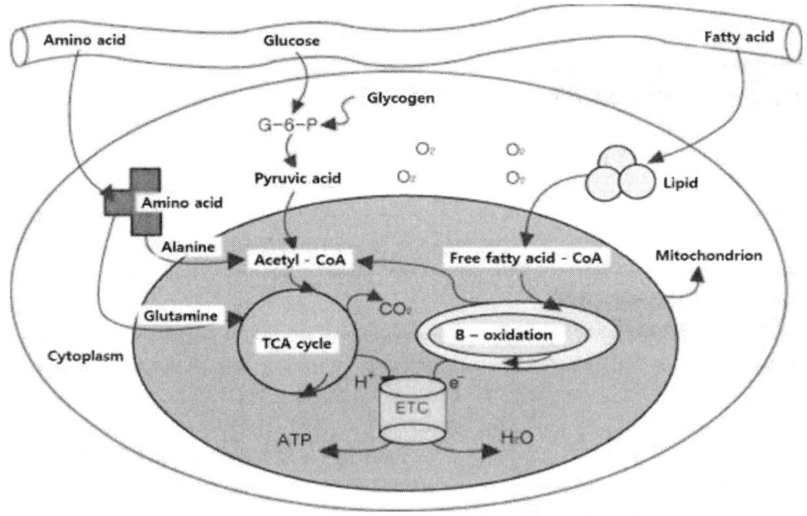

Fig. 1.5 ***Aerobic process using carbohydrates, fats and proteins***

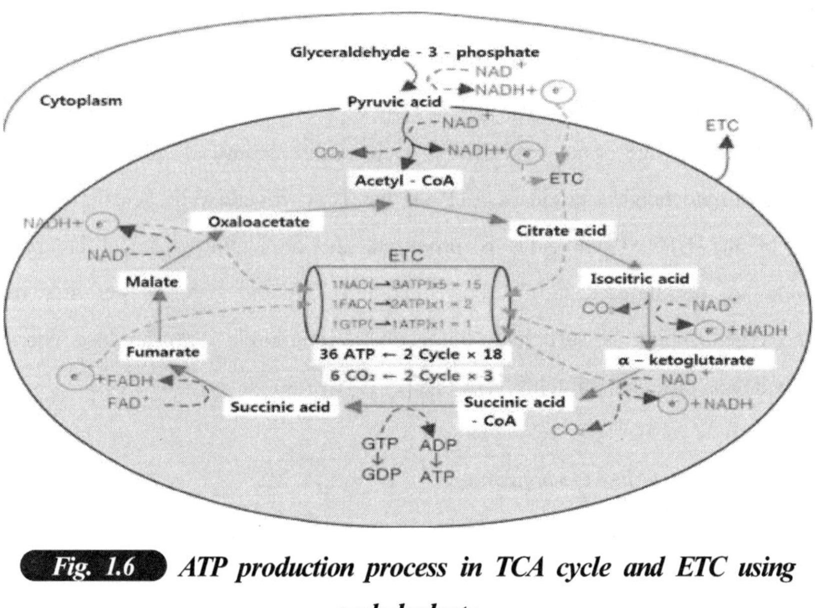

Fig. 1.6 ***ATP production process in TCA cycle and ETC using carbohydrate***

---

1) Oxidation: The process by which one molecule combines with oxygen or removes hydrogen from that material. Or a reaction in which one molecule releases electrons to increase the number of cation atoms.

The hydrogen ions and electrons released from glycolysis and the TCA cycle enter the ETC system as NADH and FADH, and ATP is obtained by the reaction of releasing electrons. The process of producing ATP by continuous oxidation in the ETC system is called oxidative phosphorylation. What happens in an ETC system is that a hydrogen ion and an electron are combined with oxygen by a series of enzymatic reactions to form water, which is a final product. That is, ATP is formed through a binding reaction when water is formed [Fig. 1.7]. For reference, in the ETC system, 3 ATP is generated when NADH is involved and 2 ATP when FADH is involved. In other words, in [Fig. 1.7], FADH generates only 2 ATP since it enters after ⓐ reaction.

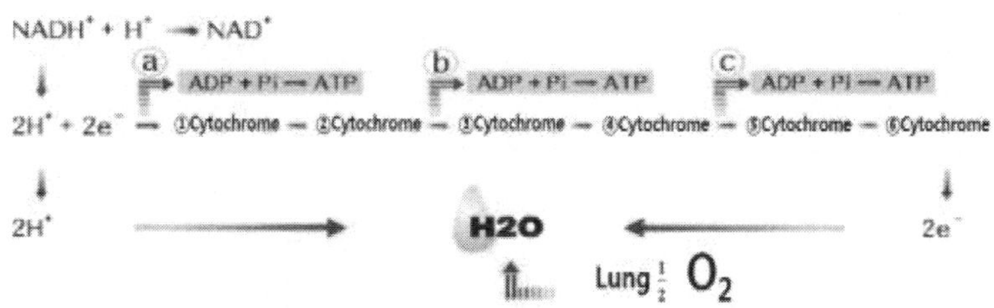

Fig. 1.7 ***Generating NADH and APT***

The cytochrome enzyme responsible for the transport of electrons (e⁻) in the ETC is a substance consisting of protein and iron.

Carbohydrate decomposition during the aerobic process is summarized in [Fig. 1.8]. For reference, the process of carbohydrate degradation can be evaluated using a gas analyzer. As shown in the diagram in [Fig. 1.8], six oxygen atoms are needed to dissolve one molecule of carbohydrate and ultimately, six carbon atoms remain. The respiratory exchange rate (RQ) can be calculated by dividing the amount of CO_2 emitted by the oxygen used, which is 1 for carbohydrates.

$$1\ C_6H_{12}O_6 + \underline{6O_2} \cdots\cdots \triangleright\ \underline{6CO_2} + 6H_2O + \underline{38ATP}$$

↓

Energy → Exercise over 3 min

Calculation of respiratory exchange rate (RQ) in gas test during GXT :

Amount of carbon dioxide (**$6CO_2$**) ÷ Amount of oxygen (**$6O_2$**) = **1**

Fig. 1.8 ***Energy release process through carbohydrates during aerobic exercise***

The Process of Using Fat

Since fat has a higher number of carbon bonds than carbohydrates, it produces a large amount of ATP, but it has to undergo as much decomposition. This decomposition process is called β-oxidation.[6] Stearic acid, which is a raw material of beef, goes through the β-oxidation cycle 8 times, using 26 oxygen atoms, and producing 147 ATP molecules [Fig. 1.9].

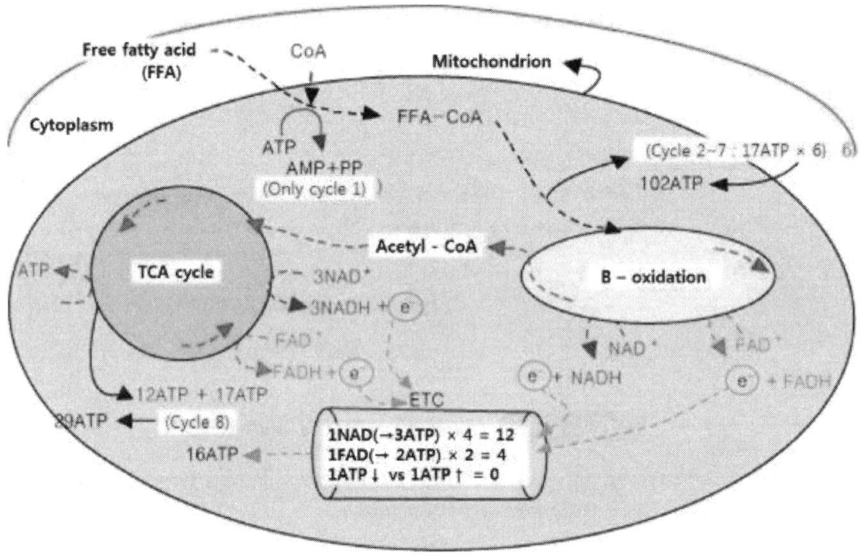

Fig. 1.9 ***ATP production in β-oxidation using fatty acids***

$$1\ CH_3(CH_2)_{16}COOH + \underline{26O_2} \cdots\cdots \triangleright\ \underline{18CO_2} + 18H_2O + \underline{147ATP}$$

↓

Exercise for a long time ← Energy

Calculation of respiratory exchange rate (RQ) in gas test during GXT :

Amount of carbon dioxide ($\mathbf{18CO_2}$) ÷ Amount of oxygen ($\mathbf{26O_2}$) = **0.7**

Fig. 1.10 ***Energy release process through fat during aerobic exercise***

As shown in [Fig. 1.9], stearic acid produces a large amount of ATP through a total of 8 β-oxidation steps. In the first cycle, 17 ATP molecules are produced in total. However, 1 ATP molecule is consumed, therefore 16 ATP molecules remain. During the second to the seventh cycles, 102 (17 × 6) ATPs are produced. In the last cycle, 29

ATPs are generated by adding 17 ATPs generated in one complete cycle and 12 ATPs generated from the TCA cycle. This is summarized in [Fig. 1.10]. For reference, the decomposition of fatty acids can be evaluated using a gas analyzer. As shown in [Fig. 1.10], 26 oxygen atoms are needed to dissolve one molecule of fatty acid and ultimately, 18 carbon atoms remain. The RQ can be calculated by dividing the amount of carbon dioxide emitted by the oxygen used, which is about 0.7 in the case of fatty acids.

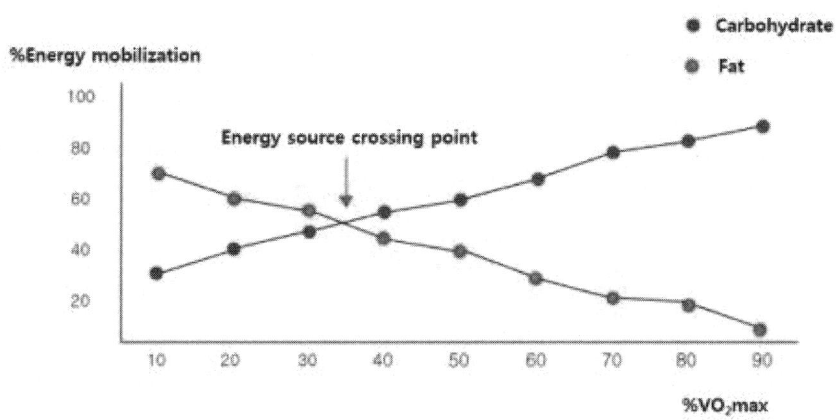

Fig. 1.11 *Crossing point of energy substrate during exercise*[12]

Fats, on the other hand, produce energy in mitochondria in myocytes when oxygen is fully supplied. It is derived from TG stored in muscle cells, adipose tissue, blood or free fatty acids sequentially. The enzyme that breaks down TG into free fatty acids and glycerol is lipase. This enzyme is activated by epinephrine, norepinephrine, and glucagon, but is inhibited by insulin. The increase in sympathetic nerves during exercise increases the hormones of epinephrine, norepinephrine, and glucagon and decreases the insulin. Lactic acid, a byproduct of strenuous exercise, also reduces lipase activity and inhibits fatty acid mobilization. Therefore, as glycolysis accelerates and lactic acid production increases during strenuous exercise, fatty acid mobilization is suppressed, so the rate of using fat as a source of energy is reduced. In other words, fatty acid mobilization increases at a low exercise intensity of less than 30% of maximum oxygen uptake ($\dot{V}O_2max$), while carbohydrate acts as the main energy substrate for exercise when $\dot{V}O_2max$ is above 70% [Fig. 1.11].

[Fig. 1.11] shows that when exercise intensity is increased, the energy substrate is converted from fat to carbohydrate, which makes it impossible to exercise for a long period of time. The theoretical causes are as follows. Firstly, high-intensity exercise stimulates Type II muscle fibers that are well adapted to explosive force among the muscle fibers. While these muscle fibers are rich in glycolytic enzymes, their mitochondria and lipolytic enzyme content are so low that exercise cannot be sustained for long durations. Secondly, as exercise intensity increases, hormones such as epinephrine increase, and glycogen in muscle is used as energy. This is the theory that it rapidly depletes the stored glycogen whilst increasing the amount of lactic acid produced, thereby inhibiting continuous exercise.

When exercise intensity is lowered and exercise duration is longer than 30 minutes, the energy substrate is converted from carbohydrate to fat. As mentioned above, fat is degraded by an enzyme called lipase, which only works when the hormones epinephrine, norepinephrine, and glucagon are activated. During low-intensity long-term exercise, the concentration of epinephrine in the blood increases, thereby increasing the lipase and accelerating lipolysis. On the other hand, insulin has a high affinity for glucose, which is a degradation product of carbohydrates, and therefore inhibits the mobilization of fatty acids when the insulin concentration in the blood is high.[7,9] For example, if a high-carbohydrate meal or drink is consumed 30 to 60 minutes before exercise, the insulin secretion is promoted in the pancreas to reduce fat metabolism, thereby preventing long-term exercise. The contribution of fat and carbohydrates to exercise duration is shown in [Fig. 1.12].

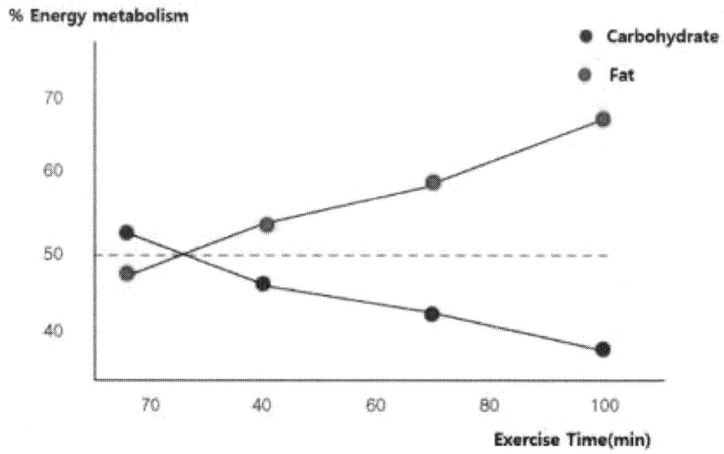

Fig. 1.12 ***Changes in carbohydrate and fat metabolism with exercise time***

The Process of Using Protein

Protein contributes as an energy source very rarely compared to carbohydrates and fats. After carbohydrates and fats are depleted as energy sources, a small amount of protein is used. The amount is approximately 16 ATP molecules, which increases by up to 15% after 1 hour of exercise.[11] Protein is also used as an energy substrate in cases of severe fasting, or in diabetic patients with abnormal carbohydrate metabolism, except when participating in extremely long-term exercise.[8]

In order for protein to be used as an energy source, it can only function as an amino acid. Amino acids are the most basic constituent of the proteins that make up the human body. Around 22 kinds of amino acids are combined with other amino acids to form all cells and organs such as hair, bones, muscles, nerve cells, and white blood cells. When protein is completely decomposed, ammonia and free amino acids are produced.[10,13] The separated amino acids are usually bonded to carbon atoms such as amino group (NH_2) and a carboxyl group (COOH) to form a general formula of R-$CHNH_2$-COOH (R is aromatic). The major amino acids constituting the protein are shown in [Table 1.1].

As shown in [Table 1.1], the main amino acids synthesized in the body are called non-essential amino acids (13 species), but amino acids that cannot be synthesized in the body and instead can only be obtained through food intake are known as essential amino acids (9 species).

Table 1.1 ***Types of amino acids***

Major amino acid(22)		Other amino acid(8)
Essential amino acid(9)	Non-essential amino acid(13)	
Valine	Glycine	β-alanine
Leucine	**Alanine**	Aminobutyric acid
Isoleucine	Serine	Ornithine
Threonine	Cysteine	Citrulline
Methionine	Cystine	Threonine
Lysine	Aspartate	Triiodotyrosine
Phenylalanine	Asparagine	Thyroxine
Tryptophan	Glutamine	Deoxyphenylalanine
Histidine : only childhood	Iodotyrosine	
	Arginine	
	Tyrosine	
	Proline	
	Oxyproline	

The main pathway in which amino acids are used as an energy substrate is when the amino group in the mitochondria binds to pyruvate to form alanine, another amino acid, which is transported to the liver to become liver glycogen. This path is called the "glucose-alanine cycle" and this process is called gluconeogenesis. In addition, many amino acids contribute to ATP production in the mitochondria through several pathways, as shown in [Fig. 1.13].

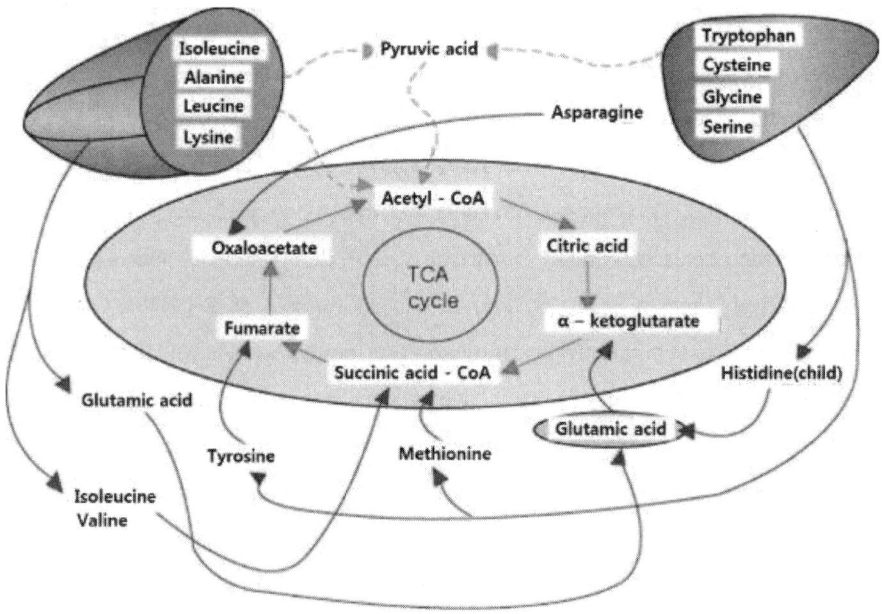

Fig. 1.13 ***Access pathway to TCA cycle for ATP generation of amino acids***

Ultimately, the three systems that supply ATP differ in the fuel used, the amount of ATP produced, the rate of ATP production, and the maximum supply capacity. This is summarized in [Table 1.2].

Table 1.2 ***Comparison of characteristics of ATP supply system***

		Fuel used	Oxygen requirement	ATP supply rate	ATP generation (molecules)
Anaerobic process	ATP-PC	PC	Non-involvement	Fast	0.7
	Glycolysis	Carbohydrate	Non-involvement	Fast	2
Aerobic process		Carbohydrate	Involvement	Slow	36
		Fat	Involvement	Slow	147
		Protein	Involvement	Slow	16

Development of Energy Systems through Training

Training and ATP-PC System

Repetitive short-term bursts of high intensity exercise (near 100% physical exertion) with an exercise-rest ratio of 1:2~1:6 develops the ATP-PC system. This form of exercise is enhanced by increasing the activity of ATPase or by increasing the mobilization of fast-twitch muscle fibers. It is important to ensure that the PC in the muscles have been fully restored by providing adequate rest between bursts. If the PC is not fully replenished during the break, glycolysis becomes the primary source of energy and lactate accumulates, which means the exercise can no longer be continued.

Training and Glycolysis

Exercise performed at around 90~95% maximum heart rate with an exercise-rest ratio of 1:1~1:2 improves "anaerobic endurance ability". On the other hand, exercise with 95~105% of the speed and exercise: rest ratio of 1:2 to 1:8 raises "lactic acid tolerance". In other words, exercise that produces a lot of lactic acid and causes severe pain in the muscles improves the tolerance of the lactic acid system.

Training and Aerobic System

The development of the ability to exercise faster without the accumulation of lactic acid is promising. This is the primary principle of the "anaerobic threshold (AT)". This is a concept where the athlete must reach the maximum intensity at which the aerobic metabolic process can be improved while remaining at the minimum intensity that can stimulate the improvement of cardiopulmonary endurance [Fig. 1.14].

To develop the aerobic system, as shown in [Fig. 1.14], an untrained person must perform long-term exercise at less than 50~60% of their maximum exercise capacity, while a trained person must exercise at less than 65~80%. This means that the distance should be between 1 km and 3 km and the total exercise time should be at least 30 minutes. Exercise with a 1:1 exercise-rest ratio can increase the $\dot{V}O_2max$, which is an index of cardiopulmonary endurance. This increase in the $\dot{V}O_2max$ is indirectly related to lifespan and is a subject of interest to researchers. Particularly, aerobic exercises are commonly prescribed for adults or elderly patients, including walking, jogging, swimming, and cycling.

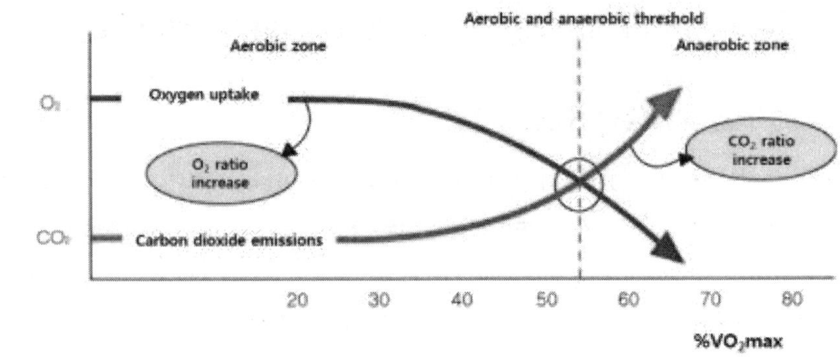

Fig. 1.14 ***Anaerobic threshold: In the general population without training, 50-60% of $\dot{V}O_2max$ and 65~80% of trainees have threshold levels***[5]

Contribution of energy system and calorie consumption during various exercises events

Physiologically, calorie calculations usually use Atwater's coefficient for simple calculations. It is calculated that proteins and carbohydrates have a calorie content of 4 kcal/g, and fat has 9 kcal/g. When we calculate calories primarily for weight control, estimating 1 kg at 7,700 kcal is mainly about the weight of fat tissue. This is because the carbohydrates are used in specific organs, including the brain, or in the muscles during intense exercise. Since protein is a constituent of the body, the fat present in the surplus energy source is mainly used to refer to weight control. In addition, since fat tissue is considered to be a major contributor to diseases when it is accumulated in the human body, calories are calculated mainly by the weight of fat tissue when referring to weight control. 86% of human fat are lipids, and 1kg of fat tissue is roughly composed of 860 g of pure fat, so the caloric value is 9 × 860 ≒ 7,700 kcal. In order to eliminate 1 kg of fat tissue, 7,700 kcal must be expended, but the fat is not burned first, so the actual amount of exercise should be far greater. Consider this in light of various exercises. [Fig. 1.15] shows how an energy system is applied to change the body when we are performing exercises or when we are about to start. In [Fig. 1.15], for example, a football player weighing 80 kg consumes 3,000 kcal per day and basal metabolic rate (BMR)2) excluding exercise or activity is assumed to be about 60% of the calorie intake.

2) BMR: Minimal energy expenditure for life support, affected by weight or body surface area. It was proposed by physiologist Rubner and is calculated by oxygen consumption and CO_2 emissions. It is measured in the lying position in the room at 18-20℃ in the morning after fasting for 12 hours. BMR is about 64.3%, among which energy consumption of muscles is 38%, liver 12.4%, stomach 7.6%, and kidney 6.3%.

The example formula in [Table 1.3] can be used. [Table 1.3] shows that when a person who has played soccer for 90 minutes performs 90 minutes of cross-country skiing, there is there are differences which are shown in [Table 1.4].

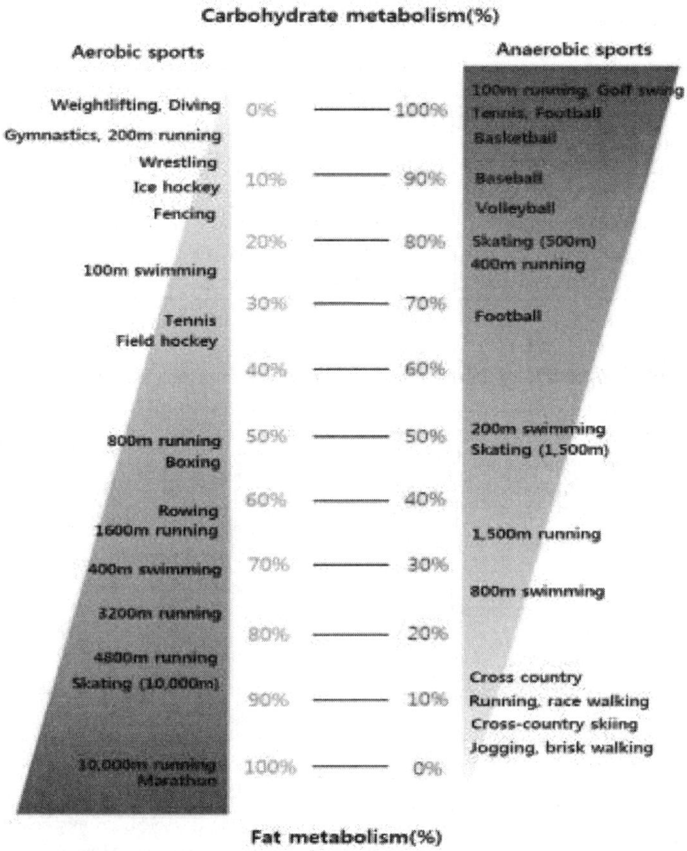

Fig. 1.15 *Contribution of energy system by sports category*

Table 1.3 ***Estimation of calorie consumption by energy contribution in soccer event***

① Calorie intake = 3,000 ㎉ ② Basal metabolic rate = 60% ③ 1㎏ body weight = 7,700 ㎉	⇨	① × ② = 1,800 ㎉ (basic metabolic rate) ▷ Remaining calories = 1,200 ㎉
④ If not play soccer and do not do any other activities at all	⇨	▷ Remaining calories accumulated in fat ▷ 7,700㎉ ÷ 1,200㎉ = 6.4 days (1㎏ body weight increase per week)
⑤ When playing soccer, a person of 80㎏ consumes 10.6 ㎉ per minute [see Table 2.1]	⇨	▷ Consumption of 954 ㎉ in 90 minutes ▷ 1,200 ㎉ - 95 4㎉ = 246 ㎉ remaining ▷ 7,700 ㎉ ÷ 246 ㎉ = 31.3 days (1㎏ increase in weight per month)
⑥ The energy consumption rate of this person who played soccer	⇨	▷ Aerobic (fat metabolism) ratio 30%: 954 ㎉ × 0.3 ≒ 286 ㎉ ▷ Anaerobic (carbohydrate metabolism) ratio 70%: 954㎉ × 0.7 ≒ 668 ㎉ ▷ Not suitable for exercise to reduce fat

Table 1.4 ***Estimation of calorie consumption by energy contribution in ski event***

① Calorie intake = 3,000 ㎉ ② Basal metabolic rate = 60% ③ 1 ㎏ body weight = 7,700 ㎉	⇨	① × ② = 1,800 ㎉ (basic metabolic rate) ▷ Remaining calories = 1,200 ㎉
④ If not play ski and do not do any other activities at all	⇨	▷ Remaining calories accumulated in fat ▷ 7,700 ㎉ ÷ 1,200 ㎉ = 6.4 days (1㎏ body weight increase per week)
⑤ When playing ski, a person of 80 ㎏ consumes 21.9 ㎉ per minute [see Table 2.1]	⇨	▷ Consumption of 1,971 ㎉ in 90 minutes ▷ 1,200 ㎉ - 1,971 ㎉ = -771 ㎉ ▷ 7,700 ㎉ ÷ 771 ㎉ = 9.9 days (1㎏ decrease in weight per 10 days)
⑥ The energy consumption rate of this person who played ski	⇨	▷ Aerobic (fat metabolism) ratio 90%: 1,971 ㎉ × 0.9 ≒ 1,774 ㎉ ▷ Anaerobic (carbohydrate metabolism) ratio 10%: 1,971 ㎉ × 0.1 ≒ 197 ㎉ ▷ Suitable for exercise to reduce fat

Physiological Changes after Training

Short-term physiological benefits of regular exercise include sleep improvement, glucose control, and increased catecholamine activity. When exercise is done regularly, as shown in [Table 1.5], improvement of cardiovascular function, cardiorespiratory function, performance, increase in strength and muscle endurance, flexibility and range of joint motion (ROM), fat reduction, and improvement of lipid composition can be cited.

Physiological responses to exercise are reported to be essentially the same, regardless of age. Specifically, the results of the studies up to now are presented in [Table 1.5]. If you do not exercise regularly and continue an inactive lifestyle, your fitness and health conditions will deteriorate. However, it can be concluded that when regular exercise is performed, physical conditions and health states improve, along with quantity of life and quality of life (2QoL).

Table 1.5 ***Differences of physiological variables between sedentary and active lifestyle***

	Functions	Sedentary lifestyle	Active lifestyle
Nervous System	• Parasympathetic tone	⇩	⬆
	• Sympathetic tone	⬆	⇩
	• Reaction time	⇩	⬆
	• Neural conduction time	⇩	⬆
	• Sensory deficit	⬆	⇩
Cardiovascular System	• Heart rate	⬆	⇩
	• SBP	⬆	⇩
	• Cardiac output	⇩	⬆
	• Stroke volume	⇩	⬆
	• Oxygen consumption	⇩	⬆
	• Left heart ventricle	⇩	⬆
	• Plasma volume	⇩	⬆
	• Capillary density	⇩	⬆
	• Myoglobin content	⇩	⬆
Respiratory System	• Vital capacity	⇩	⬆
	• Total lung volume	≈	≈
	• Respiratory frequency	⬆	⇩
Musculoskeletal System	• Bone mineral density	⇩	⬆
	• Muscle mass	⇩	⬆
	• Muscular strength	⇩	⬆
	• Muscular endurance	⇩	⬆
	• Flexibility	⇩	⬆
	• Balance	⇩	⬆
Renal System	• Renal function	⇩	⬆
	• Acid-base balance	⇩	⬆
	• Glucose tolerance	⇩	⬆
	• Drug clearance	⇩	⬆
	• Cellular water	⇩	⬆
Metabolic System	• Basal metabolic rate	⇩	⬆
	• Lean body mass	⇩	⬆
	• Fat mass	⬆	⇩
	• Triglyceride (TG)	⬆	⇩
	• Total cholesterol (TC)	⬆	⇩
	• HDL cholesterol	⇩	⬆
	• LDL cholesterol	⬆	⇩

⇩ decrease, ⬆ increase, ≈ no change

❖ Study Questions

1. A new disease caused by a decrease in physical activity is called (*hypokinetic disease*).

2. Hypokinetic disease and poor eating habits lead to (*obesity, heart disease, hypertension, stroke, diabetes, and cancer*).

3. Adult diseases progress insidiously, and have already progressed considerably if you feel (*subjective symptoms*).

4. The reason to exercise is to prevent (*adult diseases*) and increase (*quality of life*) and (*quantity of life*).

5. Energy is defined as the human body's (*capacity for work*).

6. The food we consume for energy production is stored in the form of six nutrients, but only (*carbohydrate*) and (*fat*) are used during exercise.

7. Carbohydrates are called glucose at room temperature, blood sugar in the blood, and (*glucose*) in the tissues.

8. Glucose enters tissues by (*insulin*) and is stored as (*glycogen*) when not available for energy. The storage of glycogen is (*100*) g/kg in body weight per liver and (*200~300*) g/kg in muscle.

9. All food should be converted into (*ATP*), which can be used as energy in the body.

10. The path through which ATP is supplied to the body is made by the (*anaerobic*) system and the (*aerobic*) system.

11. The anaerobic system produces ATP using only (*carbohydrates*), and the aerobic system produces ATP using (*carbohydrates*) and (*fat*).

12. The anaerobic system is divided into the (*ATP-PC*) system with little oxygen and (*glycolysis*) is used when oxygen is insufficient.

13. (*ATP-PC*) system is used when short-term, high-intensity activity and exercise are started and does not produce (*lactic acid*).

14. Phosphagen is present in large amounts in (*white muscle fibers*) compared to red muscle fibers and produces (*0.7*) ATP.

15. The process of carbohydrate degradation under oxygen deficiency is called (*glycolysis*).

16. In high-intensity exercise, ATP is supplied through (*fast*) glycolysis, whereas in moderate to high-intensity exercise, ATP is supplied through (*slow*) glycolysis. The difference between these two processes is the involvement of (*NADH*).

17. Fast glycolysis is the process of converting pyruvate to lactic acid by (*LDH*), a process that converts NADH to NAD. Lactic acid inhibits (*phosphorylase*), which converts G6P to glycogen, and (*phosphofructokinase*), which causes G6P to convert to glyceraldehyde triphosphate, preventing further high-intensity exercise.

18. NADH activated at a relatively low intensity is a substitute for oxygen and is a coenzyme that enters into (*ETC*) system for ATP production. It is the substance that starts the aerobic process.

19. After stopping exercise and entering rest, lactic acid is transferred to the liver and stored as glycogen, which is called (*Cori-cycle*).

20. The anaerobic system produces ATP in the (*cytoplasm*), whereas the aerobic system produces ATP in the (*mitochondria*).

21. If the intensity of the exercise is slow or the pace is constant, the human body will produce ATP using carbohydrates for a short time. (*Pyruvate*), the final product degraded in the cytoplasm, binds to oxygen and enters the mitochondria, circulates two (*Krebs*) cycle, and produces 18 ATPs through each (*ETC*). In other words, the production of ATP through carbohydrates is 2 in the anaerobic process, 18 in the Krebs cycle and ETC, and 18 in the other Krebs cycle and ETC, producing a total of (*38*) ATPs.

22. Carbohydrates are represented by the molecular formula ($C_6H_{12}O_6$), which uses six oxygen molecules to form six carbon dioxide molecules, six water molecules, and 38 ATPs. When a carbohydrate breaks down in a (*gas analyzer*) during graded exercise testing, the appearance of (*1*) indicates the amount calculated by dividing carbon dioxide production by the amount of oxygen needed for carbohydrate decomposition.

23. Fats produce a large amount of ATP because of the high number of (*carbon bonds*) compared to carbohydrates. This process is called (*beta oxidation*).

24. There are various types of fat, but mainly ATP production is estimated by (*stearic acid*). (*Stearic acid*) produces 18 carbon dioxide molecules, 18 water molecules, and (*147*) ATPs through 8 beta oxidation steps using 26 oxygen molecules. When fat is decomposed in the gas analyzer, (*0.7*) appears as the amount calculated by dividing the amount of CO_2 produced by the amount of oxygen required for fat decomposition.

25. Fat is stored in the form of (*triglycerides*) in the body and is used as energy when fasting, resting, lightly exercising, or exercising for a long time at a constant pace.

26. In order for fat to be converted to ATP and used as energy, triglycerides should be broken down into free (*fatty acids*) and glycerol, and free (*fatty acids*) are the source of ATP. The enzyme that breaks down TG into free (*fatty acids*) is referred to as (*lipase*).

27. Lipase is activated by (*epinephrine, norepinephrine, and glucagon*), while it is inhibited by (*insulin*). Lipase is also inhibited by (*lactic acid*) produced in glycolysis. It has been shown that fatty acid mobilization is not possible during intense exercise.

28. Fatty acids are mainly mobilized in (*less than 30*) % of the $\dot{V}O_2max$, and carbohydrates are mainly mobilized in (*more than 70*) % of the $\dot{V}O_2max$.

29. Among muscle fibers, (*white muscle fibers*) contain many enzymes necessary for glycolysis, and low (*lipase*).

30. During exercise, mainly carbohydrates and fats are used as primary sources of energy, but for (*long-term exercise*), (*severe fasting*), and (*diabetes*), protein is often used as an energy source.

31. Protein is not purely converted to ATP, but it can produce ATP by converting (*alanine*) in (*amino acid*), the constituent unit of protein, to glucose. This is called the (*glucose-alanine cycle*).

32. There are 13 kinds of (*non-essential amino acids*) that are produced by the human body and 9 kinds of (*essential amino acids*) that can be obtained only through food. Alanine is one of the (*non-essential amino acids*).

33. To develop the ATC-PC system, you should run for (*15 seconds or less*), with a (*1 : 2*) or (*1 : 6*) exercise-to-rest ratio.

34. To develop glycolysis, run at (*95~105*) % of the maximum speed, with a (*1 : 2*) or (*1 : 8*) exercise-to-rest ratio.

35. In order to develop aerobic systems, a general person should walk, trot, or jog for a long time, with (*50~60%*) of maximum capacity and less than (*65~80%*) of maximum capacity for a trained person. It is preferable to set the exercise-to-rest ratio at (*1 : 1*).

36. Since human fat is 86% lipid and 1kg fatty tissue is roughly composed of (*860*)g pure fat, (*7,700*) kcal is obtained by multiplying 9.

37. The minimum energy expenditure used to maintain life is called (*basal metabolic rate*).

38. Basal metabolic rate is approximately (*60*)%.

39. When the calorie intake is 3,000 ㎉, the calories consumed naturally for maintaining life is (*1,800*) ㎉.

40. When a person plays soccer, it depends on 30% of the anaerobic metabolic process and 70% of the anaerobic metabolic process. When this person consumes 1,000 ㎉ per day and exercises for 7 days, the fat consumed is estimated to be (*2,100*) ㎉, and when it is converted to weight, it is 2,100 ÷ 7,700, (*0.27*) kg.

Chapter 2

Exercise and Nutrition

Goals

- To understand the amount of energy consumption through exercise.
- To understand the concept of calories and the consumption of calories per minute by various exercises.
- To understand the six nutrients (carbohydrate / protein / fat / water / vitamins / minerals) for the structure and function of the human body.
- To understand the contribution of each nutrient according to exercise events.

Exercise and Energy Expenditure

The foods we eat every day become energy or fuel for our bodies. This energy varies according to the level of activity, which means that the more intensely you exercise, the more calories[3)] you will need. In fact, the amount of energy needed varies because some sports require muscle strength while others require cardiopulmonary endurance depending on the characteristics of the sport. In this context, energy expenditure per day is divided according to body weight as shown in [Table 2.1] and classified according to age, sex, weight and height as shown in [Table 2.2]. [Table 2.1] shows that the amount of energy consumed by a soccer player with a weight of 65 kg for a 45-minute match is 8.6 × 45 = 387 kcal. The amount of energy consumed when a Judo player weighing 80 kg competes for 5 minutes is 78 kcal. These energy consumption estimates can be used to suggest how much athletes need to intake prior to a match.

On the other hand, if an athlete performs a high-intensity training in preparation for a match, more calories will be required. The amount of calories required for athletes is shown in [Table 2.2], which shows calorie intake appropriate to the athlete's age. For

3) Calorie (or kcal): The unit of energy. 1 calorie means the amount of energy needed to raise 1 kg of water by 1°C.

example, a man with an average age of 17 years, a body weight of 60 kg, and a height of 174 cm is recommended to consume 3,000 kcal a day, which usually means that he should consume about 300 kcal (a bowl of rice) more than the intake for older adults.

Table 2.1 ***Calorie consumption by exercise***

Items	Weight (kg)																
	50	53	56	59	62	65	68	71	74	77	80	83	86	89	92	95	98
Volleyball	2.5	2.7	2.8	3.0	3.1	3.3	3.4	3.6	3.7	3.9	4.0	4.2	4.3	4.5	4.6	4.8	4.9
Soccer	6.6	7.0	7.4	7.8	8.2	8.6	9.0	9.4	9.8	10.2	10.6[A]	11.0	11.4	11.7	12.1	12.5	12.9
Basketball	6.9	7.3	7.7	8.1	8.6	9.0	9.4	9.8	10.2	10.6	11.0	11.5	11.9	12.3	12.7	13.1	13.5
Tennis	5.5	5.8	6.1	6.4	6.8	7.1	7.4	7.7	8.1	8.4	8.7	9.0	9.4	9.7	10.0	10.4	10.7
Swimming	6.4	6.8	7.2	7.6	7.9	8.3	8.7	9.1	9.5	9.9	10.2	10.6	11.0	11.4	11.8	12.2	12.5
Ski	13.7	14.5	15.3	16.2	17.0	17.8	18.6	19.5	20.3	21.1	21.9[B]	22.7	23.6	24.4	25.2	26.0	26.9
Cycle	5.0	5.3	5.6	5.9	6.2	6.5	6.8	7.1	7.4	7.7	8.0	8.3	8.6	8.9	9.2	9.5	9.8
Golf	4.3	4.5	4.8	5.0	5.3	5.5	5.8	6.0	6.3	6.5	6.8	7.1	7.3	7.6	7.8	8.1	8.3
Judo	9.8	10.3	10.9	11.5	12.1	12.7	13.3	13.8	14.4	15.0	15.6	16.2	16.8	17.4	17.9	18.5	19.1

Table 2.2 ***Average calorie intake***

Men				Women			
Age(yr)	Weight(kg)	Height(cm)	Calorie(kcal)	Age(yr)	Weight(kg)	Height(cm)	Calorie(kcal)
15~18	60.3	175.2	3000	15~18	53.5	165.1	2100
19~22	66.15	175.2	3000	19~22	57.6	165.1	2100
23~50	69.3	175.2	2700	23~50	57.6	165.1	2000
51+	69.3	175.2	2400	51+	57.6	165.1	1800

Exercise and Nutrition

Nutrients4) refers to the kind of foods that must be ingested to enable humans to perform their daily activities. Nutrients consist of macronutrients (such as carbohydrate, protein, fat) and micronutrients (such as mineral, vitamin, and water). The intake of these nutrients requires a balance, especially for the more active athletes. The main components of the diet should consist of carbohydrates, proteins, and fats. Nutritionists recommend 60~65% carbohydrates, 15~20% proteins, and 20~25% fats.[2,9]

On the other hand, macronutrients absorbed by the human body have different calories: carbohydrate and protein produce 4 kcal each, and fat produces 9 kcal. Fat has twice as

4) Nutrient: Nutritive value refers to food containing micronutrients.

many calories as carbohydrates and protein, so it is important for athletes to control their body weight by reducing fat intake and increasing carbohydrate and protein intake. The macronutrients and micronutrients, together, are called the six major nutrients, and their functions are as follows.

Carbohydrates

Carbohydrates are classified in the form of monosaccharides, disaccharides, and polysaccharides. Monosaccharides and disaccharides are simple carbohydrates, including fruits, juices, soft drinks, and sweeteners. Polysaccharides are complex carbohydrates, including brown rice, noodles, rice, bread, and vegetables. Carbohydrates are substances composed of carbon, hydrogen, and oxygen atoms and supply energy to the human body. However, simple carbohydrates such as soft drinks contain many sugars, but they are not nutritious. In other words, monosaccharides lack nutritional value, vitamins, and minerals, and have low calories.[10] Also, monosaccharides supply energy quickly, but they are very temporary and do not supply energy during training or games. A better source of energy is complex carbohydrates like polysaccharides, which the body decomposes into glucose and stores in the muscle tissues or liver as glycogen. Therefore, in order to exercise efficiently, it is preferable that 60~65% of consumed nutrients are polysaccharides.

Complex carbohydrates contain nutrients, vitamins and minerals, so they are rich in nutritional value, and can be consumed in large quantities with low calories. Also, it gives you a feeling of fullness for a longer time, which can be helpful in preventing the consumption of unnecessary sugars from snacks or junk food.

Protein

The protein that constitutes the muscles is not only a component of the cell protoplasm, but also a major component of enzymes, hormones, immunogens, and genes. In fact, muscle tissue consists of about 70~75% moisture and 10~25% protein. Therefore, most athletes who are active should have a total daily consumption that consists of between 10~25% protein. Daily protein intake ranges from 1~1.5 g/kg of body weight, which means that a person who is 80 kilograms should consume 80~120 g of protein per day. This can be thought of as three cups of milk, two pieces of chicken breast, and one piece of cheese.

As mentioned above, high-quality protein refers to beef, pork, poultry, fish, eggs, dairy products, etc. When an adequate amount of protein is ingested into the human body, surplus protein is stored as fat or excreted outside the body. In other words, eating a lot of protein does not mean you become physically bigger, agile, faster, or stronger. Rather, proper conditioning is more important. Complex carbohydrates, and not proteins, is a rich source of energy.

Proteins are made up of amino acids and more specifically, 22 amino acids are needed for growth and development. Thirteen of these are produced in the human body, but the other nine amino acids are called "essential amino acids" because they can only be supplied through diet.[3,12] For reference, some vegetables, including beans, are considered to be incomplete proteins.

Fats

Despite the controversy so far, fat is very important for a balanced diet. This is because fat is essential for the absorption of fat-soluble vitamins A, D, E, and K, and it constitutes the majority of human cells. In addition, fat layers identify different sections of the human body, and it also functions as a cushion for internal organs. It is recommended that fat accounts for 20~25% of meals. You do not need to purposely intake more fat. In other words, even if athletes consume all of the recommended fat intake, it is not recommended to use fat as primary calories or main energy source. Fat is contained in meat, ice cream, chocolate, whole milk, cheese, butter and so on. When these foods are consumed in large quantities, it can cause various diseases.

Water

Water is an essential nutrient for the human body. If a person is going to exercise under moderate climates, about 2,000 ㎖ of water per day is needed. This moisture is involved in the plasma concentration in the amount needed for the body to ingest, digest and excrete food, and it also softens the organs and joints. Moisture plays two important roles when exercising. First, it keeps your body temperature constant and lowers your body temperature during exercise to make you less tired. Second, it carries nutrients and transports the products into and out of cells. So, water should be ingested before, during, or after exercise.

In fact, water is a very important nutrient and occupies the largest part of the body. That is, 60% of body weight, 75% of brain and muscles, and 25% of bones are water. Excessive exercise or sweat and long exposure to hot weather will reduce the body's water content. A 10% loss of water causes dehydration, and a loss of more than 20% leads to death. During such dehydration, it is necessary to drink water with salt. The intake of water in the morning improves the ability of the gastrointestinal tract and the colon to function which has an excellent effect on stool excretion. Specific water intake tips are as follows.

- Drink water before you feel thirsty.
- Drink 6~8 cups of water daily (cider cup size).
- Take 1 cup of water 15 minutes before exercise.
- Drink 1 cup of water every 30 minutes during heavy workouts.
- If you exercise more than 2 hours or exercise strenuously for more than 1 hour, take a drink containing about 8% carbohydrates (fructose).
- After exercise, drink 2 cups of water.
- Observe changes in body weight before and after exercise (there is a risk of dehydration if body weight is reduced by more than 2 kg after exercise).
- Drink 1 cup of water within two hours if you drink coffee (diuresis, quickening dehydration).

Table 2.3 *Types and functions of fat-soluble vitamins and their daily requirements*

Types of vitamins		Functions	Daily requirements
Fat-soluble	A	• Maintain eye and skin health / prevent infection • Anti-aging involvement (provitamin A)	2000 IU
	D	• Calcium absorption and bone and tooth formation	100 IU
	E	• Prevent the destruction of vitamins and essential fatty acids • Anti-aging	400 IU
	K	• Blood clotting	-

Table 2.4 *Types and functions of water-soluble vitamins and their daily requirements*

Types of vitamins		Functions	Daily requirements
Water-soluble	C	• Strengthen somatic cells, injuries and bone therapy • Prevention of infection / anti-aging	50 mg
	B1	• Energy generation	1.0 mg
	B2	• Energy metabolism • Vision and skin protection	1~1.3 mg
	B3	• Fat, carbohydrate metabolism • Skin, nerve, digestive organ protection	-
	B6	• Protein, fat metabolism • Required for red blood cell formation	3~4 mg
	B9	• Protein metabolism • Red blood cell generation	0.2 mg
	B12	• Red blood cells and nerve tissue maintenance	0.6~1.2 mg

Because humans have irregular thirst mechanisms, they do not thirsty for a long time even when there is insufficient water. It is therefore important to develop a habit of regularly drinking water, which helps the body recover and use fat as a primary energy source after exercise.

Ultimately, when sweating during exercise, water loss occurs, and the viscosity of the blood increases. The higher the viscosity, the greater the burden on the heart to exercise and the more heat it generates. Particularly, when heat is increased, carbohydrates are used as an energy source rather than fat, so that it is impossible to perform effective physical fitness and weight management. Therefore, it is important to drink plenty of water during exercise and to drink water before thirst.

Vitamins

The body needs vitamins, but a lot of it is unnecessary. Vitamins play a special role in the proper functioning of muscles and nerves and promote the normal growth of human tissue. However, vitamins are a non-energy source, and excessive consumption can cause stomach cramps.

Table 2.5 *Types and functions of major antioxidant vitamins*

Antioxidants	Functions	Recommend amounts
Provitamin A (β-carotene)	• Single oxygen combustion • Free radical removal • Reduce the incidence of cancer	10,000~50,000 IU
Vitamin C (ascorbic acid)	• Role in blood flow and other water cells • Regeneration of vitamin E • Immune function enhancement • Antibacterial / antiviral action	250~2000 ㎎
Vitamin E (α-tocopherol)	• Membrane protection • Vitamin A and selenium protection • Protection against smoking	200~800 IU
Selenium	• Main ingredients of GPX • Concurrent function with vitamin E • Protection against cancer outbreak	50~200 mcg

Vitamins are divided into fat-soluble vitamins (A, D, E, K) and water-soluble vitamins (B, C) as shown in [Table 2.3] and [Table 2.4]. Water-soluble vitamins are not stored in the body even if they are consumed in excess. On the other hand, excessive intake of fat-soluble vitamins leads to fat accumulation. This can lead to hypervitaminosis, leading to health hazards, poor physical condition, and even toxicity.

In addition to general vitamins, vitamin-related substances associated with anti-aging and oxygen free radical elimination also affect exercise [Table 2.5]. These are called antioxidant vitamins. The toxic oxidation that occurs after intense physical activity harms and causes inflammation of the skeletal muscle, with about 2~5% being converted to peroxidic radicals and substances such as hydrogen peroxide and hydroxyl radicals. In other words, it is known that oxygen free radicals generated by excessively intense exercise have electrons that do not form an atomic structure pair and thus have a bad influence on the human body.[8]

Table 2.6 ***Types and functions of minerals and their daily requirements***

Types	Functions	Daily requirements
Calcium	• Bone and tooth formation, muscle contraction and relaxation • Nerve stimulation conduction, cell membrane function • Blood coagulation control, glycogen degradation	1000 ㎎
Iron	• Hemoglobin components for oxygen carrying	10 ㎎ (Men) 18 ㎎ (Women)
Magnesium	• Maintain normal function of heart, muscles • Energy extraction from food	350 ㎎
Phosphorus	• Bone formation, ATP component • Required when using glucose as fuel	800 ㎎
Iodine	• Normal development • Needed for reproduction and feeding	150 ㎎
Potassium	• Control moisture content in cells • Proper function of kidney, heart, and muscle	400 ㎎
Zinc	• Acts as a part of insulin with glucose to be used as energy through the cell membrane • Promoting recovery from cell division, tissue growth and damage	15 ㎎

However, all organisms that use oxygen can dilute the toxicity because they contain antioxidants, but also produce harmful oxygen. The antioxidant enzymes responsible for this defense mechanism in the body include superoxide dismutase (SOD), catalase (CAT), and glutathione peroxidase (GPX). SOD catalyzes the conversion of peroxide anions, CAT converts hydrogen peroxide to water and oxygen, and GPX acts to reduce hydrogen peroxide to water and then hydroperoxide to hydroxide. However, when the antioxidant enzyme's defense function is overwhelmed by harmful oxygen, it reacts with polyunsaturated fatty acids in the cell membrane to form new active oxygen. The newly formed peroxyl radical (ROO) binds to oxygen and causes malondialdehyde (MDA) to destroy cell membranes and protein.[8,10] The substances to supplement them are presented in [Table 2.5]. When the recommended amount is taken into consideration, it is possible to prevent aging and enhance physical strength by preventing the action of harmful oxygen.

Minerals

Minerals are substances that help regular physical activity, body organization, and metabolism. Major minerals include calcium, iodine, iron, phosphorus, magnesium, sodium, potassium and so on. These minerals are also called electrolytes. Electrolytes help muscles work to maintain normal muscle contractions for prolonged periods of time. There are more than 20 minerals in the human body, 17 of which can be obtained from food. Minerals are divided into two major categories: major-macrominerals, which require more than 100 mg per day, and trace-microminerals, which require a few contents.[11]

Athletes need more vitamins and minerals than ordinary people, and they can be supplemented by taking tablets. The easiest way is to take chewing vitamins for children. The types, functions, and requirements of minerals are shown in [Table 2.6].

Supplement foods

Supplemental foods include beverages, powders, nutrition bars, and nutrients. Some are good and others are bad, but none of them can substitute for physical activity. The human body has to move for 24 hours, but supplements are not stored in the human body, so they only play a temporary role. In other words, they cannot be used as the main fuel or energy source. This is why a balanced diet is necessary.[7]

If you have a healthy nutritional diet, your body will continue to be well fed with calories, protein, vitamins, minerals, and everything else you need. In other words, taking proper supplements to a balanced diet can improve health, prevent illness, and quickly recover from fatigue after exercise. However, since supplements are not essential, you should consider whether it is compatible with the daily recommendations of a typical diet. If you are using powdered supplements, you should mix them with water or milk, and take them between 45~60 minutes after exercise.

Exercise and Body Weight Control

The goal of body weight control should be balanced nutrition and regular exercise for a long period of time. In particular, you should choose the right method to lose or gain weight.[9] You should not control your weight through irrelevant changes in dietary intake, nor should you try to control your weight by reducing or increasing unplanned exercise. To control your body weight, receive a comprehensive checkup. If this is not possible, a body composition test (the impedance method is sufficient) should be done to check your "ideal weight", lean body mass, and fat mass. Then try to control your weight with scientific nutrition plans and exercise programs.

Weight Loss Programs

If overweight or obese patients need to lose weight, the goal of weight loss should be limited to 2~4 kg per month through prescribed nutrition and exercise. When the target amount is exceeded, the electrolytes, vitamins, and water, which are very necessary for the human body, are discharged, resulting in anemia or dehydration, and muscle mass is reduced rather than body fat. If you want to lose weight, you should make a reasonable plan on a weekly or monthly basis. As described above, it is preferable to reduce 500 g to 1 kg per week or 2~4 kg per month in combination with diet and exercise therapy.[1]

On the other hand, for the body fat reduction method, all patients should avoid fasting and reduce calorie intake by eating complex carbohydrates. In order to avoid the loss of interest in exercise, light to moderate intensity aerobic exercise (indoor cycling, walking, jogging, stair climbing, etc.) should be performed every day for 20 minutes. On the other hand, when you eat meals, you should consume low-fat, high-carbohydrates that do not contain monosaccharides and appropriate amounts of protein.

Weight Gain Programs

Excessive weight does not equate to power. Rather, exercise capacity may be deteriorated and lead to chronic diseases. However, since it is desirable for patients with lower than normal weight to reach a normal range of weight, it is necessary to perform a weight gain program. As with the goal of the weight loss program, weight gain programs should prescribe nutrition and exercise by limiting the weight gain goal to 2~4 kg per month. Weight gain should focus on diet and strength training.

First, in order to increase weight, you must take in more calories than you expend. To increase your calorie intake, you need to increase the amount of food you eat every day, and it is good to eat snacks between three meals a day. If you do not have time to increase your weight, you should reduce your activity time because you need enough rest to increase your weight. If you want to increase your weight by 500 g per week, you should consume more than 3,500 ㎉. If you want to increase your weight by 500 g per week, more than 3,500 ㎉ should be consumed. This means that you should consume more than an additional 500 ㎉ daily.

Second, the increase in the amount of food prescribed above can only cause an increase in body fat mass, so muscle mass must be increased through exercise, especially weight training. If you don't do weight training or resistance training, you should keep in mind that "fat" is not "muscle".

Exercises and Nutritional Prescription

Nutrition for Ball Games

In ball games such as soccer, basketball, handball, hockey, baseball, rugby, and tennis, functions such as dribbling, passing, and shooting, are required. Because a variety of muscles are mobilized, a personal strengthening program is necessary. If muscle strength is increased, injury can naturally be prevented. In the event that the competition time is relatively long, it is necessary to improve the maximum oxygen uptake ability and to improve the ability to process lactic acid quickly. Carbohydrates should be taken 3-4 hours before a specific game day. Carbohydrates with fast digestion and absorption are preferable, and starch must be included so that hunger does not appear during competition. Supplementing water-soluble vitamins 30 minutes to 1 hour before the game can prevent accumulation of lactic acid. A moderate amount of citric acid, sugar, and water-soluble vitamins should be taken during rest if you feel a lot of fatigue.

Nutrition for One-on-One Competitions

One-on-one competitions such as wrestling, judo, boxing, and taekwondo are high-intensity and fast-changing events. Preparation for these competitions should be aimed at improving muscle strength and stamina since individuals must fight alone and cannot depend on others. To do this, weight training and protein should be taken properly and anaerobic endurance should be developed by overloading to improve lactic acid tolerance. Because carbohydrate accumulation is important in these types of sports, it is preferable to eat 3~4 hours before the match. Eating foods high in starch (rice cake, rice, bread, noodles, etc.) and drinking orange juice that can exercise power immediately after the match. Thirty minutes before the game, taking enough vitamins for lactic acid treatment and drinking a cup of coffee to activate sympathetic nerves and energy metabolism may be a good idea. However, caution should be given because coffee can cause doping tests to indicate positive when caffeine levels of 12 μg / 10 mℓ or more is detected in urine. On the other hand, concentration is also a very important factor in one-on-one competitions, so when concentration levels are low, glucose should be taken to maintain blood sugar levels. In addition, when judgment is weakened due to stress, taking vitamin C can activate anti-stress hormones.

Nutrition for Personal Sports

Nutrients can be prescribed depending on the type of individual sports: powerful-type, powerful endurance-type, and endurance-type.

Nutrition for Powerful-type Sports

Strong muscle strength is needed in individual competitions such as athletics, gymnastics, diving, short-range swimming, table tennis, and weightlifting. Sufficient intake of protein and the secretion of growth hormones for protein utilization are needed, so plenty of sleep and naps are required. We should carefully perform weight training centered on the agonistic muscles, but also strengthen the muscles of the entire body. In the case of powerful sports, it is best to stay in top condition during the match as the game is decided in a short time. High-carbohydrates should be ingested 3-4 hours before the match and controlled so that the glycogen breakdown is most active. Before the match, it is also good to take enough vitamin C to eliminate the stress that occurs during the match. It is effective to take an appropriate amount of glucose and sugar 30 minutes before the match so that the main energy metabolism can be changed from fatty acid to glycogen since it needs to use the stored glycogen instantaneously.

Nutrition for Powerful Endurance-type Sports

Individual competitions requiring simultaneous power and endurance, such as running, road cycling, swimming more than 200-m, and 1,500-m speed skating, should focus on improving muscle endurance. During the game, a strong exercise load is required. Therefore, to improve the maximum oxygen uptake, athletes need to train for a certain period of time, such as running 100-m in 25 seconds. Protein intake, weight training, and maximum load exercises are needed to maximize power and endurance.[12] In addition to a high-fat diet, foods that can be fat-decomposed in the body should be chosen. High-carbohydrate meals are preferred 3~4 hours before the match, but fat intake should also be kept in mind. The ability to process lactic acid can be increased by supplementing vitamin C while taking soluble vitamins one hour before the game and relaxing muscles after the game.

Nutrition for Endurance-type Sports

Individual endurance events, such as middle to long distance running, marathons, race walk, cross-country skiing, etc., require training to improve their maximum oxygen uptake capacity. It is important to make the body environment favorable for the fat decomposition so that the metabolism process that the fat is used as the energy works well by habituation of the usual high-fat diet method. Individual endurance games need nutrition management during training like a real match and nutritional prescription according to individual differences such as carbohydrate accumulation should be thoroughly done. To increase the rate of fat use during the game, eat three to four hours before the game, preferably with some fat. It is good enough to eat starch, but be careful about foods that are prone to cause gas in the intestines, such as milk, burdock, and potatoes. Sports drinks containing water, juice, and carbohydrates are suitable during the game. In order to remove accumulated lactic acid, it is necessary to balance the intake of carbohydrates and to take fructose so that the energy metabolism of fat is not inhibited by saccharide.[9]

❖ Study Questions

1. The definition of calorie is the amount of heat needed to raise 1 g of water by 1°C. Because the specific heat of water varies with temperature, it is precisely defined as the amount of heat required to raise 1 g of water at (*14.5*) °C to (*15.5*) °C under 1 atmospheric pressure.

2. Nutrients, in other words, (*nutritional value*), also refers to foods containing (*micro*) nutrients.

3. Nutrients are classified into six major nutrients, the bigger ones are called (*macronutrients*), the smaller ones are called (*micronutrients*) depending on the size of the molecular weight.

4. Macronutrients are divided into (*carbohydrates*), (*fats*), and (*proteins*), and micronutrients are composed of (*minerals*), (*vitamins*), and (*water*).

5. Most recently, the recommended intake of macronutrients is (*60~65*) % carbohydrate, (*15~20*) % protein, and (*20~25*) % fat.

6. Carbohydrates are classified into two types: (*simple*) carbohydrates and (*complex*) carbohydrates.

7. Simple carbohydrates include (*monosaccharides*) such as fruits, juices and disaccharides. Complex carbohydrates refer to (*polysaccharides*) such as rice and bread.

8. Soft drinks contain many sugars, but there is no (*nutritional value*).

9. (*Complex carbohydrates*) are recommended during exercise because they have the rich nutritional value of sugars.

10. A food that is low in nutritional value and has high calories and gives the feeling of fullness even in small amounts is considered (*junk food*).

11. Muscle tissue is composed of (*70~75*) % water and (*10~25*) % protein.

12. The recommended daily intake of protein is about (*1~1.5*) g/kg of body weight. If more is consumed, it is converted to triglycerides and stored in the body.

13. Proteins that can be found in common foods include red (*meat*), white (*poultry*), egg whites, milk, and (*beans*).

14. Fat is important for a balanced diet because it is important to absorb (*fat-soluble*)

vitamins A, D, E, and K.

15. Fat is contained in a lot of the white parts of (*meat*), ice cream, chocolate, cheese, and butter.

16. When exercising, it is advisable to drink (*2,000*) mℓ of water per day.

17. The most important part of water intake during exercise is to drink water before you feel (*thirsty*).

18. Water consists of (*60*) % of body weight, (*75*) % of brain and muscles and (*25*) % of bones.

19. A (*10*) % loss of water in the body is called dehydration, and if more than (*20*) % of the body's water is lost, death occurs.

20. A difference of (*2*) kg before and after exercise is deemed to indicate dehydration.

21. (*Vitamin*) intake is important to maintain strength and nervous system function and to grow human tissue.

22. Types of vitamins are largely divided into (*fat-soluble*) vitamins and (*water-soluble*) vitamins.

23. The fat-soluble vitamin needed for eye and skin health and infection prevention is vitamin (*A*) and should be taken up to 2,000 IU.

24. The fat-soluble vitamin needed for calcium absorption and bone and tooth formation is vitamin (*D*) and should be taken up to 100 IU.

25. Anti-aging vitamins are fat-soluble vitamins (*A, E*) and water-soluble vitamin (*C*).

26. Vitamin (*B12*), a water-soluble vitamin required for the production of red blood cells and maintenance of nerve tissue, is recommended at 0.6-1.2 mg daily.

27. Vitamin (*E*), which protects cell membranes and protects against the effects of smoking, is recommended at 200-800 IU daily.

28. Antioxidant enzymes that remove harmful substances generated by harmful oxygen and protect the human body are (*SOD*), (*CAT*), (*GPX*).

29. A substance that maintains normal muscle contraction for an extended period of time is called a (*mineral*).

30. More than (*100*) mg of major-macrominerals should be consumed per day, and

trace-microminerals should be consumed in lower quantities.

31. The mineral that carries oxygen and is a component of hemoglobin is called (*iron*) in which 10 to 18 mg is required per day.

32. The mineral that promotes recovery from cell division and tissue growth and damage is called (*zinc*) in which 15 mg is required per day.

33. The mineral needed for normal growth, development, and reproduction is called (*iodine*), and 150 mg/day is recommended.

34. It is recommended that supplements are consumed between (*45~60*) minutes after exercise.

35. The target goal of weight loss or gain is preferably (*2~4*) kg per month.

36. Good nutrients for ball games should include (*carbohydrates*) with fast digestion and absorption and include starch so that hunger does not appear during the competition. In addition, the accumulation of lactic acid can be prevented by drinking (*water-soluble vitamins*) 30 to 60 minutes before the game.

37. Because power and (*stamina*) are very important for one-on-one competitions such as judo, it is important to supplement weight training with protein intake.

38. In the case of one-on-one competitions, if judgment is impaired due to stress, take (*vitamin C*) to activate anti-stress hormones.

39. In the case of quick-acting sports, high (*carbohydrates*) should be consumed. In the case of quick-acting and endurance type sports, (*protein*) intake should be emphasized.

40. Although starch intake is important for endurance type sports, the consumption of (*milk*), burdock, and potatoes that can create gas in the stomach should be avoided as much as possible.

Chapter 3

Clinical Exercise Prescription

Goals

- To understand the definition of clinical exercise prescription.
- To understand the seven principles of exercise prescription (specificity / crossover / overload / progressive / individualized / diversity / reversibility).
- To understand the five requirements of exercise prescription (exercise type / exercise intensity / exercise time / exercise frequency / exercise period).
- To understand and become acquainted with the three phases of the phase-by-phase exercise plan (daily plan / weekly plan / annual plan).
- To be able to perform warm-up, work-out, and cool-down exercise procedures of the daily exercise plan.
- To create weekly plans during the phase-by-phase exercise program, and practice them to find out the advantages and disadvantages.
- To understand the 10 steps of exercise prescription (questionnaire / pre-exercise consultation / medical examination / body composition test / exercise test / muscle function test / physical fitness test / exercise prescription / exercise start / reevaluation).

Definition of Clinical Exercise Prescription

Clinical exercise prescription is believed to have been first invented by Dr. Igao Michio from Japan in the 1960s and later by Dr. Horman from Germany. The definition of clinical exercise medicine is as follows. First, a medical examination such as body composition, blood test, ECG, radiographic test is performed in a medical clinics, and the maximum exercise ability is measured through exercise tests such as cardiopulmonary capacity, muscle function, physical fitness test. According to the results, the exercise type, exercise intensity, exercise duration, exercise frequency and exercise period are determined by determining the results of exercise medicine procedure. The above series of procedures are called clinical exercise prescription.

Principles of Exercise Prescription

Systematic and regular exercise achieves optimal health care. Therefore, to be effective in prescribing exercise, it is important to be an expert and to understand and practice the universally applied principles of exercise. This is called the constituent of exercise prescription, and its principles and elements are as follows.

Specific Principle

The specific principle is the principle that changes occur only in the muscles and related elements of the region depending on the type, intensity, and duration of exercise. In other words, when performing any exercise, not all kinds of physical elements are developed, but limitedly developed depending on the muscle used during the exercise, the load used at the time, and the mode of operation.

Neural Crossover Principle

The neural crossover effect is the principle that the limbs of the human body are dominated by the same nerve in the spinal cord and are divided into limbs so that the movement of extremities from one side affects the limbs on the other side to some extent. In other words, movements of the left arm have some effects on the right arm, and exercising the left leg can affect the right leg. This principle is often used in clinical practice to prevent muscle atrophy caused by immobilization on the injured side limb and is a principle that refutes the principle of specificity described above.[30] As a testimony to this, one study was conducted to examine the muscle function (strength, power, muscle endurance) of quadriceps and hamstring around the knee joints in 10 healthy adult men and women with isokinetic machine. Ten randomly selected subjects from 20 subjects were randomly assigned to an experimental group to perform isokinetic muscle training on one leg for 3 days per week for 7 weeks, and were compared to the other 10 subjects. Experimental results showed that the quadriceps and the hamstring muscles from training on one leg had a cross-transfer effect to the other leg, which was not involved in training. That is, the peak torque of the quadriceps muscle of the trained leg increased by 19% and the peak torque of the untrained leg increased by 11%, while the comparison group showed no change. The peak torque of the hamstring muscle also increased by 14% on the trained leg and by 5% on the untrained leg, while the comparative group decreased by 1%. On the other hand, the total workload representing the muscle endurance in the quadriceps muscle was improved by 15% on the trained side and by 7% on the non-trained side, but decreased by 1% in the control group. Hamstring muscles showed similar increases of 17%, 7%, and 3% of the trained side, untrained side, and control group, respectively.

Overload Principle

The overload principle is the principle that the applied part or the physical element develops only if the human body is given a higher load than the usual load in order to adapt to the stimulus of the exercise effectively. However, when applying the overloading principle, if the stimulation is too strong, the limit that the human body can adapt to may be exceeded, which may cause injury or serious chronic fatigue.

Progressive Principle

The progressive principle is that the load should begin light and then deliberately increase the weight or time. In other words, when a sudden strong load is applied, the human body cannot withstand it and reacts abnormally, which can result in fatigue or injury. It is, therefore, necessary to start with a light load at first and gradually increase the amount of exercise. The progressive principle gives satisfactory results when applied in a stepwise manner while taking into consideration the principle of overloading.

Individualized Principle

The individualized principle can provide safe and effective exercise by taking into consideration the individual's sex, age, family history, exercise history, fitness level, genetic factors, nutrition status, occupation type, and other personal and environmental factors. In other words, it is not the most effective method to apply a uniform program to people with different conditions and expect satisfactory results for everyone. Therefore, it is desirable to measure and evaluate an individual's fitness level to determine the type of the exercise that is most suitable.

Diverse Principle

The diverse principle states that various exercises and programs should be planned in order to increase interest in the exercise and to maximize participation. Changes in environmental factors, such as the amount of exercise and rest, combination of hard and easy, different exercise methods, and including music or TV shows, play an effective role in increasing interest and participation in exercise.

Reverse Principle

The reverse principle states that the changes in the body caused by exercise such as an increase in muscle mass, decrease in fat mass, improvement in flexibility will return to the initial state or deteriorate as soon as training is stopped. To prevent this, you should exercise at least three days a week, and not rest for at least two weeks.

Requirements for Exercise Prescription

Exercise prescription is to determine what exercise should be done to improve physical fitness for healthy people and to improve functional capacity[5)] for the sick. In other words, exercise prescription is similar to how a doctor prescribes certain medicine for a patient. It is an exercise prescription that diagnoses the physical fitness level for a certain person and prescribes the exercise suitable for the physical fitness level. The exercise type, intensity, duration, frequency, and period are the factors to be considered for exercise prescription.

Exercise Type

Exercise type refers to a specific type of sport or activity (soccer, baseball, volleyball, etc.) and may be expressed as either aerobic or anaerobic exercise. As previously mentioned in 'Part 1 Exercise and Health' section, aerobic exercise refers to a long duration type of exercise using a steady amount of oxygen, namely walking, jogging, running, cycling, swimming and so on. Anaerobic exercise refers to weight training, 100-meter running, diving, etc., in which the rate of using oxygen is low and the exercise ends in a short amount of time. However, in the field of exercise prescription, the exercise type is classified into physical fitness areas, that is, the physical activity factors necessary for health-related fitness and the sports factors necessary for technical

5) Functional capacity: It refers to the most basic and independent ability in daily activities (such as dressing, going to the toilet, eating, etc.) and a higher physical fitness factor. This can be assessed as a metabolic equivalent (MET), and running over walking requires a functional capacity above 5MET.

fitness. There are five elements of health-related physical fitness: cardiopulmonary endurance, strength, muscle endurance, flexibility, and body composition. The types of exercise to develop these elements are walking, brisk walking, jogging, running, cycling, swimming, climbing, weight training, stretching, and so on. There are also five elements of skill-related physical fitness: power, speed, agility, balance and coordination (cooperative or interdependent). The types of exercise to develop these elements are listed as high jump, long jump, sidestep, balance beam exercise, soccer, basketball, volleyball, baseball, tennis and so on. These physical factors (health-related and skill-related physical fitness) are interrelated and affect the selection of certain exercises. Prescribing the items related to health-related fitness should be periodized over those related to skill-related fitness, since the purpose of clinical exercise prescription for the health promotion of patients and the general public.

Exercise Intensity

Exercise intensity is a measure of how difficult an exercise is. In the case of aerobic exercise such as running, $\dot{V}O_2max$, maximal heart rate (HRmax), maximal systolic blood pressure (SBPmax), and RPE (ratings of perceived exertion or Borg Scale)[9] are used to indicate exercise intensity. For anaerobic weight-bearing exercises such as weight training, one repetition maximum (1RM) is expressed as the intensity. In the case of patients with muscle rehabilitation, exercise intensity is expressed using peak torque, average power, and total work.[4,5] This chapter deals with the setting of exercise intensity to prescribe aerobic exercise patterns, while setting the intensity of anaerobic weight exercise is covered in the fitness test section.

Table 3.1 ***Aerobic exercise prescription formula***

Items	Target exercise range		Formula
$\dot{V}O_2R$ formula	Target VO_2	=	(Prescribed intensity) × (VO_2max - 3.5) + 3.5
HR_{max} formula	Target HR	=	(Prescribed intensity) × HR_{max} (220 - age)
HR reserve formula	Target HR	=	(Prescribed intensity) × (HR_{max} − HR_{rest}) + HR_{rest}
SBP reserve formula	Target SBP	=	(Prescribed intensity) × (SBP_{max} − SBP_{rest}) + SBP_{rest}

※ Reserve means the amount at which the minimum value is subtracted from the maximum value. In other words, it is easy to think of the amount of energy saved. For example, when comparing the reserves of an athlete and an elderly person (resting heart rate is equal to 60 bpm), the reserve heart rate of a 20 year old athlete is {(220-20 years) - 60} = 140 bpm. On the other hand, the reserve heart rate of a 70-year-old is {(220-70) - 60} = 90 bpm. The difference is about 50 bpm. In other words, the young athlete has a saving rate that can make 50 bpm more.

Exercise intensity is the most important factor to maximize the physiological effect that can be obtained from the human body. It is more important to prescribe exercise based on the data derived from the exercise test by visiting a doctor directly [Appendix B]. However, if you cannot receive a direct exercise test, you should use the "220-age" formula to calculate the maximum heart rate and exercise within the target exercise zone (TEZ) based on the calculated data. This is a better way to do exercises without planning. However, it may be an exception for patients with disease. On the other hand, exercise prescribers use the $\dot{V}O_2max$, maximum heart rate, and maximal systolic blood pressure by direct examination, and maximum heart rate obtained by the indirect formula with the aerobic exercise prescription formulas presented in [Table 3.1]. It is necessary to set the TEZ within a safe limit and effective range.[37,53]

Using the HRR formula for aerobic exercise prescription shown in [Table 3.1], let's set the TEZ for a man whose age is 50 years and whose resting heart rate is 70 bpm. The exercise intensity for the effective limit is 60% and the exercise intensity for the safe limit is 85% [Fig. 3.1].

- HRmax : 220-50 (yr) = 170 bpm
- HRR : 170 bpm - 70 bpm = 100 bpm
- Effective limit : [100 bpm × 60%] + 70 bpm = 130 bpm
  - If converted to 10 seconds (130÷6 = 22 beats/10sec)
- Safe limit : [100 bpm × 85%] + 70 bpm = 155 bpm
  - If converted to 10 seconds (155÷6 = 25 beats/10sec)

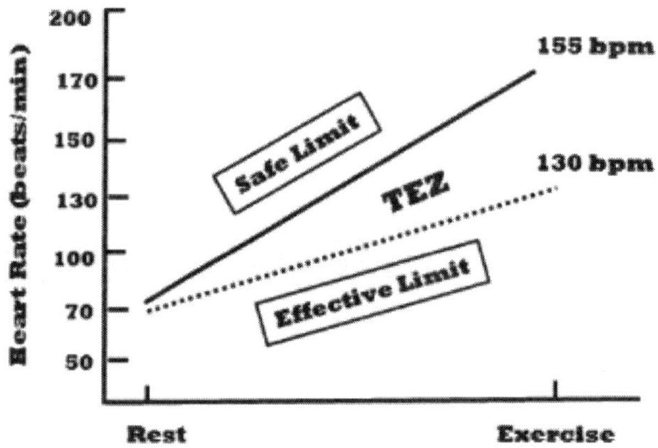

Fig. 3.1 *Target exercise zone*

For effective exercise, the above person should at least reach a heart rate of 130 bpm during exercise, and when considering for safety, the heart rate should not exceed 155 bpm during exercise. In particular, exercises with an intensity of up to 90% may impair the heart or may be accompanied by musculoskeletal disorders. Therefore, in order to perform exercise that is safe and effective, exercise intensity should be kept within the TEZ.

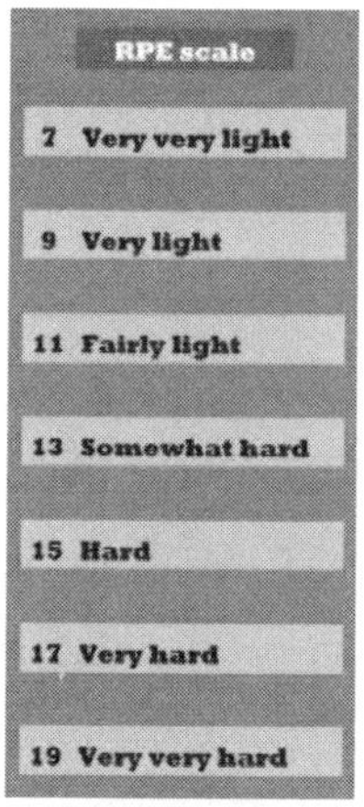

RPE scale
7 Very very light
9 Very light
11 Fairly light
13 Somewhat hard
15 Hard
17 Very hard
19 Very very hard

Fig. 3.2

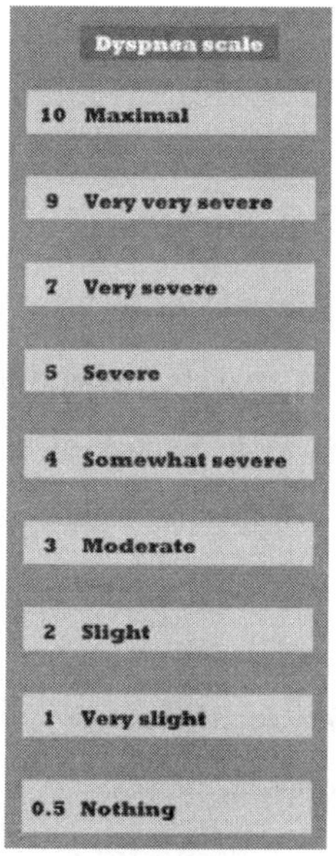

Fig. 3.3

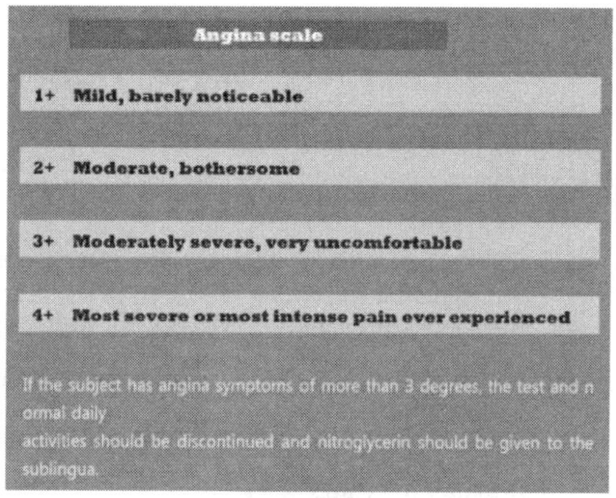

Fig. 3.4

Exercise intensity may be derived from physiological factors such as $\dot{V}O_2max$ and heart rate, but exercise intensity may also be determined by detecting the state of psychological fatigue. This is called RPE [Fig. 3.2]. RPE is based on the assumption that physiological fitness and psychological health conditions do not match. In addition, patients with unstable pulmonary disease use the Dyspnea scale [Fig. 3.3], and patients with angina or myocardial infarction who need rehabilitation therapy use the Angina scale [Fig. 3.4]. This can be used to set the end point for exercise tests or TEZ for exercise prescription [Appendix A].

According to the ACSM, RPE is related to the ratio of exercise intensity to $\dot{V}O_2$ Reserve, HRmax and HR Reserve, and it is possible to switch among them [Table 3.2].[2] Since the target intensity of the above example was 60~85%, the corresponding range of RPE is 14 (between 'somewhat hard' and 'hard') to 17 ('very hard').

Table 3.2 ***Relationship between RPE, $\dot{V}O_2R$, HRR and HRmax***

RPE	%$\dot{V}O_2R$	%HRR	%HRmax
12	40%	40%	64%
13	50%	50%	71%
14	60%	60%	77%
15	70%	70%	84%
16	80%	80%	91%
17	85%	85%	94%

Exercise Duration

Exercise duration or exercise time refers to the duration of a single exercise session. In the case of running, it can be expressed in seconds, minutes and hours, while in the case of weight training, it can be expressed as a number of sets and repetitions. For those who visit a clinic for the first time, the exercise durations can be set using the formula in [Table 3.3].

Table 3.3 ***Calculation of exercise time by METs***

① Maximal METs (㎉/kg/hr) × Intensity ≒ X ㎉/kg/hr
② X ㎉/㎏/hr × Weight ㎏ = Y ㎉/hr
③ Y ㎉/hr ÷ 60 = Z ㎉/min
④ Calories to fit the fitness level ㎉ ÷ Z ㎉/min ≒ Exercise time (min)

※ Fitness and calorie prescription levels

Low	Mid	High
5~8 METs	8~13 METs	≥ 13 METs
≤ 200 ㎉	200~400 ㎉	≥ 400 ㎉

※ The body weight is calculated in units of ㎏ for the exercise time. Calculate the VO_2max or maximal METs (㎉/kg/hr) derived from the graded exercise test. Next, select a calorie amount that matches the fitness level and substitute it into the formula.

- Gender : male
- Age: 32 years old
- Height / Weight : 175 ㎝ / 75㎏
- Maximum MET : 13 METs (㎉/kg/hr)
- Fitness level : 200 ㎉ ~ 400 ㎉
- Exercise intensity : 50%
- Exercise time :
  ① 13 METs × 0.5 ≒ 7 MET (Jogging at 8.0 km/h on the treadmill)
  ② 7 METs × 75 ㎏ = 525 ㎉/hr
  ③ 525 ㎉/hr ÷ 60 = 8.75 ㎉/min
  ④ 200 ㎉ ÷ 8.75 ㎉/min ≒ 23 min
  ⑤ 400 ㎉ ÷ 8.75 ㎉/min ≒ 45 min

[Table 3.3] can be used to set the exercise time for the following patient who is a 32-year-old male with a height and weight of 175 ㎝ and 75 ㎏, respectively. Suppose that the maximum MET value derived from the exercise test is 13 METs, which indicates a moderate fitness level. If the initial exercise intensity for this patient is set at 50% and the patient is instructed to jog at 8.0 km/h on the treadmill (around 7 METs), it will take 23 minutes to consume 200 ㎉ and 45 minutes to consume 400 ㎉.

ACSM recommends 20~60 minutes of caloric consumption through aerobic exercise, excluding warm-up and cool-down.[2] However, in the case of a person with a specific illness, as shown in the example above, it is preferable to set the exercise time accurately considering the oxygen uptake ability or MET of the person rather than the approximate exercise time. Patients who are to be rehabilitated after a heart attack or stroke should be encouraged to repeat the procedure several times with an aerobic exercise time of less than 20 minutes. The reason for strictly keeping the exercise time in such a way is due to the injury rate that can occur in the muscle joints. For this, 15 minutes, 30 minutes, and 45 minutes of daily exercise time were applied to compare the increases in the rate of $\dot{V}O_2max$ and injury rate of muscle joints [Fig. 3.5]. According to the results, $\dot{V}O_2max$ was slightly less than 8% for 15 minutes of daily exercise, while the injury rate was about 20%. On the other hand, when exercising 30 minutes daily, the $\dot{V}O_2max$ increased by more than 15% and the injury rate was 25%. The $\dot{V}O_2max$ was increased by 17% in the case of exercising for 45 minutes per day, but the injury rate was as high as 55%. From these results, it appears that the most desirable exercise time is 30 minutes per day.

However, the results of that study on exercise time and injury rate refer to the short term. After the body adapts to the exercise time to a certain degree, it should be increased to 60 minutes based on the progressive principle of exercise prescription. The extension of this exercise time is effective when the patient does not show signs of excessive fatigue or injury to the prescribed exercise [Appendix C] and is observed to have fully adapted. Usually, this point is less than 2 weeks for athletes with excellent physical fitness, 4 weeks for normal adults with moderate fitness, and about 4 weeks or more for the elderly or weaker patients.

On the other hand, in addition to the above-mentioned aerobic exercise, the duration of cardiopulmonary exercise and muscle endurance exercise should be less than 60 minutes per day and muscle strength exercise should amount to less than 60 minutes per day, while flexibility exercise should be maintained for 10~30 seconds per event [Table 3.4].

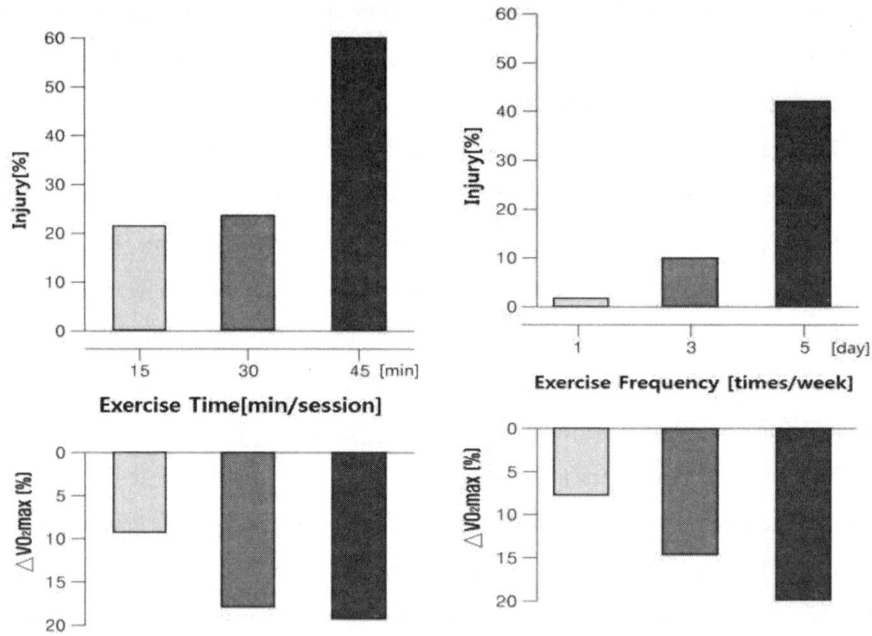

Fig. 3.5 *Comparison between $\dot{V}O_2max$ and injury rate based on exercise time and frequency*

Exercise Frequency

Exercise frequency is a process that considers how many times a day or week exercise should be performed. All of these processes provide the baseline data for developing the following step-by-step exercise plans. As with all procedures, exercise frequency should be prescribed according to the health status and fitness levels of the subjects. Using MET is recommended when considering exercise frequency. According to ACSM's report, which is consistent with the contents in this textbook, a person with a physical fitness level of less than 8 METs must have a professional supervisor. Severe patients with a physical fitness level of less than 5 METs have been reported to differ in their guidelines, depending on their conditions. However, if the physical fitness level of an adult who does not have a specific disease is about 5~8 METs, exercise frequency is recommended to be 3 days per week on alternate days. It may be extended up to 5 days after considering whether the fitness level should be increased.[2] The reason why exercise frequency should be strictly maintained is because of the risk of injury that can occur in the muscle joints. The exercise frequency of 1 day per week, 3 days per week, and 5 days per week was applied to compare the rate of increase in $\dot{V}O_2max$ with that of muscle joints [Fig. 3.5]. According to the results, the $\dot{V}O_2max$ increased by less than

Table 3.4 ***Exercise prescription requirements***

Items	Type	Intensity	Time	Frequency	Period
▪ Cardiopulmonary exercise	▪ Major muscle activity ▪ Continuous motion ▪ Dynamic motion	▪ VO_2R 40~85% ▪ HRR 40~85% ▪ HR_{max} 64~94% ▪ RPE 12~17	▪ 20~60 min ※ In the case of patients, intermittent segmentation	▪ 3~5 days/week ※ For patients, differentiation	▪ More than 12 weeks ※ For patients, until successful rehabilitation
▪ Muscular endurance exercise ※ Circuit training	▪ Target muscle group ▪ Full ROM range ▪ High-speed muscle contraction	▪ 1RM 40~50% ※ Light weight	▪ Less than 60 min ▪ Items : 9~12 ▪ Times : 40~100 ▪ Set : 1~4	▪ 2~3 days/week ▪ Every other day	▪ 8 ~ 12 weeks or more ※ Patient's third stage rehabilitation program
▪ Strength exercise (Muscular hypertrophy improvement)	▪ Major muscle group ▪ Full ROM range ▪ Medium-speed muscle contraction	▪ 1RM 60~80% ※ Moderate weight	▪ Less than 60 min ▪ Items : 8~10 ▪ Times : 10~25 ▪ Set : 1~4	▪ 2~3 days/week ▪ Every other day	▪ 8 ~ 12 weeks or more ※ Patient's second stage rehabilitation program
▪ Strength exercise (Neuromuscle improvement)	▪ Major muscle group ▪ Full ROM range ▪ Low-speed muscle contraction	▪ 1RM 80~95% ※ 1RM 100% is the development of muscle power	▪ Less than 60 min ▪ Items : 8~10 ▪ Times : 1~10 ▪ Set : 1~4	▪ 2~3 days/week ▪ Every other day	▪ 8 ~ 12 weeks or more ※ Patient's first stage rehabilitation program
▪ Flexibility exercise	▪ Static stretching ▪ Dynamic stretching ▪ PNF	▪ Mild discomfort	▪ Time : 10~30sec ▪ Set : 3~4	▪ More than 2~3 days/week	▪ More than 8 weeks

10% when exercise was performed for 1 day per week, while the injury rate was less than 5%. On the other hand, when exercising for 3 days per week, the $\dot{V}O_2max$ was increased by 15% and the injury rate was less than 10%. In the case of exercising 5 days per week, the $\dot{V}O_2max$ increased by 18% and the injury rate was as high as about 40%. In other words, the most effective exercise frequency has been shown to be 3 days per week.

However, the frequency of exercise and injury rates mentioned above refer to the short term. After the adapts to the exercise frequency to a certain degree, it should be increased to 5 days based on the progressive principle of exercise prescription. The increase in exercise frequency is similar to the increase in exercise time suggested above, and should be applied only when the subject has fully adapted without showing signs of excessive fatigue and injury to the prescribed exercise. In addition to the above mentioned aerobic exercise, the recommended frequency of cardiopulmonary exercise and muscle endurance exercise is 2~3 days per week, muscle strength exercise is preferably 2~3 days per week, while flexibility exercise is 2~3 days per week as shown in [Table 3.4].

Exercise Period

Exercise period refers to a length of time in terms of weeks or months in which an exercise is expected to produce an effect. This process is the basis for preparing a 'step-by-step exercise plan', and it is recommended to prescribe the exercise period based on the individualized principle of exercise prescription.

It is important to note that the recommended exercise period reported so far varies according to fitness level, but generally, 4~8 weeks is prescribed. A period of 12 weeks is best to observe changes in fitness level. Of course, this does not mean that exercise can be stopped after 12 weeks. Recall that based on the reverse principle of exercise prescription, if exercise is stopped for more than 2 weeks, the health state or fitness level reverts back to the initial level. Therefore, it is recommended to exercise for a lifetime under a specific plan. For example, adult diseases are called 'incurable diseases' or 'life-long illnesses' and are difficult to manage. Also, since adult diseases cannot be found if it is well managed at a young age, exercise should be lifelong. Ultimately, the requirements of exercise prescription described so far are listed according to fitness factors [Table 3.4].

Exercise Planning

Daily Plan

In order to successfully achieve the goals of the exercise prescribed, it is recommended to plan daily exercise time effectively. In other words, most people want to participate in exercise, but on the other hand, they do not have the time and can miss the opportunity to participate, so exercise time and daily activities should be properly coordinated. Therefore, a daily plan should be designed to find the most appropriate time for exercise and then prescribe an exercise program for that time. Typically, daily exercise plans include warm-up, work-out, and cool-down.

Warm-up

A warm-up is literally a pre-exercise that lasts 10~15 minutes. The reason is that warm-up do not exceed 15 minutes is because it may prevent the subject from performing the main exercise.[41] Specifically, warm-up refer to the stage before sweating, which is the process of warming and softening each joint or muscle by raising the heat of the entire body. On the kinematic side, warm-up is also referred to as a step of raising the body temperature (rectal temperature) by about 1°C above the stable state. Types of warm-up may include flexibility exercises to soften joints with appropriate stretching, or simple exercises such as standing walks. The sequence of warm-up is as follows, and it is performed about 8~10 times twice per motion.

The below warm-up consists of 12 steps and includes breathing at the end. In addition, warm-up help prevent shocks by starting from the most distant ankle and gradually reaching the heart.

Work-out

A work-out consists of aerobic exercises such as walking or biking, and resistance exercises such as weight training or elastic bands. In general, those with moderate fitness levels who want to enjoy sports can play tennis, table tennis, volleyball, basketball, go bowling, or swimming. The exercise duration of a workout should be less than 60 minutes of aerobic exercise and 50 minutes of weight training. Therefore, when both types of exercises are to be performed, gender, age, physical condition, and mobility, should be taken into consideration. It is recommended for the average person or beginner to carry out aerobic exercise every day and resistance exercise every other day.

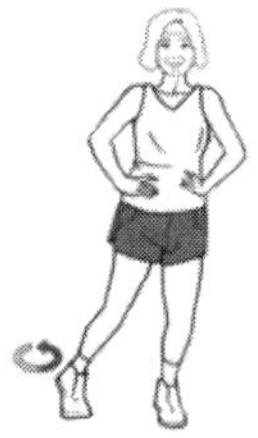

Ankle rotation

Stand naturally. Raise your ankle and rotate it slightly larger than normal ROM. Perform two sets of 8 to 10 times.

Knee rotation

Bring your legs and bend your knees slightly. Turn your knee 8 times from left to right and 8 times from right to left.

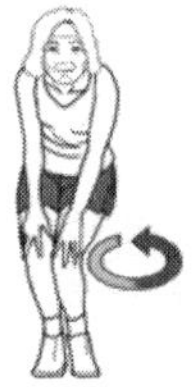

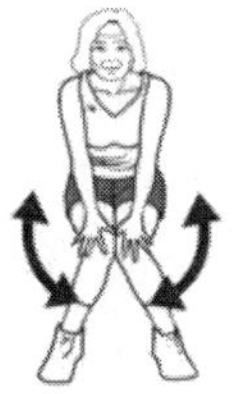

Knee cross rotation

Stand your knees wide with your shoulders wide and rotate them from in to out, from out to in, 8 times each.

Hip anterior / posterior rotation

Lift one leg and rotate it from front to back and from back to front 8 times.

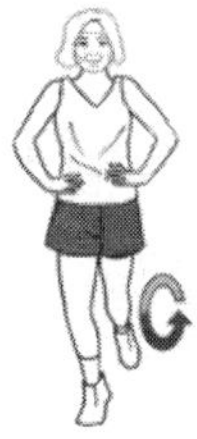

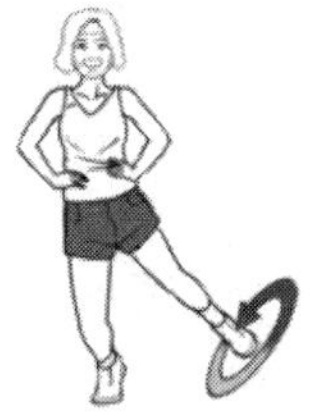

Hip side rotation

Spread one side of the legs on the side and turn it inside out, and from outside to inside 8 times. Do the same on the opposite side.

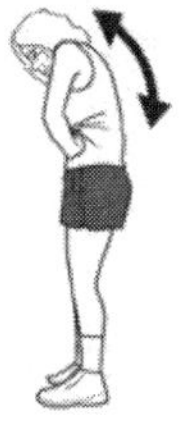

Trunk flexion

Attach the jaw to the chest as much as possible, keeping the back bent like a whale for 10 seconds. This is done in two sets.

Trunk extension

Strike your head back as far as possible, hold your back for 10 seconds with your back extended. This is done in two sets.

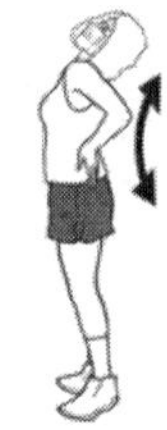

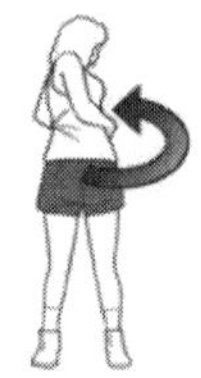

Trunk lateral rotation

Cross your hands back and forth a wrap your waist. Keep your eyes far back as possible for 10 secon Do the same on the opposite side.

Shoulder rotation

With your elbows in line with your shoulders, rotate your elbows from inside to outside, from outside to inside, 8 times each.

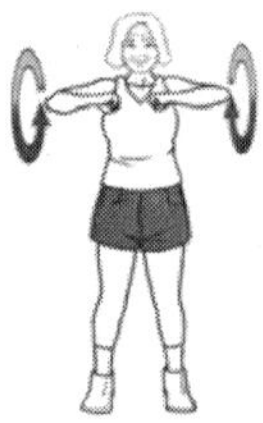

Elbow rotation

Turn your elbows 90 degrees from outside to inside 8 times. This is done in two sets.

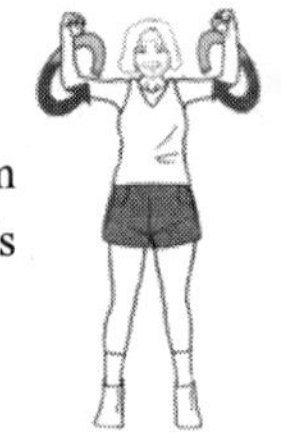

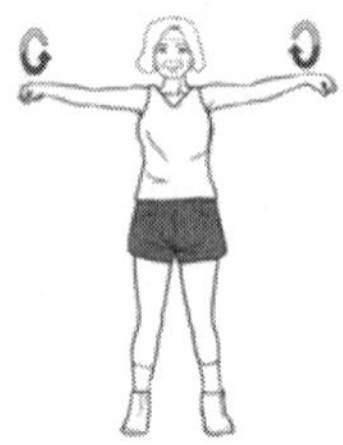

Wrist rotation

Stand with your arms open sideways and rotate the small circles of the shoulder joints in and out, out and in, eight times each.

Neck rotation

Pull down your head and lower it. Hold your waist with both hands and turn your head slowly from left to right and right to left 8 times.

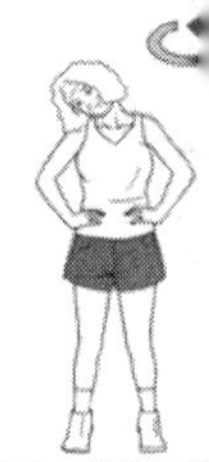

Cool-down

It is recommended that cool-down exercises should be performed for 10-15 minutes after the main exercise. However, in the case of the elderly, it takes about 30 minutes without any time limitation to increase the vein return to help the fatigue recovery. In summary, cool-down refers to the process of relieving tension and fatigue accumulated in the body during exercise by performing light exercises at a constant tempo or stretching. Cool-down means to return the body temperature to a stable state by lowering the body temperature by 1°C in contrast to the warm-up concept. Cool-down is based on stretching as follows. It is desirable to keep 2 repetitions and 10 seconds in one motion. The 18 cool-down steps are shown below. As opposed to warm-up exercises, cool-down exercises start with the head, closest to the heart, and gradually reach the distal parts to help relieve fatigue.

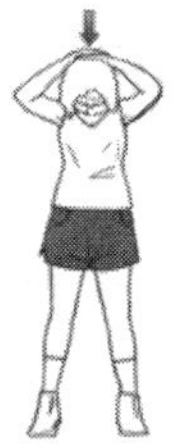

Neck flexion

Place both hands on the parietal bone and apply light pressure. Keep breathing out for 10 seconds. Perform two sets.

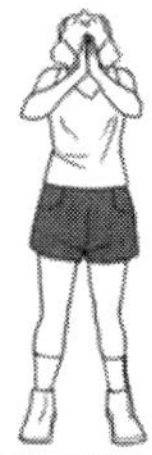

Neck hyperextension

Put both hands on your chin and push lightly. Keep breathing out for 10 seconds. Perform two sets.

Neck lateral extension

The head is on the side and one hand holds the temporal bone of the opposite side and the neck is extended. This is done in two sets for 10 seconds.

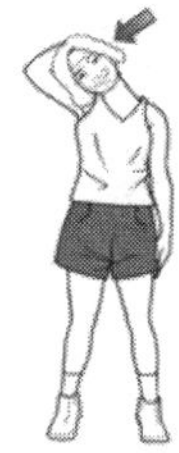

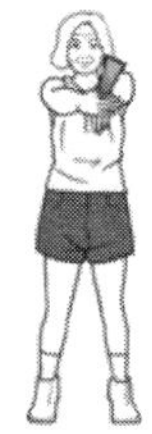

Wrist flexion

Stretch one hand forward, lightly stretch your back with one hand. This is done in two sets for 10 seconds.

Shoulder flexion

Clasp hands and lift arms up. At this time, the breath is spit, and it is done for two sets for 10 seconds.

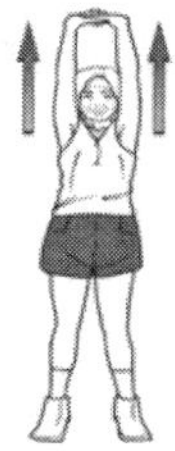

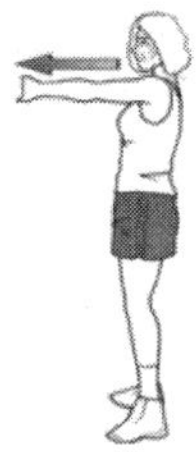

Shoulder protraction

Clasp hands and push arms forward. At this time, the breath is spit, and it is done for two sets for 10 seconds.

Shoulder overextension

Put your hand pod behind your back and lift it up slightly. At this time, the breath is spit, and it is done for two sets for 10 seconds.

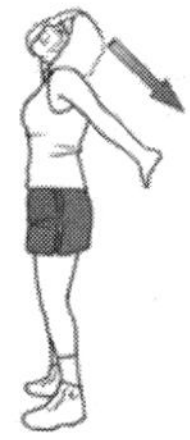

Shoulder horizontal adduction

With one arm pointing sideways, press the elbow with the opposite arm. The head is reversed and two sets are carried out for 10 seconds.

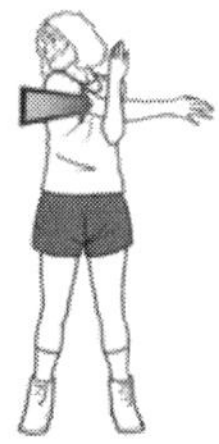

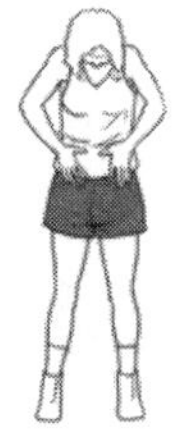

Trunk flexion

Keep your jaw on your chest as much as possible, and keep your back for 10 seconds with your back bent like a whale. This is done in two sets.

Trunk extension

Strike your head back as far as possible, and hold your back for 10 seconds with your back extended like a bow. This is done in two sets.

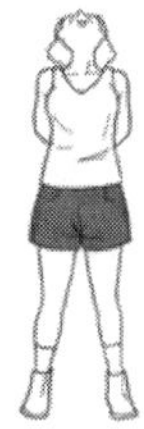

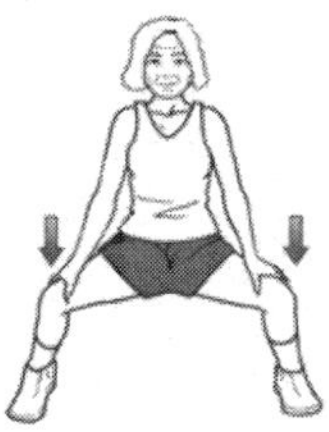

Pelvic extension

Make your legs wide and your knees 90°. Lean your arms on both thighs and hold them for 10 seconds.

Hip abduction

Sit with one leg extended to the side with both hands on the waist. Hold for 10 sec and perform two sets.

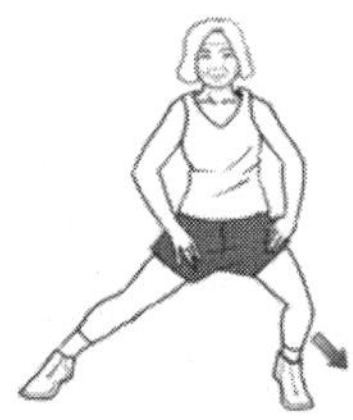

Forward lunge motion

Sit one leg forward and stretch it so that your knee is 90°. Keep this for 10 seconds and repeat 2 sets.

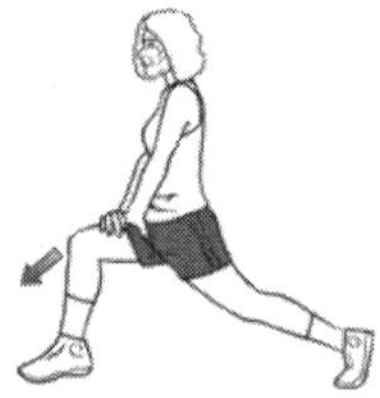

Hamstring extension

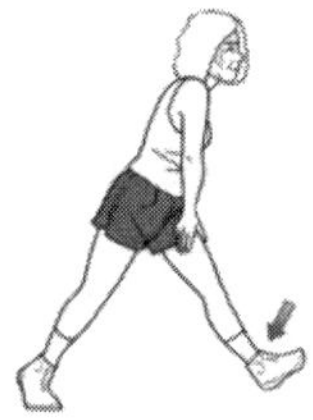

Stretch one leg forward, and put weight behind. Keep this for 10 seconds and repeat 2 sets.

Quadriceps extension

Fold one leg back and hold your forefeet with one hand for 10 seconds. This is done in two sets.

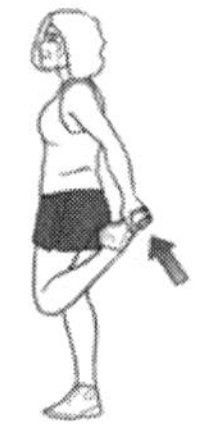

Ankle eversion

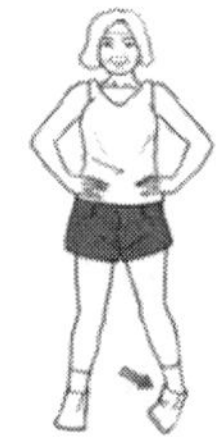

Lightly bend one of the ankles outward. Two sets are performed for 10 seconds, and the opposite side is performed in the same manner.

Ankle eversion

Lightly bend one of the ankles outward. Applying too much weight can put strain on your ankle.

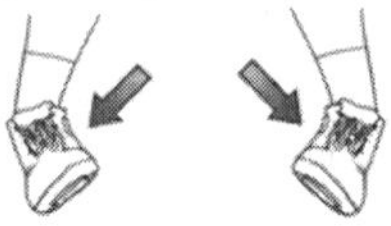

Ankle dorsiflexion / plantarflexion

Put pressure on the forefoot and heel in the right or left sides. Repeat this two sets of 10 seconds each.

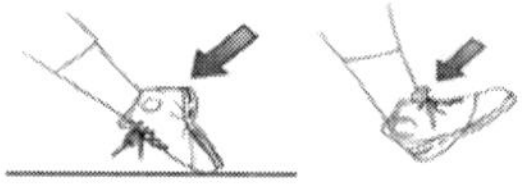

Weekly Plan

It is ideal to create a weekly exercise plan. While exercising daily is beneficial, it is impossible to carry out many exercises in one day. On the other hand, planning on a monthly basis is too broad to grasp physiological exercise effects. Therefore, it is desirable to create an exercise plan on a weekly basis. An example of a weekly exercise plan is shown in [Table 3.5].

Table 3.5 ***Example of an afternoon weekly plan***

	Monday	Tuesday	Wednesday	Thursday	Friday	Saturday
7:00~7:15	Warm up	Warm up	Warm up	Warm up	Warm up	Warm up
7:15~7:45	Walking on a treadmill	Swimming	Walking on a treadmill	Swimming	Walking on a treadmill	Badminton
7:45~7:50	5 minutes break	Cool down	5 minutes break	Cool down	5 minutes break	Cool down
7:50~8:20	Resistance exercise	Shower	Resistance exercise	Shower / clothes	Resistance exercise	Shower
8:20~8:30	Cool down		Cool down		Cool down	
8:30~8:40	Shower		Shower		Shower	

Annual Plan

An annual plan is the best tool that an exercise specialist can use to set direction and guide a subject for a year. The annual plan is based on the concept of the periodization principle. It is divided into a conditioning phase, an improvement phase, and a maintenance phase.

Conditioning Phase

The conditioning phase is the initial process of the exercise program designed to adapt the human body to exercise, minimize the side effects that may occur during exercise, and improve the muscles and human organs necessary for exercise. The conditioning phase must be included for those who have not had any exercise experience or have not exercised for a long time, especially for patients with chronic diseases. The exercise program in this phase emphasizes warm-up and cool-down and starts with an intensity and duration that is 10% less than the prescribed exercise program. For example, if a hypertensive patient is prescribed exercise to reduce blood pressure which is set at 160/90 mmHg during exercise, then a range of 145/81 mmHg, which is 10% lower, would be appropriate. The duration of the conditioning phase depends on age, severity of disease, and physical fitness level of the participant, but generally, about 4 weeks is recommended.

Improvement Phase

The improvement phase is the most important step for achieving the maximum exercise effect in the exercise program. In this phase, the exercise program should be structured in consideration of exercise intensity, time, and frequency according to the components of exercise prescription. In the case of the hypertensive patient presented above, the blood pressure during exercise was 145/81 mmHg which lasted for 4 weeks. Therefore, from the 5th week, the exercise intensity should be increased by 2% per week

Phase	Jan		Feb	Mar	Apr	May	Jun	Jul	Aug	Sep	Oct	Nov	Dec
	0wk	~4wk	~4wk	~4wk	~4wk	~4wk	~4wk	~4wk	~4wk	~4wk	~4wk	~4wk	~4wk
Conditioning	Test	RT											
Improvement							RT						
Maintenance													RT

RT(Retest) : It is recommended that the retest be performed at a time point of 1 month / 6 months / 12 months after starting of the exercise.

Fig. 3.6 ***Annual plan for clinical exercise prescription***

so that the final 160/90 ㎜Hg should be reached and maintained. That is, the blood pressure level on the 5th week (× 2%) should be 148/83 ㎜Hg, 150/84 ㎜Hg on the 6th week (× 4%) and 154/86 ㎜Hg on the 7th week. After reaching 157/87 ㎜Hg on the 8th week (× 8%), exercise should be performed at 160/90 ㎜Hg, which is the original prescription strength from the 9th week (× 10%). After this process lasts more over one month, it is recommended to intermittently include a program reaching a SBP of 180 ㎜Hg to increase resistance to blood vessel elasticity. The period of such an improvement phase is usually set for about 24 weeks.

Maintenance Phase

The maintenance phase is the last phase of an exercise program and is performed after 24 weeks to maintain an improved fitness level. Considering that the maintenance phase should be continued over a long period of time, it is recommended to set the exercise intensity, time, and frequency of the improvement phase 5~10% lower. In other words, it must be decided whether the exercises will continue to attract interest in the future.

Ultimately, the annual plan for the conditioning, improvement and maintenance phases is shown in [Fig. 3.6]. Reevaluation should be conducted periodically, such as one month or six months, depending on the characteristics of the patient or athlete. The results have a major impact on the motivation of the subjects.

Procedure and Pre-examination of Exercise Prescription

Exercise offers many benefits for everyone. This includes not only lowering cardiovascular risk factors, but also lowering the prevalence of coronary heart disease and increasing psychological well-being.[8,16,54] However, in spite of these benefits, past experts who have tried to implement exercise programs often provided incomplete and inaccurate information to patients.[7,22] If the factors and procedures for exercise prescription are learned and understood, an improvement of physical activity can be expected. For this, pre-test factors for exercise prescription should be obtained through questionnaires, pre-exercise consultations, medical examinations, body composition tests, exercise tests, muscle function tests, and physical fitness tests. Based on the results of the tests, exercise prescription (exercise type, intensity, time, and frequency) should be followed and the subject should be continuously encouraged to participate in a full-scale exercise program. The pre-test provides important information for assessing not only the presence or absence of diseases, but also the risk factors for disease onset. [Fig. 3.7] shows the pre-examination flow chart according to exercise prescription procedures [Appendix D].

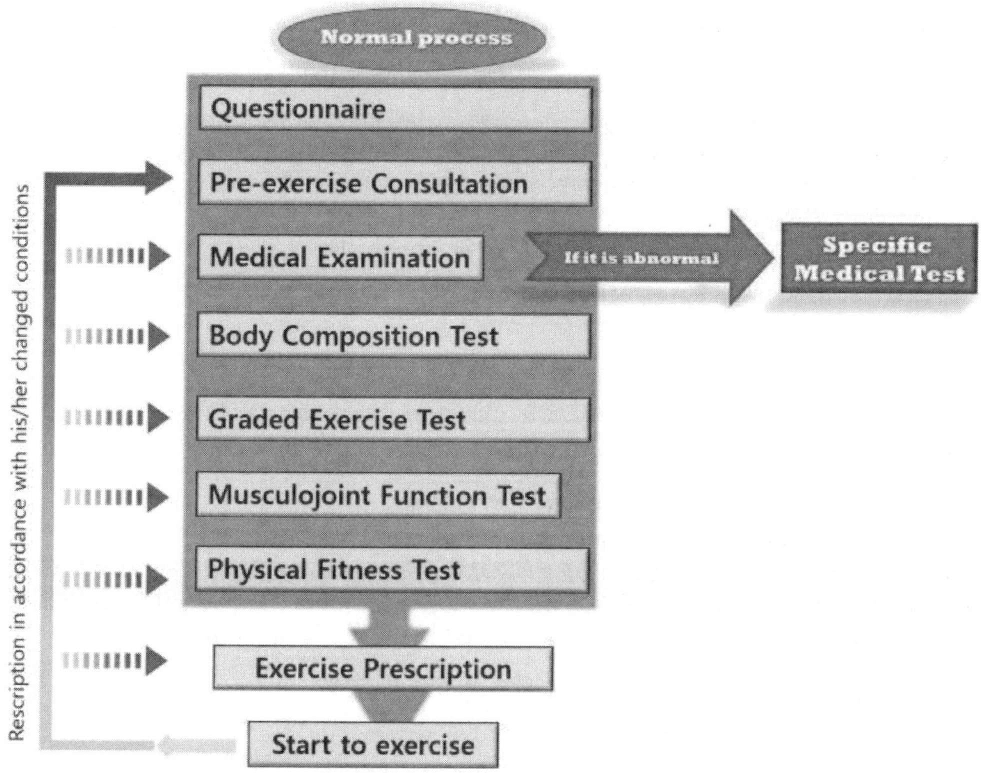

Fig. 3.7 *Procedure of exercise prescription*

Questionnaire

When a patient visits a clinic, he or she is seated in a comfortable chair and is guided to fill out a health questionnaire and personal record form. This is the minimum required information to know a patient's physical characteristics, including consciousness of health [Table 3.6]. This should include age, occupation, past medical history, past exercise habits, current exercise activities, current health condition, diet, sleep patterns, digestive issues, drinking habits, smoking habits, and the type of medication being used. In other words, the pre-exercise prescription questionnaire is to determine the 'eligibility condition' of exercise availability (see Tables 3.6a, 3.6b, and 3.6c).

Refer to [Appendix C] for information on injuries during exercise that are not listed in [Table 3.6c], and be well-acquainted with the treatment methods and preventative measures. Refer to [Table 3.6] and classify the subjects according to [Table 3.7]. It is advisable to give accurate information on the type of exercise tests and the types of exercise programs recommended for the categorized patients.[2]

Table 3.6 ***ACSM Screening Tests*** ** When you agree with this case, mark ✔ in the judgment box ▢*

Name/ Age :	Gender (M / F) :	Height (m) / Weight (kg) :	Occupation :

	I. Risk factor (Two or more belong to moderate risk group)	✔
1.	Have any of the parents/siblings died of heart-related surgery or sudden death before the age of 55 (male relative) or 65 years (female relative)?	▢
2.	Have you ever smoked before the past six months? ※ Please fill in current smoker	▢
3.	Is normal blood pressure greater than 140/90 mmHg? ※ Even if you take hypotensive agents at present	▢
4.	What about your cholesterol level? ※ LDL > 130 mg/dℓ, TC > 200 mg/dℓ, HDL < 40 mg/dℓ is dangerous. However, when HDL > 60 mg/dℓ, one point is cut from the risk factor.	▢
5.	What about your fasting glucose level (≥ 100 mg/dℓ or ≤ 125 mg/dℓ) or postprandial 2 hour glucose level (≥ 140 mg/dℓ or ≤ 199 mg/dℓ) ?	▢
6.	What is the height / weight (BMI ≥ 30kg/m²) and waist circumference (male > 102 cm (40 in) and female > 80 cm (35 in)?	▢
7.	Do you have 30 minutes of physical activity more than 3 times per week?	▢
	II. Symptom factor (One or more belong to high risk group)	✔
8.	Have you experienced pain or discomfort in or around your chest?	▢
9.	Have you experienced fainting or dizziness other than when you wake up quickly?	▢
10.	Have you ever felt difficulty breathing when sitting down or sleeping?	▢
11.	Have you ever experienced an ankle swelling other than standing for a long time?	▢
12.	Have you ever felt the chest pounding or a rapid pulse?	▢
13.	Have you ever experienced leg pain such as intermittent claudication?	▢
14.	Have you ever heard of a heart murmur?	▢
15.	Have you ever experienced breathing difficulty or an unusual fatigue with routine activities?	▢
	III. Other factor (According to the standard value of each item)	✔
16.	How old are you now? ※ Male 45 years old, female 55 years or older belong to the risk group.	▢
17.	Do you have problems with worsening bones or joints when you exercise? If yes, postpone the test or apply the modified test	▢
18.	Do you currently have a cold or other infection? If yes, postpone the test or apply the modified test	▢
19.	Are you pregnant now? If yes, postpone the test.	▢
20.	Do you have other problems that make vigorous exercise difficult? If yes, postpone the test or apply the modified test	▢
21.	Do you have any of these diseases? Heart disease, Peripheral blood vessel, Cerebrovascular disease, COPD, Asthma, Lung disease, Cystic fibrosis, Diabetes, Thyroid, Kidney, Liver diseases, If yes, you belong to high risk group.	▢

Table 3.6a ***Evaluation and judgment of ACSM Screening Tests***

I. Risk factor (Two or more belong to moderate risk group)

	Yes	Unknown	No
1. Have any of the parents/siblings died of heart-related surgery or sudden death before the age of 55 (male relative) or 65 years (female relative)?	(①)	(②)	(③)

① If you have a relative who died of heart disease, you are encouraged to visit a clinic and have a close examination.
② If you do not know your cardiovascular history, you will be judged as normal, but you should be careful if you are 45 years old and 55 years old or older.
③ In the absence of heart disease, it is normal and indicates a healthy condition.

	Yes	Unknown	No
2. Have you ever smoked before the past six months?	(①)	(②)	(③)

① Smoking may cause cardiovascular and cerebrovascular disease, so no smoking should be encouraged.
② If you do not know the period of no smoking, it is recommended to be careful if you are 45 years old or older and 55 years old or older.
③ If you do not have any smoking experience, it is normal and your health condition is good.

	Yes	Unknown	No
3. Is normal blood pressure greater than 140/90 mmHg?	(①)	(②)	(③)

① High blood pressure can cause cardiovascular and cerebrovascular disease, and it is recommended that you receive regular checkups.
② If you do not know the figures, you are considered to be at risk. Men 45 years old / women 55 years or older should be careful.
③ Low blood pressure is normal and indicates good health. ※ The optimum level is 115 / 75 mmHg.

	Yes	Unknown	No
4. What is cholesterol level?	(①)	(②)	(③)

① High cholesterol may cause cardiovascular and cerebrovascular disease, and it is recommended that you have regular checkups.
② If the numerical value is not known, it is considered to be abnormal. Men 45 years old / women 55 years or older should be careful.
③ Low cholesterol levels are normal and indicate good health.

	Yes	Unknown	No
5. What is fasting glucose(≥110mg/dℓ)?	(①)	(②)	(③)

① In the case of hyperglycemia, it may cause diabetic complications, so it should be regularly diagnosed and treated.
② If you do not know the figures, you are considered to be at risk. Men 45 years old / women 55 years or older should be careful.
③ If the blood glucose level is normal, it means that the health condition is good.

	Yes	Unknown	No
6. What is the height / weight (BMI≥30kg/m²) and waist circumference (male>90cm, female>85cm)?	(①)	(②)	(③)

① If the BMI is ≥ 30kg/m² and the waist circumference is > 102 cm for men and > 88 cm for women, treatment is required because it is abdominal obesity.
② If you do not know the figures, you are considered to be at risk. Men 45 years old / women 55 years or older should be careful.
③ If the BMI is 18.5~24.9 kg/m², or if the waist circumference is 102 cm or less and 88 cm or less, it means that the health condition is good.

	Yes	Unknown	No
7. Do you have 30 minutes of physical activity more than 3 times per week?	(①)	(②)	(③)

① It provides a very significant effect on the cardiovascular and musculoskeletal system and means that the current health condition is good.
② If you do not know the regularity of exercise, it is considered abnormal and you are recommended to have a graded exercise test.
③ If you do not exercise regularly, it is abnormal and may cause adverse health effects.

Table 3.6b ***Evaluation and judgment of ACSM Screening Tests***

II. Symptom factor (more than one belongs to high risk group)

8. Have you experienced pain or discomfort in or around your chest?	Yes (①)	Unknown (②)	No (③)

① If you feel pain often, it is dangerous. It is recommended that you visit the clinic and have a close examination.
② If you do not feel pain, it is normal. If you are 45 or over, you must take a graded exercise test.
③ If you do not feel any pain, it is normal and your health is good.

9. Have you experienced fainting or dizziness other than when you wake up quickly?	Yes (①)	Unknown (②)	No (③)

① If you feel dizziness frequently, it is dangerous. It is recommended that you visit the clinic and have a close examination.
② If you do not feel dizziness, it is normal, but if the man is 45 years old / woman is 55 years old or older, you should get graded exercise test.
③ If you do not feel dizziness, it is normal and it means your health is good.

10. Have you ever felt difficulty breathing when sitting down or sleeping?	Yes (①)	Unknown (②)	No (③)

① If you have difficulty breathing, it is dangerous. It is recommended that you visit the clinic and have a close examination.
② If you do not feel difficulty breathing is normal. However, more attention is given to men over 45 years old and women over 55 years old.
③ If you do not feel difficulty breathing, it is normal and it means your health condition is good.

11. Have you ever experienced an ankle swelling other than standing for a long time?	Yes (①)	Unknown (②)	No (③)

① If your legs swell frequently, it is recommended that you visit your clinic and have a close examination because it is a health signal.
② It is normal if you do not know that your legs are swollen. However, more attention is given to men over 45 years old and women over 55 years old.
③ If the leg is not swollen, it is normal and it means that the health condition is good.

12. Have you ever felt the chest pounding or a rapid pulse?	Yes (①)	Unknown (②)	No (③)

① It is dangerous to experience frequent pounding, so it is recommended that you visit the clinic and have a close examination.
② It is normal if you do not feel pounding. However, more attention is given to men over 45 years old and women over 55 years old.
③ If you do not feel pounding, it is normal and means your health is good.

13. Have you ever experienced leg pain such as intermittent claudication?	Yes (①)	Unknown (②)	No (③)

① It is dangerous to experience frequent leg numbness, so it is recommended that you visit your clinic and have a close examination.
② If you do not feel leg numbness, it is normal. However, more attention is given to men over 45 years old and women over 55 years old.
③ If you do not feel the leg numbness, it is normal and the condition is good.

14. Have you ever heard of a heart murmur?	Yes (①)	Unknown (②)	No (③)

① If you have been told that your heart is weak, you are encouraged to have a close examination.
② It is normal if you do not know if your heart is weak. However, more attention is given to men over 45 years old and women over 55 years old.
③ If you have not heard that your heart is weak, it is normal and means you are in good health.

15. Have you ever experienced breathing difficulty or an unusual fatigue with routine activities?	Yes (①)	Unknown (②)	No (③)

① Severe breathing difficulties and fatigue are health threats, so it is recommended that you visit your clinic and have a close examination.
② It is normal if you do not know dyspnea and fatigue. However, more attention is given to men over 45 years old and women over 55 years old.
③ If you do not feel dyspnea and fatigue, it is normal and it means that your health condition is good.

Table 3.6c ***Evaluation and judgment of ACSM Screening Tests***

III. Other factor (According to each item, only item 21 is delivered to the patient)

21. Do you have any of these diseases? Heart disease, Peripheral blood vessel, Cerebrovascular disease, COPD, Asthma, Interstitial lung disease, Cystic fibrosis, Diabetes, Thyroid, Kidney, Liver diseases

□ Hospital diagnosis history

Item	Check	Item	Check
1. Heart disease	(①)	6. Diabetes	(⑥)
2. Peripheral vascular disease	(②)	7. Thyroid disease	(⑦)
3. Cerebrovascular disease	(③)	8. Renal disease	(⑧)
4. Pulmonary disease	(④)	9. Liver disease	(⑨)
5. Asthma	(⑤)	10. Other (musculoskeletal disease)	(⑩)

① If you are experiencing heart disease, but you are receiving treatment, you may be able to exercise safely while consulting with an expert.
② If you are experiencing peripheral vascular disease, but you are receiving treatment, you may be able to exercise safely while consulting with an expert.
③ If you are experiencing peripheral cerebrovascular disease, but you are receiving treatment, you may be able to exercise safely while consulting with an expert.
④ If you are experiencing peripheral pulmonary disease, but you are receiving treatment, you may be able to exercise safely while consulting with an expert.
⑤ If you are experiencing peripheral asthma, but you are receiving treatment, you may be able to exercise safely while consulting with an expert.
⑥ If you are experiencing diabetes, but you are receiving treatment, you may be able to exercise safely while consulting with an expert.
⑦ If you are experiencing thyroid disease, but you are receiving treatment, you may be able to exercise safely while consulting with an expert.
⑧ If you are experiencing renal disease, but you are receiving treatment, you may be able to exercise safely while consulting with an expert.
⑨ If you are experiencing liver disease, but you are receiving treatment, you may be able to exercise safely while consulting with an expert.
⑩ If you are experiencing musculoskeletal disease, but you are receiving treatment, you may be able to exercise safely while consulting with an expert.

Pre-exercise Consultation

Based on the questionnaire completed by the patient, a brief explanation of the medical examination, exercise prescription, type of examinations, and the kind of exercises that the patients are wondering about should be given. In addition, the atmosphere of the consultation room should be calm and designed to convey professionalism. During the consultation, a sign should be attached indicating that consultation is in progress to prevent possible interruptions. Furniture should be neatly arranged with simple, uniform colors so that the consultant and the patient can concentrate as much as possible. The consultant's appearance should be neat and professional. In addition, postprandial brushing should be performed [Fig. 3.8].

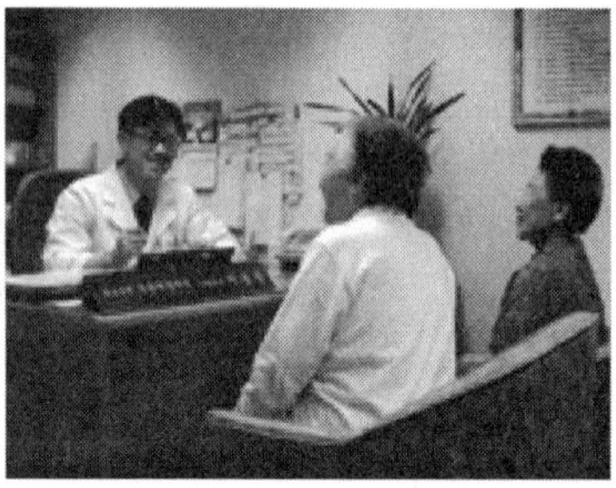

- Explanation of medical examination and exercise prescription based on questionnaires.
- Explanation of test type and kind of exercise.
- The atmosphere of the counseling room is made calm.
- Attaching a sign to inform counseling.
- The counselor clean up the appearance and clean the mouth.
- If pre-exercise testing is required, apply [Table 3.8].
- Be familiar with the simple questionnaire (PAR-Q) and ask questions and counseling.

Fig. 3.8 ***Pre-exercise consultation***

Table 3.7 ***Category of recommended exercise tests and prescriptions based on risk level of health status***

	Risk condition and degree	Recommended exercise tests and prescription categories
Low Risk Level (Normal group)	■ Middle-aged or younger (male 45 years / female 55 years or younger) ■ No coronary heart disease risk factor or less than 1 ■ No other diseases or symptoms ■ Metabolic ability of ***13 METs*** or more	■ Maximum exercise test available ■ Consumable over 400 ㎉ ■ 5 days or more per week ■ Outdoor exercise such as tennis
Moderate Risk Level (Abnormal possible group)	■ Middle-aged or older (male 45 years / female 55 years or older) ■ 2 or more of coronary heart disease risk factors ■ Metabolic ability of ***8~13 METs***	■ Submaximal (85%) exercise test possible ■ Consumable 200~400 ㎉ ■ Indoor exercise is desirable
High Risk Level (Abnormal group)	■ One or more symptoms of heart and lung disease ■ With cardiovascular / pulmonary / metabolic diseases ■ Metabolic ability of ***5~8 METs***	■ Unable to test without a doctor ■ Exercise with experts to less than 200 ㎉ ■ Indoor exercise (with experts)

Keep in mind that it is very dangerous for people who have long led sedentary lifestyles to suddenly become physically active. To prevent this, it is very important to identify the increased risk of negative cardiovascular responses during exercise. In order to identify those who are likely to be exposed to these risk factors, the ACSM has made a classification table as shown in [Table 3.7] to determine whether inspection and evaluation are necessary.[2]

As shown in [Table 3.8], the three risk categories include the patient's age, coronary risk factors, and those exposed to coronary heart disease. The patient's age must be assessed by an expert before starting an exercise program. Patients of a certain age have less negative reactions to exercise. In other words, those categorized in the healthy group can exercise without supervision and only receive initial training based on the principles of exercise prescription.

Table 3.8 ***Ages that require pre-exercise testing****

Risk category†		Age (yr)	Reference
Health group‡	Male	≥ 45	*Direct measurement is necessary for abnormalities in the cardiopulmonary / peripheral blood vessel / musculoskeletal / metabolic / endocrine system. †Classification of ACSM (1988). ‡Health group refers to groups without risk factors for CAD. §A group with one or more risk factors for CAD (hypertension, diabetes, familial history of CAD before age 50, obesity, smoking, hypercholesterolemia, sedentary lifestyle). ¶A group with or suffering from heart or lung disease.
	Female	≥ 50	
Risk group§	Male	≥ 35	
	Female	≥ 40	
Disease group¶		All ages	

Table 3.9 ***Physical Activity Readiness Questionnaire: PAR-Q***

1. Heart problems : Have you ever heard of a doctor having a heart problem?
2. Chest pain : Do you often feel chest pain?
3. Faint or dizziness : Have you ever had the feeling of sitting down or experiencing severe dizziness?
4. Hypertension : Have you ever heard your doctor tell you your blood pressure is too high?
5. Bone or joint problems : Are there any arthritic diseases that are caused or exacerbated during exercise?
6. Physical reason : Do you have any special causes that prevent you from exercising?
7. Aging : Are you older than 65 or are not used to heavy exercise?

As an alternative method to identify risk groups, seven questionnaire items (PAR-Q) were created as shown in [Table 3.9].[12] These questionnaires were designed to be easily applied in clinical as well as community clubs. In other words, if a patient were to answer 'yes' to any question, professional counseling should be sought from a specialist before beginning the exercise program.

Medical Examination

Medical examinations consist of X-ray, physical, body composition, and biochemical contents of blood tests. The results of the medical examination help determine the requirements for the next step of the examination and contraindications. For medical examinations it is advisable to consult a doctor and proceed to the next step after receiving approval if the following conditions are present: Resting heart rate is more than 100 bpm, SBP is 160 ㎜Hg or more, DBP is 90 ㎜Hg or more, TC is 260 ㎎/dℓ or more, Blood glucose is 300 ㎎/dℓ, and Any abnormalities found from ECG.

Blood and biochemical tests are the simplest and most important indicators in diagnosing and treating diseases, so these tests need to be checked thoroughly. These tests are recommended so that healthy people, as well as patients, can have confidence in their health and become more aware of their lifestyle.

Abnormal results in medical examinations

- A resting heart rate of 100 bpm or more (tachycardia)
- SBP of 160 ㎜Hg / DBP of 90 ㎜Hg or more
- Total cholesterol greater than 260 ㎎/dl
- Blood glucose level over 300 ㎎/dl
- Abnormal reactions on the ECG
  (arrhythmia, conduction disorder, cardiomyopathy, myocardial ischemia, myocardial infarction)

Components and Interpretation of Blood Tests

Blood is a fluid tissue that circulates in the blood vessels. Between the blood vessels and tissue membranes, there is a various exchange of materials, so that the internal environment of the body is constantly maintained. Blood volume accounts for 8% of body weight. In general, as shown in [Fig. 3.9], when blood is drawn into a 100-㎖ test tube, an anti-coagulant is added and the mixture is centrifuged at 3,000 rpm for about 10 minutes, which results in cell components with a high molecular weight to move to the bottom while components with a low molecular weight move to the top. The percentage of cellular components in these isolated components is called hematocrit. Specific ingredients are listed below.

■ *Albumin*

Albumin, used to assess liver function, controls the balance of osmotic pressure between blood and tissue. The ratio of albumin and globulin and the total protein test together can be used to evaluate renal function and malnutrition. The reference value is 3.5~5.3 g/dℓ.

■ *Bilirubin*

Bilirubin, which is used to evaluate liver function, is a degradation product of hemoglobin. It is used to measure liver function as it is released from the liver into the blood. Bilirubin also causes signs of jaundice and is an indicator for evaluating cirrhosis, gallbladder, pancreatic disease, and erythropoietic jaundice. The reference value is 0.1~1.2 mg/dℓ.

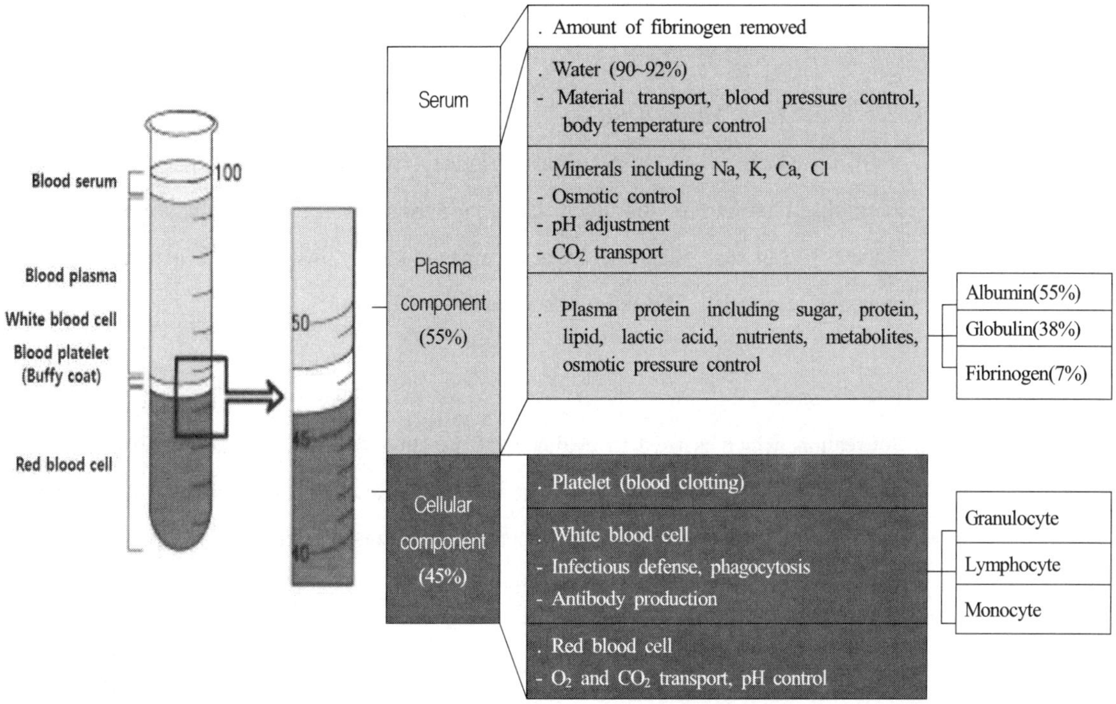

Fig. 3.9 ***Composition and function of blood***

■ *Total Protein*

The protein used to evaluate liver function is a compound that contains nitrogen in the blood. Serum proteins include fibrinogen, albumin, alpha globulin, and beta globulin, all of which are produced in the liver. Albumin, a major component of blood proteins, contributes to the balance of osmotic pressure while also producing antibodies. On the other hand, total protein decreases when there is liver and kidney disease, and increases when there is myeloma. Other body functions also affect total protein concentration. The reference value is 6.3~8.0 g/dℓ.

■ *GOT and GPT*

Glutamic oxalactic transaminases (GOT) or aspartate aminotransferase (AST) and glutamic pyruvic transaminases (GPT) or alanine aminotransferase (ALT), which are used to evaluate liver function, are enzymes found in the heart, liver, muscle, kidney and pancreas. If high levels of GOT and GPT are detected in the serum, the organ is considered to have a disease. In other words, when the cells of an organ are necrotic or damaged, GOT and GPT are released into the serum and results in higher concentrations. The reference value is 8~40 IU[6]/L for GOT and 4~44 IU/L for GPT.

■ *Blood Urea Nitrogen (BUN)*

BUN, which is used to evaluate kidney function, is the final product of the metabolized protein in the liver. Urea, a nitrogen source, is a major effluent of the kidney. It can also diagnose kidney damage, kidney disease, and hepatic dysfunction (hepatitis, cirrhosis). The reference value is 8~22 mg/dℓ.

■ *Creatine*

Creatine, which is used to evaluate the function of the kidneys, is a substance that is made by the breakdown of muscle creatine phosphate. That is, if there is a high level of creatine in the blood, kidney function and blood pressure are considered to be abnormal. The reference value is 0.5~1.3 mg/dℓ.

■ *Uric Acid*

Uric acid, which is used to evaluate the function of kidneys, is a purine body that is mainly released from muscle cells. It Increased in the case of high uric acid levels in ventilation and leukemia, pneumonia, intoxication, and kidney damage. It also diagnoses alcohol poisoning, stress, and liver damage caused by adrenal function. The reference value is 2.2~9.0 mg/dℓ.

■ *Calcium*

Calcium is used to assess the function of bone metabolism and is essential for bone

---

6) IU: Abbreviation for International Unit. As an international unit of enzyme, the amount of enzyme required to convert 1 μmol of substrate per minute to the product under optimum conditions is called 1 unit (1 IU or 1 μmol/min). Usually, the concentration of the enzyme is expressed as 1 mℓ or 1 L. For example, IU/mℓ, IU/L, or m IU/L.

tissue, muscle activity, and blood coagulation mechanisms. Calcium assesses thyroid function, bone cancer, rickets, and malnutrition. The reference value is 8.5~10.1 ㎎/dℓ.

■ *Phosphorus*

Phosphorus, which is used to evaluate the function of bone metabolism, is essential for energy storage and degradation and for the intermediate metabolism of carbohydrates and lipids. Phosphorus in the blood increases in the presence of kidney disease, hypoparathyroidism, and over-vitamin intake, while it decreases when rickets, hyperparathyroidism, and kidney disease are present. In other words, it can diagnose liver disease, bone disease, and thyroid function. The reference value is 2.4~4.7 ㎎/dℓ.

■ *Cholesterol and Triglycerides*

Cholesterol, which is used to assess atherosclerosis and cardiac function, is an alcohol derived from lipolysis in the liver. Because the liver plays a major role in the metabolism and secretion of cholesterol, this test can also be used as part of the liver function test. The test results may be used to assess dietary habits and lifestyle, as well as the risk of atherosclerosis and ischemic heart disease. The reference value is 50~160 ㎎/dℓ for low-density lipoprotein (LDL), 35~80 ㎎/dℓ for HDL-C, 140~240 ㎎/dℓ for TC, and 70~200 ㎎/dℓ for TG. TG, including cholesterol, are used as a criterion for evaluating the risk of heart disease.

• TG ≤ 150 ㎎/dl	• TC ≤ 240 ㎎/dl	• LDL-C ≤ 160 ㎎/dl
• HDL-C ≥ 35 ㎎/dl	• TC / HDL ≤ 5.0	

※ A patient can participate in exercise program after returning normal values.

■ *Lactic dehydrogenase*

LDH, which is used to evaluate the state of lipid metabolism, is an enzyme in serum and various organs that promotes the conversion of pyruvic acid to lactic acid. LDH is found in almost every cell that requires metabolism, but there are high LDH concentrations in the liver, heart, skeletal muscle, and red blood cells. Therefore, when these tissues are damaged, LDH concentrations increase. The reference value is 100~450 IU/L.

■ *Glucose*

Glucose is used to assess the status of glycometabolism. The use of glucose in muscles and other organs is regulated by insulin. This suggests that if insulin concentration in the body is not sufficient, glucose concentration will increase. Therefore, glucose is used to diagnose diabetes. The reference value is 60~110 ㎎/㎗, however, the fasting blood sugar reference value is 60~140 ㎎/㎗, and the glycated hemoglobin (HbA1c) is 4.4~6.3%.

■ *Sodium*[7)]

Also called natrium, it is an important mineral to maintain equilibrium in the body. If you intake too much salt, excess sodium is released from your kidneys into the bladder. Too much salt can cause cardiovascular disease. Also, the lack of sodium can cause diarrhea, heat stroke, and kidney disease. The reference value is 136~142 meq/ℓ.

■ *Thyroxine*

Thyroxine is involved in the development, growth, and deformation of the skeleton by facilitating metabolic functions and increasing the oxygen consumption of tissues. Typically, hyperthyroidism is Basedow disease (weight loss) caused by excessive secretion of hormones. Hypothyroidism is a myxedema (weight gain) caused by hormone secretion deficiency. The thyroid gland, thyroid cancer, and thyroiditis are thyroid-related diseases. The reference values are 0.58~1.65 ng/㎖ for triiodothyronine (T3), 0.70~1.48 ng/㎖ for thyroxine (T4), and 0.35~4.94 μU/㎖ for thyroid-stimulating hormone (TSH).

■ *Hematocrit*

Hematocrit means separated blood, which is the result of sorting elements of various cells from plasma by a centrifuge. The hematocrit level represents the number of red blood cells in the plasma. It is used to diagnose blood diseases and anemia. The reference values are about 45% (36~47 ㎎/㎗) for men, and 40% (40~54 ㎎/㎗) for women.

■ *Hemoglobin*

Hemoglobin is composed of hemp (an iron complex), and globin (a protein). This facilitates breathing by binding with oxygen or carbon dioxide. When problems occur, red blood cells and hemoglobin levels decrease and anemia occurs. Reference values are

---

7) Sodium: It is also called Na^+, and ingestion of food rich in sodium may cause heart disease such as hypertension.

12~16 g/dℓ for men and 14~18 g/dℓ for women.

■ *White blood cell (WBC)*

Proteins that have phagocytosis (granulocyte, monocyte) and immune function (lymphocyte β, γ) play a very important role as disease defense mechanisms. It is used to diagnose leukemia, respiratory diseases, and stress. The reference value is 5,000~10,000 numbers/㎣ (about 7,000 numbers/㎣) without gender differences.

■ *Red blood cells (RBC)*

Three-month-old red blood cells are degraded in the liver and spleen. At this time, hemoglobin is also decomposed and reused to make new red blood cells. It is used to diagnose anemia. The reference values are 4.4~5.5 million (approx. 5 million/㎣) for men and the 3.8~5.2 million (approx. 4.5 million/㎣) for women [Fig. 3.10].

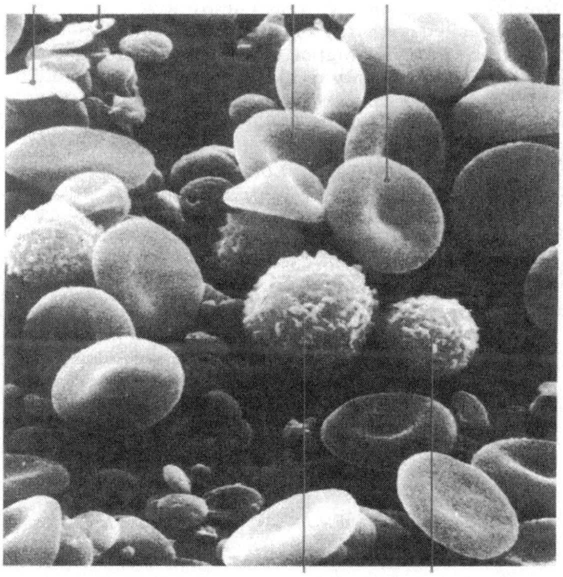
Photograph of blood cell component seen by electron microscope
Platelet
Red blood cells
White blood cell

Fig. 3.10 ***A microscopic blood cell component***

Components and Interpretation in Urinalysis

Urinalysis refers to the process of analyzing chemicals in the urine. Because the kidney is a place to filter out extra water and various substances from the blood, urine can be said to represent the functional state of the kidney. Urinalysis tests urine color, concentration, and acidity, and detects chemicals that are not found in normal cases, such as ketones, sugars, proteins, hematuria, bile pigment, and microorganisms.

■ *Ketone*

Ketone, a product of fat metabolism, is commonly used as an energy source in muscle tissue. However, when an abnormally large amount of fat is metabolized in the body, the muscles cannot use all of the ketone bodies, leading to ketone acidosis. The reference value is negative.

■ *Urine color*

Normal urine ranges from pale yellow to dark gold. The color of urine varies depending on the concentration of the dissolved substance. Therefore, the change in urine color is a pathological sign. For example, when blood is mixed with urine, the urine color becomes red or brown.

■ *Glucose in urine*

There is no sugar in normal urine. However, when the concentration of glucose in the blood becomes too high, sugar mixes with urine, which is a sign of diabetes. The reference value is 1~15 mg%.

■ *Protein*

If there is an obstruction in the kidney, albumin and globulin are detected in urine. The urine protein test is the most important test for the diagnosis of kidney disease. The reference value is negative.

■ *Specific gravity*

It is an inspection method for evaluating the ability of the kidney to remove waste products by examining the amount of dissolved substances in the urine. It diagnoses diabetes and kidney function, and the reference value is 1,003~1,020.

■ *Acidity (pH)*

Urine is mildly acidic, but acidity in the urine increases when the body's acid concentration is high (Acidosis). The pH levels can be used to diagnoses diabetes and kidney dysfunction. The reference value is 4.8~7.5.

Body Composition Test

A body composition test can easily use bioelectrical impedance analysis (BIA) to examine the body's proportion of muscle, fat, and moisture, as well as analyze individual basal metabolic rate and ideal body weight [Fig. 3.11].

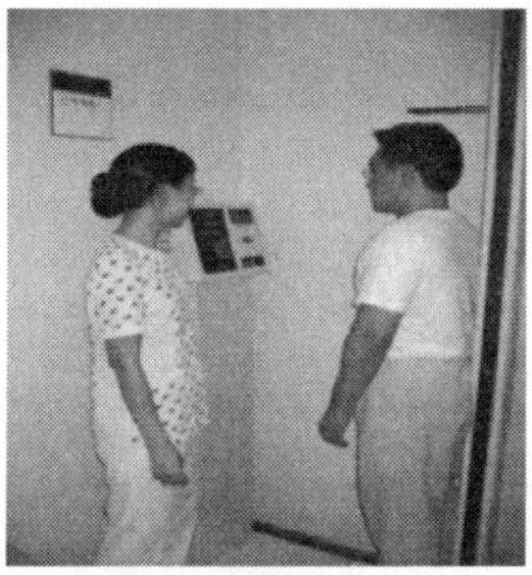

- Do not eat food 4 hours before the test.
- Stop drinking 48 hours before the test.
- Do not exercise 12 hours before the test.
- Do not take diuretics 7 days before the test.
- Be sure to urinate 30 minutes before the test.

Fig. 3.11 ***Body composition test***

The BIA can trace fat mass by conducting high-frequency harmless harmonics (500~800 KHz) and calculating the difference of electric resistance between fat tissue and non-fat tissue. This measuring instrument is highly convenient and safe and has been officially recognized by the US FAD. However, this method has an error of about 3%, obesity is underestimated, while tall subjects may be overestimated. Therefore, it is advised to observe the following items in order to minimize measurement error after considering the gender and age of the subject.

Graded Exercise Test

Necessity and Purpose of Graded Exercise Test

The graded exercise test (GXT) is a close-up test to measure ECG and respiratory gas (O_2 and CO_2 concentrations) while walking or running on a treadmill or peddling on a fixed cycle as shown in [Fig. 3.12]. This test observes the $\dot{V}O_2max$, blood pressure, heart rate, electrocardiographic waveform, and respiratory gas parameters during exercise using appropriate protocols for individual patients. These data help to predict the risk of cardiopulmonary dysfunction that may occur during exercise, even though current evaluations are normal. In addition, the exercise capacity of the heart and lung ventilation ability are evaluated, and the individual exercise intensity corresponding to the evaluation value can be set. Particularly, exercise tests should be performed because middle-aged and older adults who have not exercised in the past, and adults with hyperlipidemia and hypertension who smoke, have diabetes, and are obese may have impaired motor function.

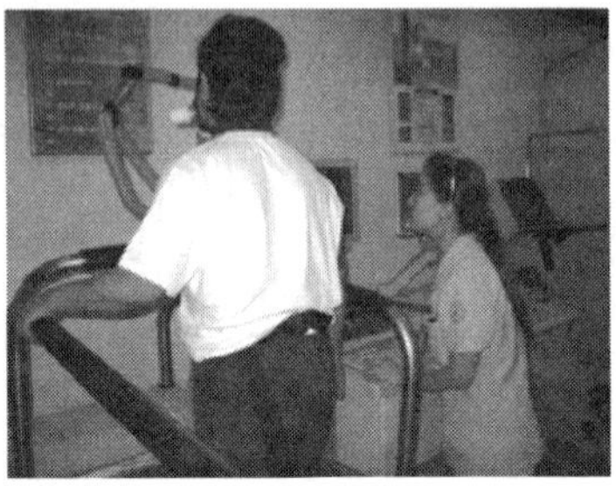

- Predicting potential cardiovascular risk during exercise
- Evaluation of exercise capacity
- Pulmonary ventilation ability of heart
- Setting of Individual exercise intensity
- Highly recommended for patients with adult diseases
- Highly recommended for middle-aged and elderly patients

Fig. 3.12 ***Graded Exercise Test***

The main reasons why exercise testing should be recommended are listed in the following seven categories. First, healthy people participating in regular exercise are provided with positive feedback regarding the preventive effects against diseases. Second, it allows early detection of coronary artery stenosis and coronary atherosclerosis. Third, the changes in the ECG (i.e., the changes in the ST segment, blood pressure response, and the size and shape of P, Q, R, S, T) make it possible to detect myocardial ischemia and arrhythmia. Fourth, unstable hypertension may be found. Fifth, it reveals the results of surgery (e.g., coronary bypass surgery) on heart-related patients or the health status of the heart. In the case of angioplasty, the possibility of vascular restenosis is predicted. Sixth, as an evaluation of the treatment process, it is also used to determine the efficacy of a drug when it plays a role in relieving ischemic symptoms or controlling arrhythmia and hypertension. Finally, it can be used as basic exercise prescription data for safe and effective exercise [Appendix B].

Protocols of GXT

The protocols of the GXT in the laboratory should be determined in advance whether to proceed with a maximal or submaximal test depending on the condition of the patient or subject. The general protocol increases by more than 2 METs, but it increases by less than 2 METs for severely ill patients and the elderly. During this process, the patient's signs, symptoms, heart rate, blood pressure or angina, and dyspnea scale should be utilized. Of course, the environmental aspects must be taken into account to ensure safe and accurate testing.

- Determine in advance whether a maximal or submaximal test should be performed.
- The general protocol increases the load by more than 2 METs, while for severe patients and the elderly, the load increases by less than 2 METs.
- Use patient symptoms, heart rate, blood pressure, RPE, angina pectoris, and dyspnea scale.
- The environmental aspects (temperature 20~22°C, humidity 50~60%) must be considered to perform the inspection correctly.
- Use the maximum predicted heart rate (220 - age) formula for the maximum or submaximal test.
- Understand the 10 different treadmill protocols.
- Understand the four cycle protocols.

On the other hand, the protocol to be determined according to the patient's condition proceeds to the maximum or submaximal test as described above, and the criterion for this is the 'predicted maximal heart rate (220 - age)' formula. First, the maximal exercise test is a method of continuing the test to an all-out condition where the patient is no longer able to continue exercising and until the heart rate reaches its limit. The submaximal exercise test is a method of ending the test before the patient reaches their maximum exercise level, and is a method of estimating the maximum level using their body reaction. The end point of the submaximal test is 85% of the predicted maximum heart rate. The methods and precautions of the exercise test are as follows: First, allow the subject to sit in a chair and rest for about 5 minutes. Then briefly explain the test method. Second, explain about the RPE which is a method of communicating with the examinee (angina scale or dyspnea scale can be used selectively). Third, after ECG leads and an automatic blood pressure monitor for electrocardiography are fixed to the subjects, the ECG should be printed. Fourth, to check the respiratory gas, it is necessary to fix the mask on the mouth and nose and to confirm that there are gaps. Finally, while recording the gas readings at rest, a protocol that can be applied to subjects during exercise should be selected.

GXT Equipment and Protocols

The equipments used for exercise testing are a treadmill, a cycle ergometer, and an arm ergometer. The treadmill has the advantage of shortening the adaptation time because walking and running, which is a common type of activity, is used as a stress. On the other hand, there is a disadvantage in that accurate electrocardiographic examinations and blood pressure measurements may be difficult due to the movement of the upper body. On the other hand, the cycle ergometer is a device that adjusts the exercise intensity via wheel speed and tension applied to the pedal. Because the upper body is fixed, the advantage is that ECG and blood pressure measurements are accurate. On the other hand, since it uses only the lower body, a disadvantage is the premature termination of the examination due to local fatigue.

How to Calculate the Treadmill Inclination in Ratio

The inclination of the treadmill is expressed in percent (%). This can be easily obtained by multiplying the tangent by 100, but since the measurement of the inclination angle is not easy and accurate, it is necessary to consider the height and the length of the belt as shown in [Fig. 3.13]. It is considered more accurate to multiply the value by 100. When using the tangent equation, we cannot consider the change in the oblique angle of the right triangle because we consider only the change in height with respect to the ground. Therefore, it is more appropriate to calculate the inclination angle and the % slope by the sign formula, which is recommended.

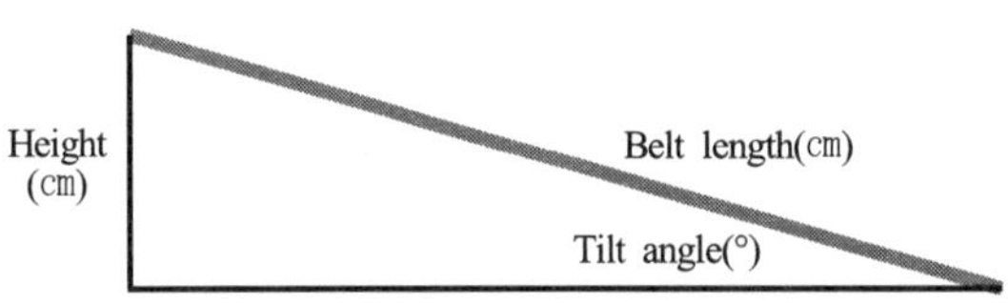

- $\sin\delta$ = (Height / Belt length)
- δ = Tilt angle(°)
- Ex] When the height is 8 cm and the belt length is 58 cm
- $\sin\delta$= (8/58) = 0.1379 [δ = 7.9°]
- % inclination = 0.1379 × 100 = **13.8%**

Fig. 3.13 ***How to calculate the inclination of the treadmill as percent***

Considerations when selecting Protocols

Exercise testing using a treadmill or cycle will identify cardiac functions such as heart rate, blood pressure, ECG type, and lung function, such as respiratory quotient, oxygen uptake, carbon dioxide emissions, and ventilation threshold. These variables will vary if they are examined by different protocols. Therefore, testing using a certain form of the protocol will yield consistent results, so that comparison with others will be accurate. In Korea, Bruce protocol is used the most, which increases the slope by 2% every three minutes. However, since the speed is not constant, it may not be appropriate to apply it to patients or the elderly. Instead, the Bruce protocol is appropriate for people who regularly exercise or young people who are not exercising. On the other hand, the Balke/Ware protocol or the Modified Bruce protocol, which has a somewhat smaller increase in exercise load, is suitable for the elderly or patients with cardiovascular disease. The selection and protocol of the subjects are shown in [Fig. 3.14~3.16].

▪ Modified Bruce Protocol

- Load type : Continuous
- Test subject : High risk group
- Initial load : Speed 1.7mph
  Grade 0~5%/ 3minutes stage

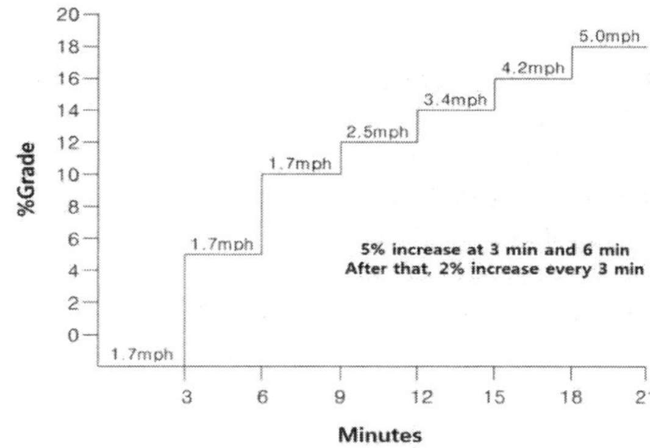

▪ Bruce Protocol

- Load type : Continuous
- Test subject : Normal group
- Initial load : Speed 1.7mph
  Grade 10%/3minutes stage

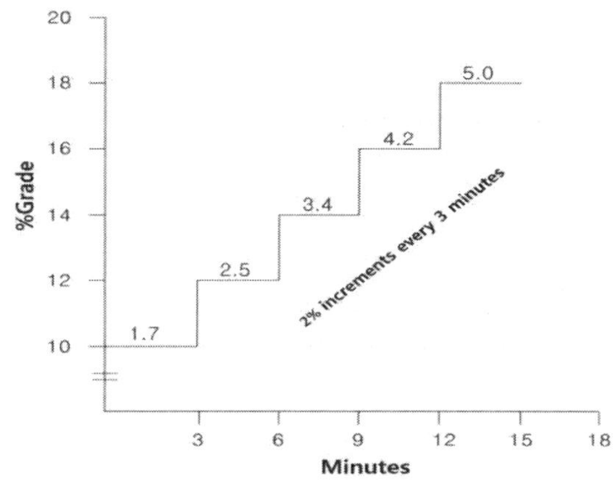

▪ Costill / Fox Protocol

- Load type : Continuous
- Test subject : Trained group
- Warm-up : 10 minutes walking
  or running
- Initial load : Speed 8.9mph
  Grade 0%/ 2minutes stage

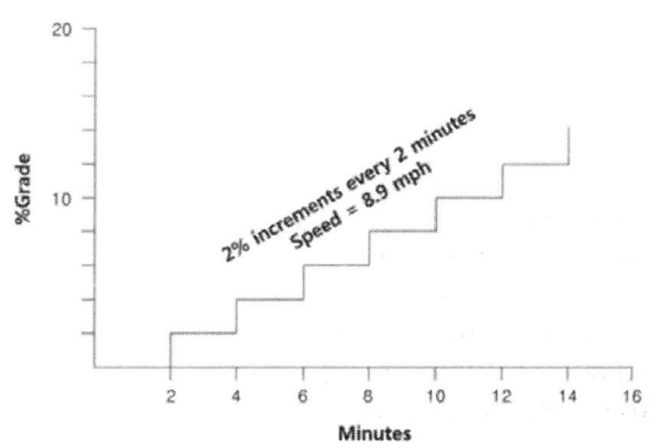

Fig. 3.14 ***Treadmill protocol***

■ *Maksud / Coutts Protocol*
- Load type : Continuous
- Test subject : Trained group
- Warm-up : Speed 3.5mph
  Walk 10 minutes at Grade 0%
- Initial load : Speed 7mph
  Grade 0%/2minutes stage

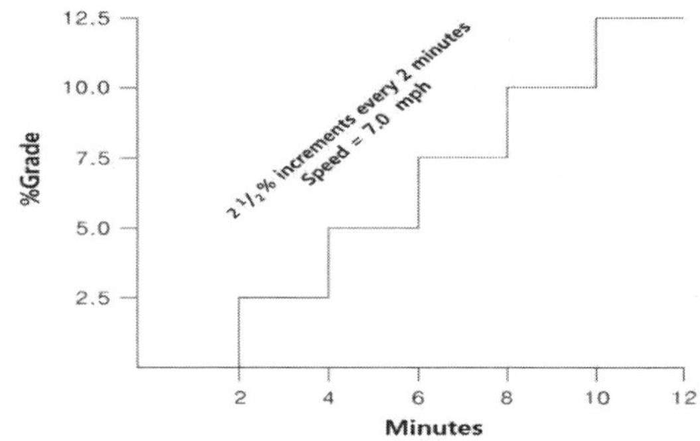

■ *Modified Astrand Protocol*
- Load type : Continuous
- Test subject : Trained group
- Warm-up : 5 minutes walking
  or jogging
- Initial load : Speed 5~8mph
  Grade 0%/ 3minutes stage

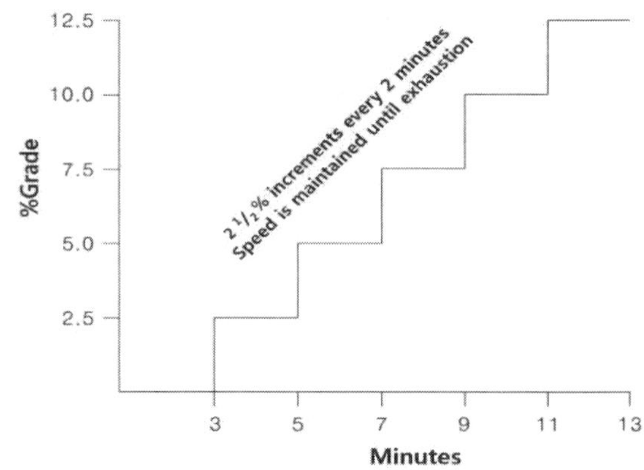

■ *Naughton Protocol*
- Load type : Continuous
- Test subject : Heart disease
  or high risk group
- Initial load : Speed 1.0mph
  Grade 0%/2minutes stage

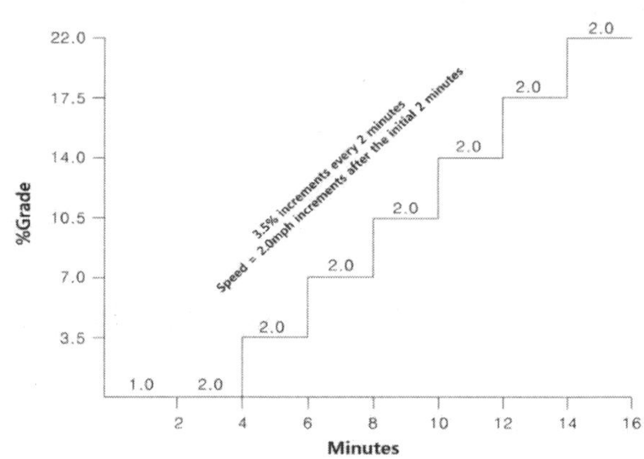

Fig. 3.14 ***Treadmill protocol (continued)***

- ***Wilson Protocol***
- **Load type : Continuous**
- **Test subject : Heart disease or high risk group**
- **Initial load : Speed 1.5mph Grade 0%/3minutes stage**

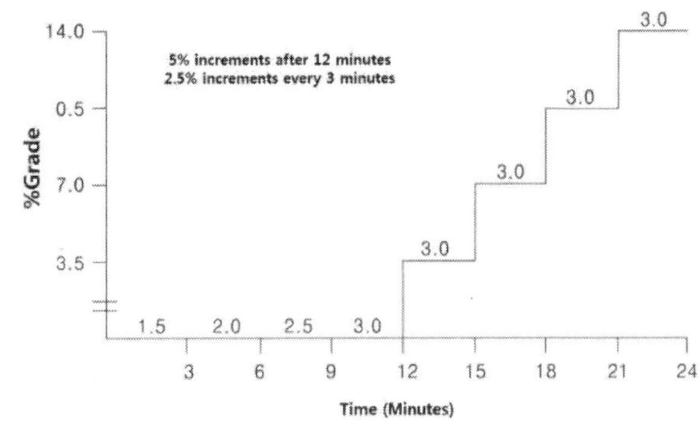

- ***Taylor Protocol***
- **Load type : Intermittent**
- **Test subject : Trained group**
- **Warm-up : Speed 3.5mph Walking / jogging for 10 minutes with grade 10%**
- **Initial load : Speed 7mph Grade 0%/3minutes stage**

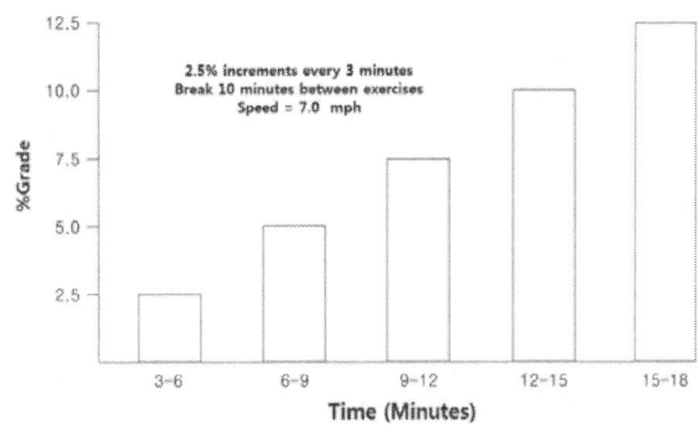

- ***Balke/Ware Protocol***
- **Load type : Continuous**
- **Test subject : Normal group and risk group**
- **Initial load : Speed 3.4mph Grade 0%/1minute stage**

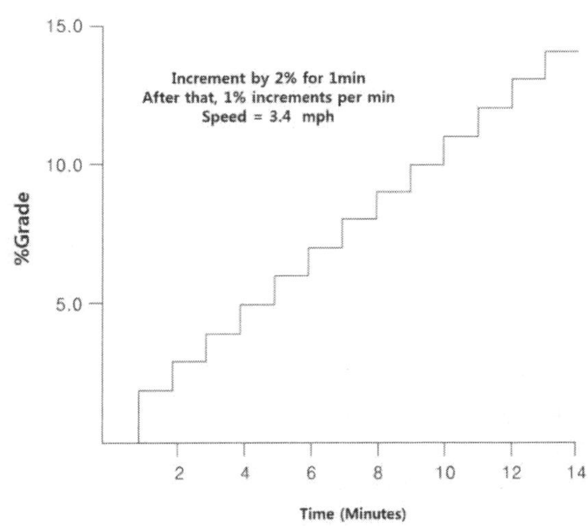

Fig. 3.14 *Treadmill protocol (continued)*

- ***Kattus Protocol***
- Load type : Continuous
- Test subject : Heart disease or high risk group
- Initial load : Speed 1.5mph Grade 10%/3minutes stage

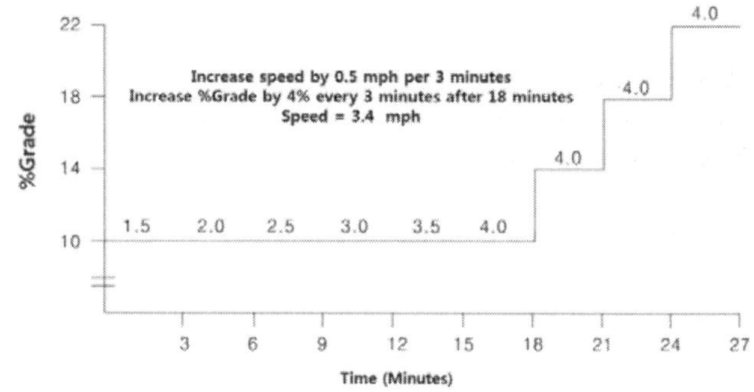

Fig. 3.14 *Treadmill protocol (continued)*

- ***Åstrand Protocol***
- Load type : Continuous
- Test subject : Normal group and risk group
- Initial load : Men 600kgm(100W)
  Women 300kgm(50W)

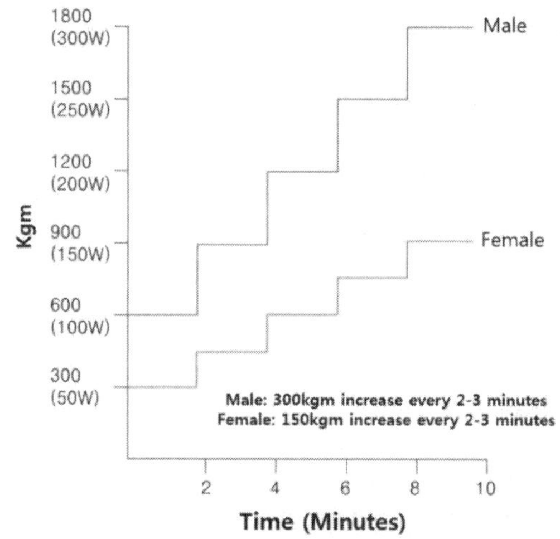

- ***Åstrand Protocol***
- Load type : Intermittent
- Test subject : Normal group and risk group
- Initial load : 720kgm(120W)

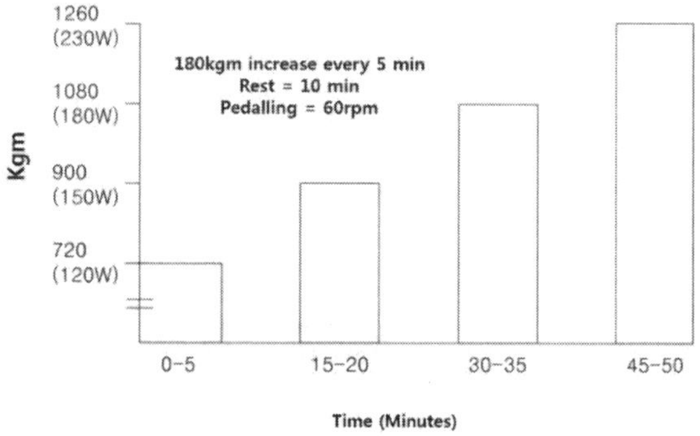

Fig. 3.15 *Bicycle protocol*

■ ***McArdle Protocol***
■ Load type : Continuous
■ Test subject : Normal group and risk group
■ Initial load : 900kgm(150W)

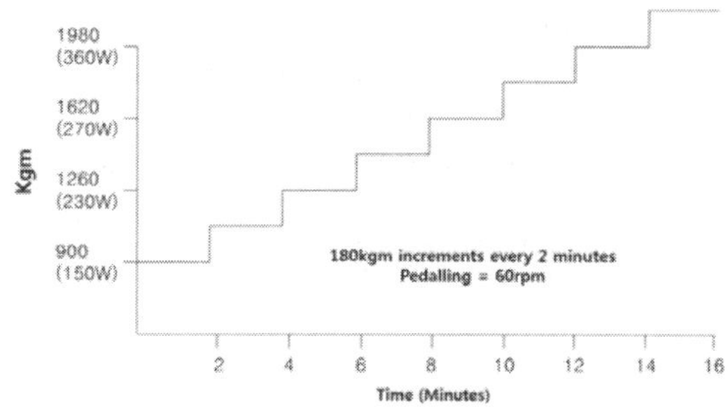

■ ***Fox Protocol***
■ Load type : Intermittent
■ Test subject : Normal group and risk group
■ Initial load : Men 750~900kgm (125~150W)
Women 450~600kgm (75~100W)

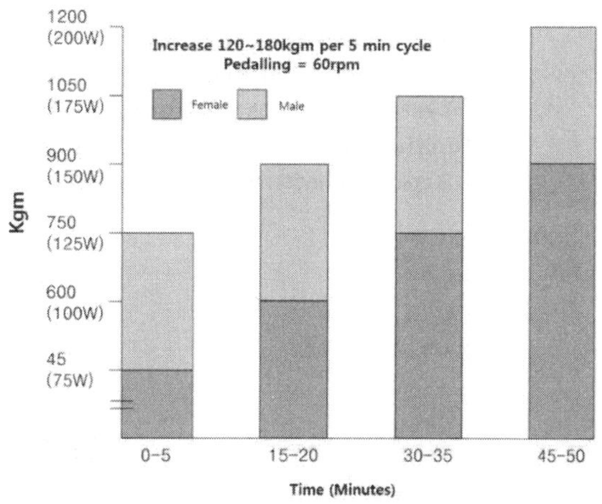

Fig. 3.15 *Bicycle protocol (continued)*

Arm Ergometry

Arm ergometer testing is used for patients who have difficulty performing a treadmill or cycle ergometer due to injuries in the lower limbs or skeletal muscle disorders (mainly paraplegic patients). Sometimes it is used to evaluate athletic ability in the upper extremity (rowers such as canoeing or kayaking) [Fig. 3.16]. The upper extremities test using an arm ergometer is similar to the lower extremities test method, but has fewer mobilized muscle masses and fewer motor units used at the beginning of the exercise. Compared to leg muscles, there is a lack of aerobic enzymes, which is 20~30% less than the $\dot{V}O_2max$ derived from the treadmill test, and the maximum heart rate is also low.

- ***Arm ergometer protocol-I***
- **Load type : Continuous**
- **Test subject :**
  Cardiovascular disease group
- **Initial load :**
  50rpm, 5W increments every 3 minutes

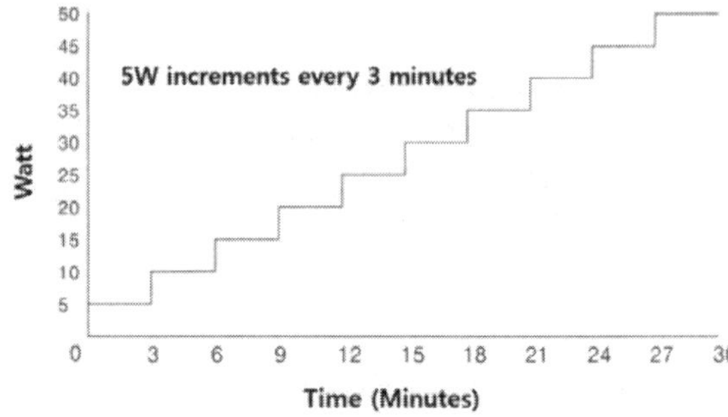

- ***Arm ergometer protocol-II***
- **Load type : Continuous**
- **Test subject : Normal group**
- **Initial load :**
  60rpm, 25W increments every 2 minutes

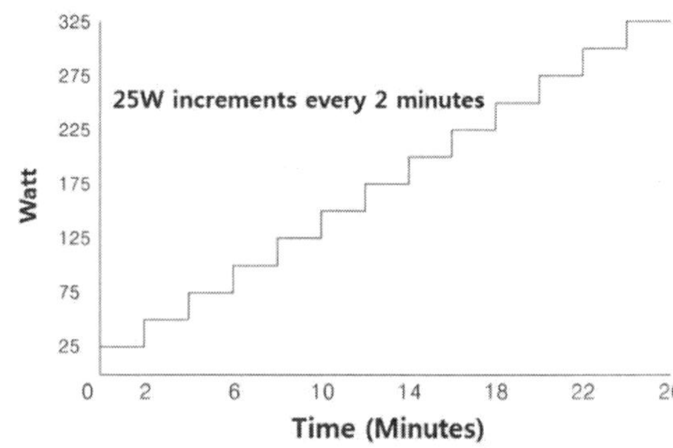

Fig. 3.16 *Arm ergometer protocol*

Utilization of GXT Results

The GXT is used to diagnose cardiac dysfunction through 12 ECG leads during rest, exercise, and recovery after exercise. The $\dot{V}O_2max$ and ventilation threshold are calculated through respiratory gas equipment and is used to determine the intensity of exercise accordingly. The variables to be observed are the change in blood pressure, heart rate, and ECG waves derived from ECG equipment [Fig. 3.17a], oxygen intake, ventilation, ventilation threshold, respiratory exchange rate, MET derived from respiratory gas equipment [Fig. 3.17b], and RPE, angina and dyspnea scales derived from observation scales such as psychological fatigue.

The protocol performed in [Fig. 3.17a] is the Bruce protocol in which the result of the numerical value of the ECG changes. Specifically, HR represents the heart rate, which is a basic indicator of the body's response to exercise and cardiac function, which refers to the number of times the heart has been beating for one minute to supply blood to each tissue in the body. Depending on the load of the Bruce protocol, the heart rate generally increases, but a person with good physical fitness has a lower heart rate. BP is an abbreviation for blood pressure of the blood vessels, which is an indicator of heart and circulatory function. The value in front refers to the pressure at which the aorta of the heart contracts, which is SBP, while the value shown in back is the pressure when the aortic contraction ability decreases with the increase in the filling pressure of the left ventricle, which is diastolic blood pressure (DBP). HR × BP represents the rate pressure product (RPP) of the myocardium, which is an estimate of how much oxygen the heart muscle consumes. Finally, ST LEVEL (II, V_2, V_5) quantitatively shows changes in the ST segment of electrocardiographic waves observed in limb lead II and chest lead V_2, V_5. Here, lead II represents the vertical slope of the heart, chest lead V_2 represents the degree of electrical excitation of the atrium, and chest lead V_5 represents the electrical excitation of the ventricle. A decrease of more than 2 ㎜ around the baseline of the sitting posture can be interpreted as a significant ischemic heart. The respiratory gas analysis performed simultaneously with the ECG examination is shown in [Fig. 3.17b].

EVENT	TIME	SPEED (mph)	GRADE (%)	HR (bpm)	ER (bpm)	BP (mm Hg)	HR×BP	ST LEVEL (mm) II	ST LEVEL (mm) V_2	ST LEVEL (mm) V_5
REST	SITTING	-	-	75	0	115 / 75	8625	1.1	1.2	1.1
	01:00	1.7	10.0	135		117 / 66	15795	0.7	1.2	0.8
Stage 1	02:00	1.7	10.0	138	0	122 / 68	16836	0.6	1.3	0.9
	03:00	1.7	10.0	141		128 / 69	18048	0.4	1.1	1.0
	01:00	2.5	12.0	145		132 / 68	19140	0.6	0.9	0.9
Stage 2	02:00	2.5	12.0	156	0	136 / 66	21216	0.5	0.7	0.7
	03:00	2.5	12.0	163		139 / 70	22657	0.4	1.0	1.1
	01:00	3.4	14.0	166		151 / 73	25066	1.1	1.1	0.9
Stage 3	02:00	3.4	14.0	165	0	156 / 70	25740	0.9	1.0	1.2
	03:00	3.4	14.0	171		155 / 69	26505	0.8	0.9	0.8

Fig. 3.17a ***Part of the results from the ECG analyzer***

Test Time	Speed MPH	Grade %	Heart Rate	VO_2 STPD	VO_2 /KG	VCO_2 STPD	R	VT BTPS	VE BTPS	RR /min	METs	kcal /min	Work Watts	VEO_2	$VECO_2$	SBP	DBP	RPE
0:30	0.0	0.0	75	0.30	3.5	0.29	0.77	0.45	11.0	16	1	1	0	30	36	115	75	-
1:00	1.7	10.0	135	0.37	5.3	0.31	0.83	0.47	12.0	26	2	2	0	29	35	117	66	7
:	:	:	:	:	:	:	:	:	:	:	:	:	:	:	:	:	:	:
6:00	2.5	12.0	163	0.58	8.5	0.50	0.86	0.64	16.3	26	2	3	0	28	33	139	70	11
7:00	3.4	14.0	166	0.60	9.0	0.53	0.91	0.65	17.0	27	3	3	0	27	32	151	73	13

Fig. 3.17b ***Part of the results from the respiratory gas analyzer***

The main variables observed in [Fig. 3.17b] are $\dot{V}O_2$/kg (oxygen uptake per body weight), R (respiratory exchange rate), $\dot{V}E$ (ventilation rate) and MET (energy metabolism). First, the oxygen uptake per body weight refers to the oxygen uptake ability of the individual body weight required for rest and exercise and is an index of exercise intensity. This variable is called the $\dot{V}O_2max$, which is obtained immediately after the maximal exercise and termination. The higher the level, the better the cardiopulmonary function. For reference, there are five factors that determine $\dot{V}O_2max$. First, there is no increase in oxygen intake despite increased exercise intensity. Second, the heart rate does not increase despite the increase in exercise intensity when the maximum heart rate has reached 95%. Third, the respiratory exchange rate is more than 1.15[8]. Fourth, blood lactate concentration is more than 8 mmol/ℓ, and Fifth, subjective exercise intensity is 17 or more on the RPE scale. Of course, the determinants of the $\dot{V}O_2max$ are only for normal individuals. It is desirable to estimate the $\dot{V}O_2max$ by considering 15% after completion of the test because severe patients, weak and elderly people will get oxygen intake by submaximal exercise load test. In [Fig. 3.17b], R is the respiratory quotient (RQ or R) and is the ratio of the amount of CO_2 expelled to the amount of oxygen inhaled during the test ($\dot{V}CO_2/\dot{V}O_2$). It is a variable indirectly showing the degree of energy utilization. For reference, if the R is close to 1, it is estimated that carbohydrates are used as an energy source, and fat is used as an energy source when the value is close to 0.7. $\dot{V}E$ refers to minute ventilation, which refers to the amount of air inspired during one minute during rest and exercise. $\dot{V}E$ is related to the ability to supply air through the lungs, but is more relevant to physical size and is therefore not an accurate indicator of cardiopulmonary function. METs is an index representing Metabolic EquivalenT, which refers to the degree of calorie consumption per body weight per hour, in units of ㎉/kg/hr. The amount of oxygen consumed at rest is 3.5 mℓ/kg/min, which equals 1 MET. If a patient reaches 13 METs immediately after maximal exercise testing, the oxygen consumption is 45.5 mℓ/kg/min. RPE refers to ratings of perceived exertion and is an indicator of psychological fatigue and exercise intensity during exercise testing. This seems to be preferable when measuring exercise intensity of any patients with chronic disease. Finally, though not shown in [Fig. 3.17b], the ventilation threshold (VT) is considered to determine the degree of improvement in endurance exercise capacity. VT is one of the anaerobic thresholds and is an index to determine the degree of bodily

8) Reasons for stopping the GXT when R value is greater than 1.15: It refers to the level that occurs when carbohydrates are completely consumed by increased exercise intensity in the GXT, and resynthesizes carbohydrates from protein and lactate in 'liver' to use energy. In other words, the level of 1.15 refers to the point at which the test should be discontinued because the ability of the liver to resynthesize can not proceed further and may cause liver damage in the future.

fatigue using respiratory gas parameters. VT is determined at the time when the ventilation rate increases sharply compared to oxygen intake. Higher levels mean less fatigue to the exercise load, which indicates good cardiopulmonary function.

Termination of GXT

The time for terminating the exercise test should be as follows: when reaching the target heart rate in the maximal test, reaching 85% in the submaximal test, reaching R value of 1.15, a blood pressure of 260/115 ㎜Hg or more, or the subjects' request to stop. It is advisable to perform a 1 to 2-minute walking exercise even after the test is completed. Patients with potential heart disease should have a recovery phase of 5 minutes or more because adverse reactions often appear during the recovery period. At this stage, if the patient exhibits severe dyspnea or a pale face, have them sit down on a chair to rest because lying down worsens breathing recovery. In addition to the above, other criteria for terminating the GXT due to abnormal reactions are shown in [Table 3.10] [Appendix B and C].

GXT may be stopped during the test as shown in [Table 3.10], but there are contraindications that must be followed before starting the test as shown in [Table 3.11]. However, among these contraindications, it is also necessary to comply with the relative contraindications in cases where abnormal reactions may be considered to some extent and may not lead to an emergency situation.

Table 3.10 ***Contraindications for terminating GXT*** [2]

Absolute contraindication	Relative contraindication
■ Drop in SBP of ≥10 mm Hg with an increase in work rate, or it SBP decreases below the value obtained in the same position prior to testing when accompanied by other evidence of ischemia ■ Moderately severe angina (defined as 3 on standard scale) ■ Increasing nervous system symptoms (e.g., ataxia, dizziness, or near syncope) ■ Signs of poor perfusion (cyanosis or pallor) ■ Technical difficulties monitoring the ECG or SBP ■ Subject's desire to stop ■ Sustained ventricular tachycardia ■ ST elevation (+1.0 mm) in leads without diagnositc Q waves (other than V_1 or aVR)	■ Drop in SBP of ≥10 mm Hg with an increase in work rate, or if SBP below the value obtained in the same position prior to testing ■ ST or QRS changes such as excessive ST depression (>2 mm horizontal or downsloping ST-segment depression) or marked axis shift ■ Arrhythmias other than sustained ventricular tachycardia, including multifocal PVCs, triplets of PVCs, supraventricular tachycardia, heart block, or bradyarrhythmias ■ Fatigue, shortness of breath, wheezing, leg cramps, or claudication ■ Development of bundle-branch block or intraventricular conduction delay that cannot be distinguished from ventricular tachycardia ■ Increasing chest pain[46] ■ Hypertensive response (SBP of >250 ㎜Hg and/or a DBP of >115 ㎜Hg)

Table 3.11 ***Contraindications before GXT***[2]

Absolute contraindication	Relative contraindication
▪ A recent significant change in the resting ECG suggesting ischemia, myocardial infarction within 2 days before, or other acute cardiac event ▪ Unstable angina. ▪ Uncontrolled cardiac dysrhythmias causing symptoms or hemodynamic compromise ▪ Symptomatic severe aortic stenosis ▪ Uncontrolled symptomatic heart failure ▪ Acute pulmonary embolus or pulmonary infarction ▪ Acute myocarditis or pericarditis ▪ Suspected or known dissecting aneurysm ▪ Acute systematic infection accompanied by fever, body aches, or swollen lymph glands	▪ Left main coronary artery stenosis ▪ Moderate stenotic valvular heart disease ▪ Electrolyte abnormalities (e.g., hypokalemia / hypomagnesemia) ▪ Severe arterial hypertension (SBP and/or DBP is over 200 and/or 110㎜Hg) at rest ▪ Tachycardia (over 100 bpm of RHR) or bradycardia (under 50 bpm of RHR) ▪ Hypertropic cardiomyopathy and other forms of blood outflow tract obstruction ▪ Neuromotor, musculoskeletal, or rheumatoid disorders that are exacerbated by exercise ▪ High-degree atrioventricular block ▪ Ventricular aneurysm ▪ Uncontrolled metabolic diseases (e.g., diabetes mellitus / thyrotoxicosis / myxedema) ▪ Chronic infectious diseases (e.g., mononucleosis / hepatitis / AIDS) ▪ Mental or physical impairment leading to inability to exercise adequately

Sensitivity and Specificity of Electrocardiography of GXT

It is important to know how clinically precise and sensitive the exercise ECG is before analyzing the results. In other words, exercise electrocardiography is intended to accurately diagnose abnormalities of ischemic heart disease or coronary artery disease (CAD) but is not always accurate. Thus, for the reliability of ECG, sensitivity and specificity must be known. The formula for calculating the sensitivity and specificity is shown in [Table 3.12].

Table 3.12 ***Sensitivity and specificity calculation formula of GXT***

$\text{Sensitivity} = \dfrac{\text{True positive}}{\text{True positive} + \text{False negative}}$	▪ True positive: The patient was unable to perform the exercise until the end due to the ST segment abnormality and was judged to have a actual CAD. ▪ False negative: If the test is completed without any adverse reactions, but it is likely that the patient is actually a CAD patient.
$\text{Specificity} = \dfrac{\text{False positive}}{\text{False positive} + \text{True negative}}$	▪ True negative: If the test is performed until the end without any adverse reactions and there is a high probability that there is no actual CAD. ▪ False positive: The patient was not able to complete the test because of the ST-segment abnormality, but was actually judged to have no CAD.

Specifically, sensitivity refers to the probability that an adverse reaction will occur when a patient with a heart disease receives an exercise test. In other words, it is the probability that a patient can be identified as a patient. Specificity refers to the probability that a normal person will appear normal for an exercise test, or the "probability that a healthy person can be identified to be healthy". The inside of the body is negative (-) when it is stable, and is considered "normal". On the other hand, when the inside of the human body is unstable, it is positive (+) and is considered "abnormal". For ease of understanding, the flow of sensitivity and specificity can be expressed as shown in [Fig. 3.18]. True positive means "real abnormal" and false positive means "false abnormal" or "normal". Also, true negative means "real normal" and false negative means "false normal" or "abnormal". A study of 112 patients with heart disease reported that the positive response (likely to be a patient) of exercise electrocardiography was proportionally increased as the coronary artery stenosis exceeded 75%. Specifically, in patients with single vessel damage (i.e., right or left circumflex coronary arteries), 44% had a positive electrocardiographic response. On the other hand, the positive electrocardiographic response of the patients with left anterior descending coronary artery was 77%. Furthermore, this prevalence is reported to be 91% when two vessels are damaged and 100% when three or more vessels are seriously damaged. In other words, since the accuracy (sensitivity) of the exercise ECG is higher in patients with more than moderate severity, it is necessary to positively recommend an ECG test.

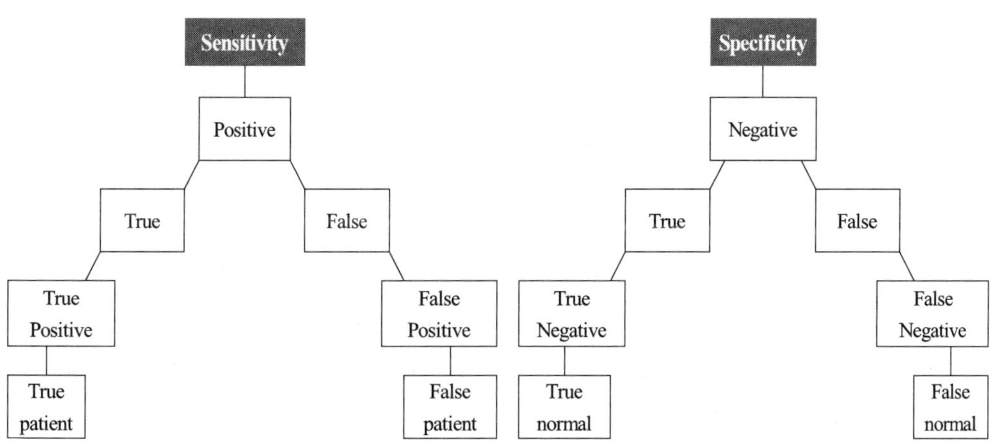

Fig. 3.18 ***Flow of sensitivity and specificity on GXT***

When the inside of the body is stable, it is negative (-) and it is said to be normal. When it is unstable, it is positive (+) and it is said to be abnormal.

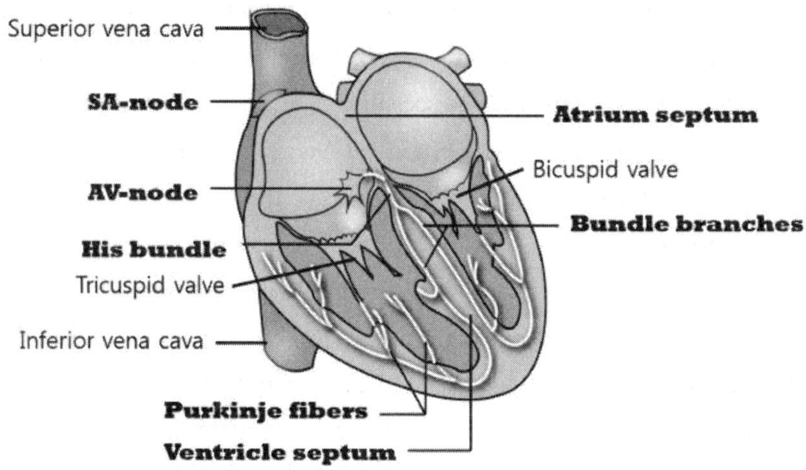

Fig. 3.19 *Nerve conduction system of the heart*

Nerve Conduction System of the Heart

The heart carries blood throughout the whole body through rhythmic contraction and relaxation of the cardiac muscle. Specifically, when the blood (vein) returned from each organ enters the ventricle, it enters the lungs and turns into clear blood, which causes blood to flow to each part of the body and lungs. This step is called systole. Diastole is the stage in which blood flows into the atria and ventricles from the lungs and body parts. The contraction and relaxation of the myocardium are possible by the nerves inside the myocardium. As shown in [Fig. 3.19], the contraction starts by the autonomic excitation of the sinoatrial node (SA-node) located at the entrance of the superior vein inside the right atrium. This area is also called the pacemaker because it is the starting point of autonomic excitement.

On the other hand, excitation stimulation in the SA-node excites the entire atrium along the right atrium wall. This excitation is transmitted to the His bundle via the atrioventricular node (AV node). It spreads throughout the ventricle along Purkinje fibers distributed on left and right ventricular wall. The electrical activity that takes place in this conduction system can be derived from the surface of the skin and is called an ECG.

Electrophysiological Mechanism of the Heart

To understand the principle of electrocardiography, we must understand the activity of nerve cells in the myocardium. Cardiac neurons can generate and conduct electrical stimulation to constrict and relax the heart muscle. This electrical stimulation occurs because the cations (Na^+, K^+, Ca^{++}) move rapidly through the cell membrane of the heart in both directions. The difference in cation concentration in the cell membrane is called the potential difference (measured in ㎷). The potential difference is called the resting state, in which the waveform is not drawn while maintaining the equipotential line on the ECG. This is also called resting membrane potential. On the other hand, the state in which the waveform is drawn up or down on the ECG is called depolarization (including repolarization) and is caused by a change in potential difference.[39]

In order for depolarization to take place, repolarization with a certain level of potential leads to the contraction of the myocardial cells, which is called the threshold potential. Let's take a closer look at the explanation below to understand the electrophysiological mechanism of the heart.

Resting state

When myocardial cells are in a resting state, the Na^+ concentration is high outside the cell while the K^+ concentration is high inside the cell. Na^+ and K^+ around the cell membrane tend to maintain the concentration difference through diffusion [Fig. 3.20].

On the other hand, K^+ has high permeability to the cell membrane, so it is free to move out of the cell. On the other hand, Na^+ is low in permeability and is slow to migrate from the outside of the cell to the inside. For this reason, the cell membrane consumes energy (ATP), causing Na^+ to move out of the cell and K^+ to move into the cell. However, since K^+ is moved out of the cell at a higher rate than Na^+, the extracellular space has positive electrodes and the inside of the cell has negative electrodes so that the inside of the cell membrane has a negative potential. This state is called polarization. In other words, the resting membrane potential is the potential difference of the resting cardiac muscle cells. The resting membrane potential of the atria and ventricles is −90 ㎷, and the resting membrane potential of the SA-node and AV-node is −70 ㎷.

Depolarization and Repolarization

When depolarized myocardial cell membranes are excited, Na^+ ions penetrate into the cells, which causes a slight decrease in the negative charge. In other words, when there is drop from −90 ㎷ to −70 ㎷, the sodium passage opens instantaneously and Na^+ permeates the cell membrane and enters the cell. As a result, the outside of the cell becomes negatively charged, and the inside of the cell turns into a positive electric charge and becomes depolarized.

On the other hand, SA-node and AV-node have a slow calcium-sodium channel that opens when the membrane potential drops from -70 ㎷ to -50 ㎷. This pathway allows the positive charge of Ca^{++} and Na^{+} to slowly enter the cell during depolarization. When myocardial cells depolarize, K^{+} moves out of the cell, stabilizing the cells and initiating the process of returning to a polarized state. This is called repolarization. The depolarization of myocardial cells is represented by P waves and QRS waves on the ECG, and the repolarization is represented by T waves.

Threshold Potential

Myocardial cells are either depolarized by −70 ㎷ or depolarized by −30 ㎷ (SA-node and AV-node), rather than being depolarized only after being fully depolarized with −90 ㎷. In other words, the cell has to be repolarized to depolarize again. This is called the threshold potential, and if this level is not reached, the action potential in the myocardium does not occur.

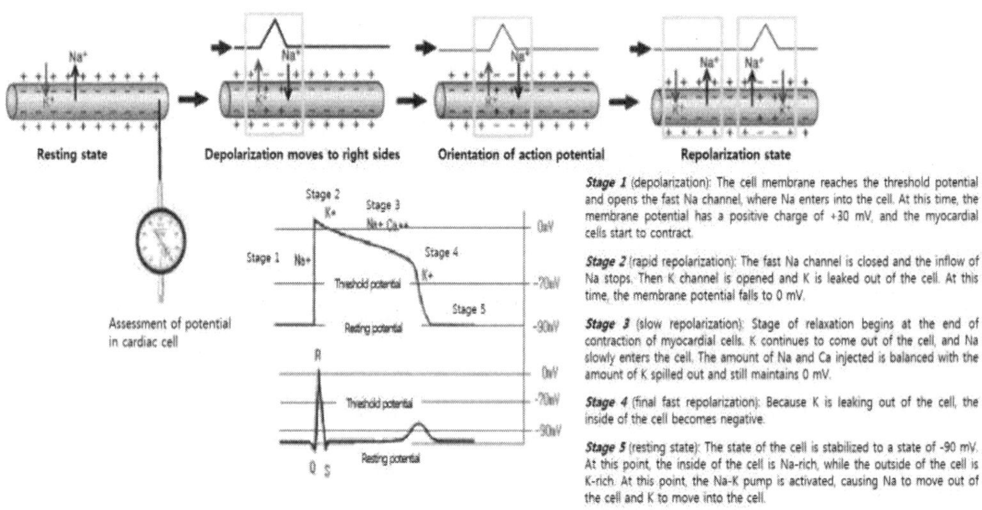

Fig. 3.20 ***Electrophysiological Mechanism of the Heart***

Action Potential

The action potential in myocardial cells is the process of changing the membrane potential during depolarization and repolarization. This is divided into five steps as shown in [Fig. 3.20].

The first stage (depolarization stage) is the stage where the cell membrane reaches the threshold potential and opens up a fast sodium passage in which Na^+ enters the cell. At this time, the membrane potential has a positive charge of +30 mV, and the myocardial cells start to contract. In stage 2 (fast repolarization stage), the fast sodium passage is closed and the inflow of Na^+ is stopped. The potassium channel then opens and K^+ spills out of the cell. At this time, the membrane potential drops to 0 mV. The third stage (slow repolarization stage) is the stage at which relaxation begins at the end of myocardial cell contraction. K^+ continues to flow out of the cell as Na^+ moves slowly into the cell. The amount of incoming Na^+ and Ca^{++} is balanced with the amount of K^+ released and remains at 0 mV. In stage 4 (the last fast repolarization step), the inside of the cell becomes negative because K^+ flows out of the cell. In the last stage (resting state), the inside of the cell becomes -90 mV, resulting in resting membrane potential. However, Na^+ is still present inside the cell, whereas K^+ is present outside the cell. At this point, the sodium-potassium pump is activated, causing Na^+ to move out of the cell and K^+ to move into the cell.

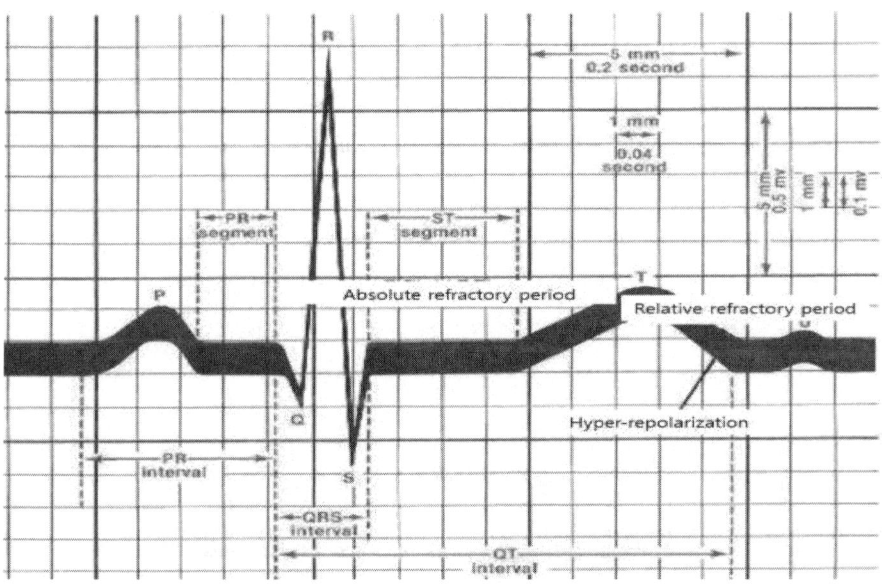

Fig. 3.21 ***Refractory period and transient steady state***

Refractory Period

At the beginning of depolarization and at the end of repolarization, another depolarization does not occur even when other electrical stimuli appear. This point is called refractory period (absolute or relative refractory period). Depolarization may be induced by mild stimulation rather than normal stimulation immediately before returning to the stable membrane potential of myocardial cells, which is the last part of the T wave. This is called transient steady state [Fig. 3.21].

ECG Leads

The electrical activity generated in the stimulation conduction system of the heart is obtained through 10 leads as shown in [Fig. 3.22]. Since the heart cannot be explained by plain view, it is recorded separately as a vertical conduction system and a horizontal conduction system. The vertical conduction system produces limb leads (I, II, III) through RA (right arm), LA (left arm), RL (right leg) and LL (left leg). The augmented leads (aVL, aVR, aVF) are produced through the center electrode of the cathode and the limbs of the anode. The horizontal conduction system draws chest leads (V_1, V_2, V_3, V_4, V_5 and V_6) through six leads.

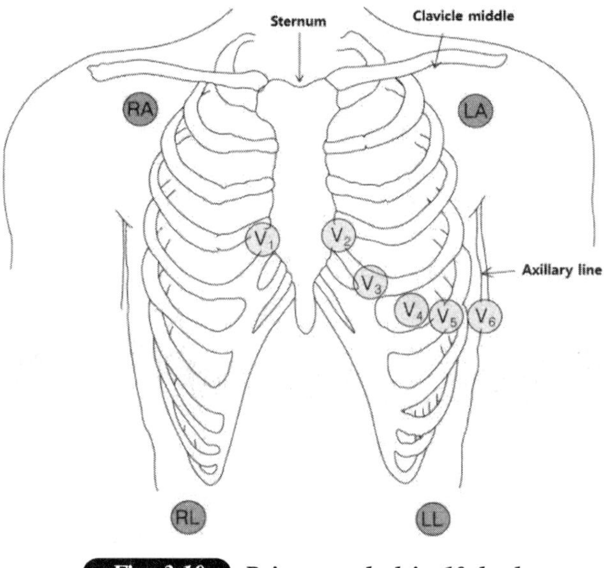

Fig. 3.10 ***Points attached in 10 leads***

The limb lead, the augmented lead, and the chest lead total 12 leads, so this is called a 12-lead ECG. 12 leads are obtained by using positive and negative electrodes, respectively, and the ground electrode is attached to the right foot or another part to absorb the current disturbance in the body. There are three cases where depolarization is depicted in the ECG. First, depolarization waves approaching the anode are recorded as positive waves (⌒). Second, depolarization waves away from the anode are recorded as negative waves (~). The depolarization wave in the direction perpendicular to the electrode is recorded with no waveform or a small waveform (-). The contents are as follows.

Limb Leads

The limb leads are bipolar leads, which measure the electrical change at two points and record the difference. As shown in [Fig. 3.22], Lead I is from RA lead (-) on the right infraclavicular region to LA lead (+) on the left infraclavicular region, Lead II is from RA lead (-) on the right infraclavicular region to LL lead (+) on the bottom left of the 12th rib, and Lead III is from LA lead (-) on the left infraclavicular region to LL lead (+) on the bottom left of the 12th rib. The limb leads record the electrical difference between each of two leads. RL lead attached to the bottom right of the 12th rib is grounded.

Augmented Leads

The augmented lead is a unipolar lead and obtained with the central terminal as the cathode and the other limb as the anode.

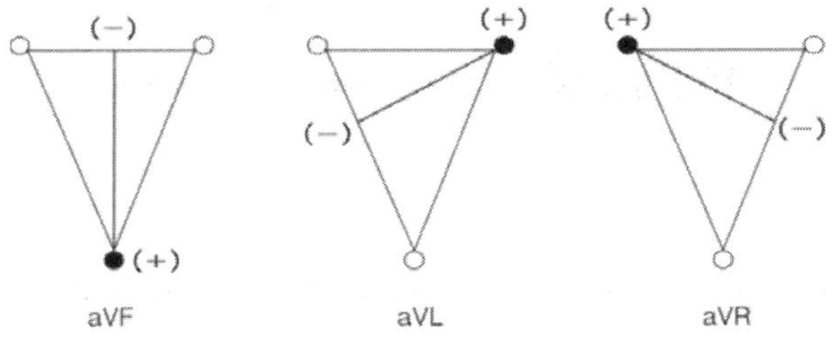

Fig. 3.23 *Augmented lead*

The augmented leads were originally VR, VL, and VF because they were obtained by connecting the central terminal of the unipolar lead to the right foot, left arm, and left foot.[38] However, the waveform and group were lower because the connection was disconnected from the central terminal. Augmented leads were developed to greatly enhance this. Since the central terminal increases the size of the waveform and group in the ECG, the unipolar leads are called "augmented" and named aVR, aVL, and aVF, respectively. aVR is obtained by attaching an anode to the right arm and a cathode to the central terminal (left arm and left foot). aVL is obtained by attaching the anode to the left arm and the cathode to the central terminal (right arm and left foot). The aVF is obtained by attaching the anode to the left foot and the cathode to the central terminal (right arm and left foot) [Fig. 3.23].

The three-axis reference diagram generated in the longitudinal plane by the axes of the three augmented leads is 60° apart from the neighboring lead, such as limb leads. However, it has a lead axis that is oriented at slightly different angles around the zero reference point.[38] A three-axis augmented leads to limb leads form a six-axis reference diagram when the reference plane is overlaid. Since each augmented lead is perpendicular to the limb lead, the lead axis is 30° apart [Fig. 3.24].

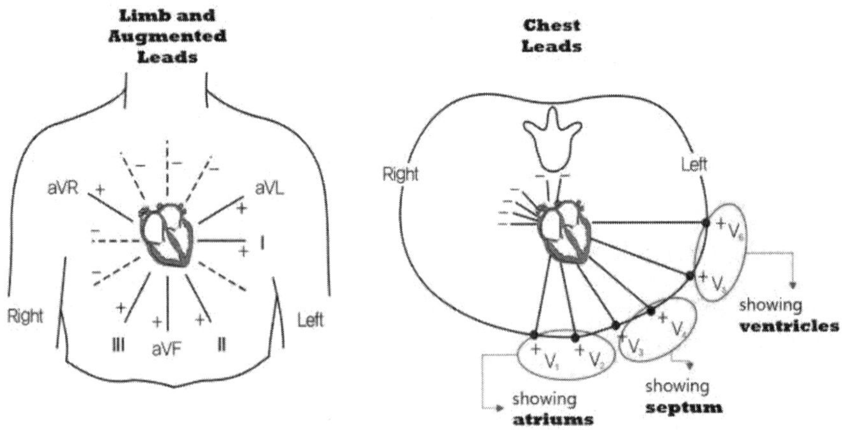

Fig. 3.24 *12 lead's anode and cathode*

Chest Leads

The chest leads represent the horizontal conduction of the heart, which is drawn through six leads (V_1, V_2, V_3, V_4, V_5, and V_6). V_1 to V_6 connect to the anode on the anterior chest wall with the central terminal formed by connecting the right arm, left arm, and left limb as the cathode. This chest lead measures the electrical load difference between the central terminal and the chest electrode. Chest electrodes are placed along the anterior chest wall from right to left, so they are located on the anterolateral side of the right ventricle, ventricular septum, and the left ventricle [Fig. 3.24]. The position of the electrodes are shown in [Fig. 3.22], and the specific locations are as follows.

V_1: Fourth intercostal space just to the right of the sternal border
V_2: Fourth intercostal space just to the left of the sternal border
V_3: At the midpoint between V_2 and V_4
V_4: On the midclavicular line in the 5th intercostal space
V_5: On the anterior axillary line and on the horizontal plane through V_4
V_6: On the midaxillary line and on the horizontal plane through V_4 and V_5

Axis of the Heart

The axis of the heart is used to determine whether the tilt is normal or deviated to the left or to the right. For each lead, the direction from the cathode to the anode is called the lead axis. The coordinate system in which 3 limb leads and 3 augmented leads are crossed is called a 6-axis coordinate system [Fig. 3.25]. On the other hand, it may be common for left and right deviations to appear, but the axis mostly changes due to disease.[38]

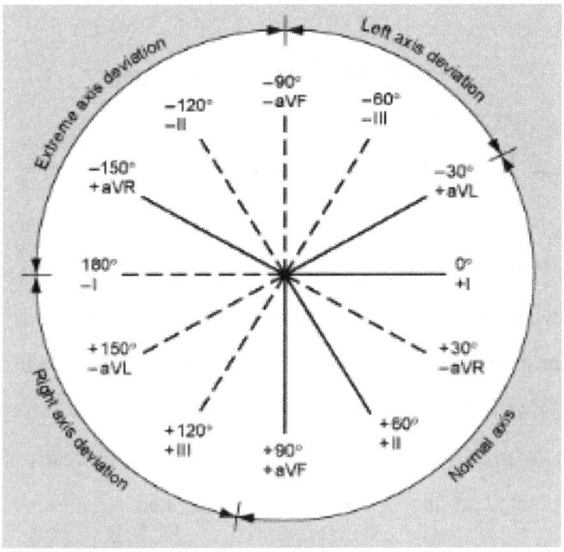

Fig. 3.25 *Axis of heart of 6 axis coordinate system*

ECG Recording

The waveforms and beats of the heart are drawn on the recording paper so that the characteristics can be grasped. However, the recording paper has specific promises. First, the horizontal line represents the time (sec), and the vertical line represents the amplitude (㎜) [Fig. 3.26]. The horizontal line of each square is calculated as 0.04 seconds, and the vertical line of each square is calculated as 1 ㎜. For reference, the speed of standard recording paper is measured at 25 ㎜ per second.

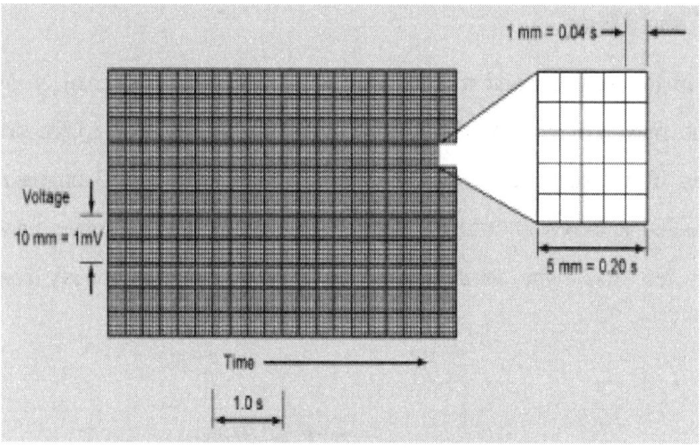

Fig. 3.26 ***ECG recording***

Generation of ECG Waveforms and Intervals

As described above, the electrical activity from the excitation generated at the SA-node to the spreading to the whole heart forms P, Q, R, S, T and U waves [Fig. 3.27]. In fact, the heart beats even when it is taken out of the body. The heart has a pacemaker inside, which enables atrial contraction, ventricular contraction, and ventricular relaxation without external nerves. This is called myogenic rhythmicity.

The order in which the heartbeats are drawn on the chart is as follows: First, electricity is generated at the SA-node and propagated to the AV-node. This process completes the following order ①, ②, ③ as shown in [Fig. 3.27]. Specifically, ① the right atrial contraction starts, ② the left atrium contracts, and ③ atrial contraction is completed. That is, a P wave is drawn on the ECG recording paper. After this process, latency occurs. This is the time for the blood in the atrium to be sent to the ventricle after the atrium has contracted, and is the point at which the PR interval appears. Subsequent electrical excitation passes through the AV-node and spreads to Purkinje fibers through His bundles and bundle branches located in the ventricular septum. That is, ⑤ the ventricular contraction starts and ⑥ the ventricular contraction is completed, and a QRS wave is formed on the recording paper. Thereafter, ⑦ a T wave is formed, which represents the time when the excitation of the ventricle settles and the diastolic phase begins. However, since the diastolic phase of the ventricle begins at the end of the S wave, the diastolic phase of the ventricle must be called the ST wave. On the other hand, a point called J point is formed in the interval where the ST wave is formed. Severe elevation or depression of this point can indicate myocardial infarction or myocardial ischemia, cardiomegaly, conduction block, and drug abuse.[9] On the other hand, the RR interval represents the heart rate. The PR interval during exercise is shortened, and irregularities are drawn in the case of arrhythmia with disease. These waves and intervals can be used as a basis for diagnosing heart diseases.

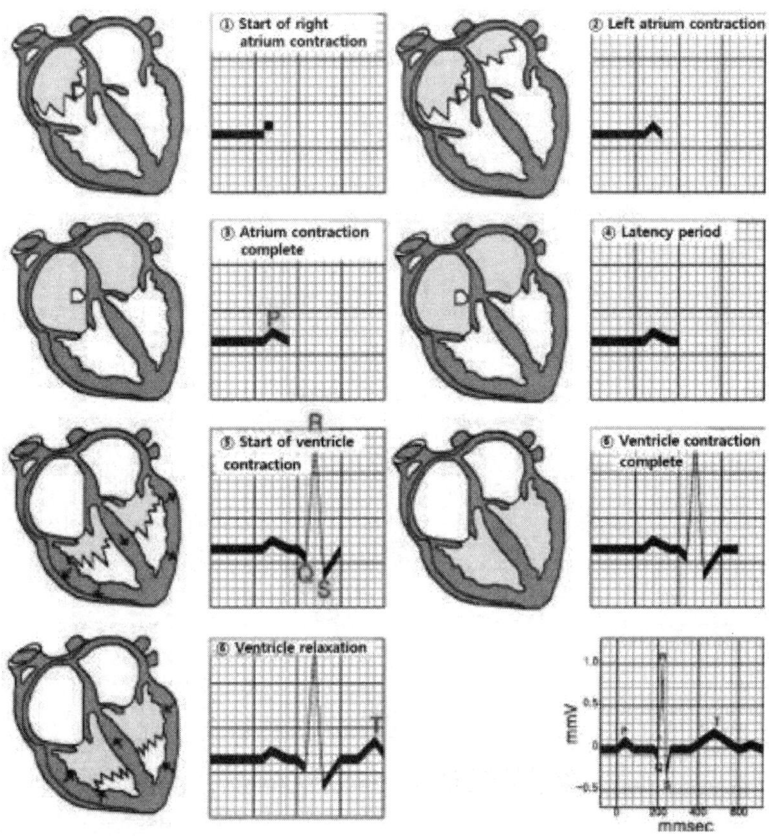

Fig. 3.27 *A flowchart of the creation of an ECG waves*

ECG Reading Method

There are many ways to read ECG, but it is ideal to analyze the whole waveform with 12 leads. [Fig. 3.28] is the actual recording sheet of a 51-year-old woman sitting on a chair before the GXT and recording the state of the ECG at rest. The recording paper is obtained at 10 ㎜/㎷, and the speed is recorded at 25 ㎜/sec. The Bruce protocol was used

9) Usefulness of ECG: Although it is not possible to know all of heart abnormalities by ECG, it is useful for diagnosing angina, myocardial infarction, ischemic heart disease, ventricular hypertrophy, myocarditis, or arrhythmia. GXT, which is currently being performed in the clinic, gives the stress of exercise to observe potential abnormalities.

for GXT. The current heart rate is 71 bpm, resting SBP is 129 ㎜Hg, and resting DBP is 88 ㎜Hg. The target HR recorded at the upper left corner is 144 bpm, which is the value obtained by calculating the maximal HR, {(220-51 years)×0.85}. For reference, maximal load (100% all-out) should be performed to determine if this person experiences adverse events when exercising (i.e., stressing the heart). However, 85% submaximal testing is accepted globally because it is similar to the results obtained with the maximal load.

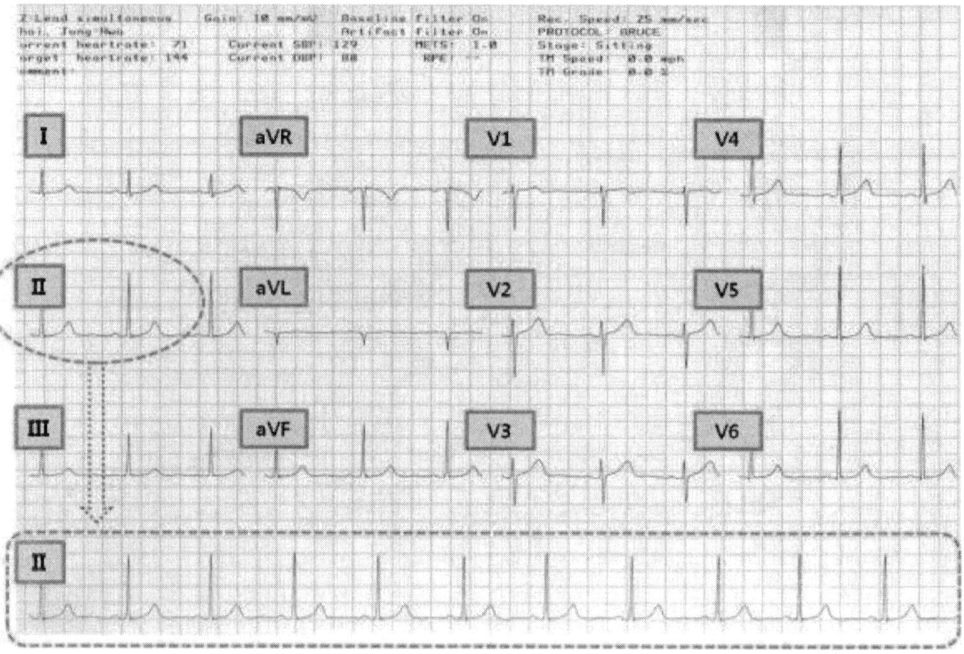

Fig. 3.28 ***12 lead test results***

As mentioned above, 12 leads have their respective meanings. Lead I and aVL represent the anterior wall of the left ventricle, leads II, III, aVF represent the lower and posterior walls of the ventricle, and aVR represents the ventricular lumen. V_1 and V_2 represent the right ventricle, V_3 and V_4 represent the ventricular septum, and V_5 and V_6 represent the left ventricle. If the height, length, and direction are different for any of the 12 leads that show each position in the ECG waves shown in [Fig. 3.28], it can be read as 'abnormal'. The easiest way to figure out an ECG is to become familiar with the normal ECG. In order to systematically analyze ECG, it should be done based on the following:

① Heart axis ② Heart rate/rhythm ③ P wave ④ PR interval ⑤ QRS wave
⑥ Q wave ⑦ ST segment ⑧ T wave ⑨ U wave ⑩ QT interval

Table 3.13 ***Electric axis reading by limb lead***

	I	III
Normal axis	anode (⌃)	anode (⌃)
Left axis deviation	anode (⌃)	cathode (⌄)
Right axis deviation	cathode (⌄)	cathode (⌄) or anode (⌃)

※ ⌃, ⌄ indicate the level of QRS.

Reading the Heart Axis

The axis of the heart uses QRS waves, and the normal axis is screened using a six-axis coordinate system. The normal QRS axis lies between -30° and +90° from the front. Starting from the range of the normal axis, QRS of the limb leads I, II, and III all show positive (+). The aVR is in the direction of -150° from the unipolar center. That is, since the opposite side of the positive direction is the range of the normal axis, the QRS axis becomes negative (-). Since the aVL lies in the direction of -30° from the unipolar center, the QRS axis becomes negative (-). Since the aVF is at +90° from the unipolar center, the QRS axis becomes positive (+). On the other hand, reading normal heart axis can be understood simply by QRS heights of limb leads I and III [Table 3.13].

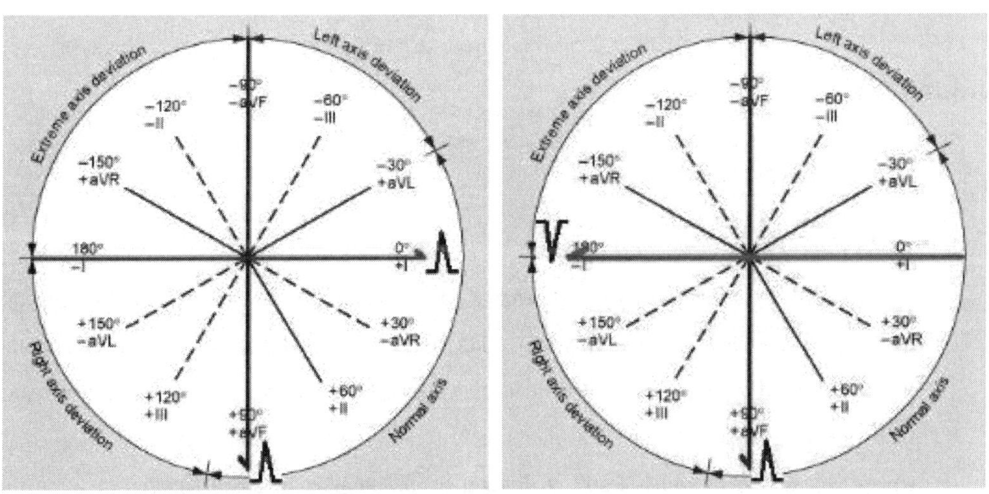

Fig. 3.29 ***Normal axis (left) and right axis deviation (right)***

For example, a QRS axis of +90° to 180°, which is not the normal axis, is considered a right axis deviation (RAD) and a QRS axis of -30° to -90° is considered a left axis deviation (LAD) [Fig. 3.25]. On the other hand, the QRS complex with LAD is always regarded as abnormal. The QRS group with RAD may be regarded as normal according to the patient's age or physique, but RAD in adulthood may indicate heart disease or lung disease. The causes of LAD and RAD are summarized in [Table 3.14]. The heart axis can be more specifically analyzed by selecting an arbitrary axis and confirming whether the QRS wave of the axis is positive or negative. If a common area is determined by looking for an axis drawn at 90° with respect to the arbitrary axis, the angle is read from the circular axis [Fig. 3.29].

On the left side of [Fig. 3.29], since the QRS wave is positive in lead I and aVF, the range of overlap is 0° to +90°, which indicates the normal axis. On the other hand, the right side of [Fig. 3.29] indicates RAD, since the QRS wave is negative in lead I and is positive in aVF with a range between -180° and +90°.

Table 3.14 ***Causes of left and right axis deviation***

Classification	Cause (diagnosis)	Axis
Left axis deviation	· Left ventricular hypertrophy (hypertension, aortic stenosis, ischemic heart disease) · Left bundle brunch blocks (ischemic heart disease, aortic valve stenosis, rheumatic disease, pericarditis, myocarditis) · Left anterior fascicular block	· LAD(left axis deviation) aVL -30° ~ aVF -90°
Right axis deviation	· Right ventricular hypertrophy (chronic obstructive pulmonary disease, preclosure, hypertension, pulmonary heart, congenital heart disease) · Right bundle brunch blocks (chronic coronary artery, hypertensive heart disease, acute heart failure, pericarditis, myocarditis) · Left posterior fascicular block	· RAD(right axis deviation) aVF +90° ~ I -180° · EAD(extreme axis deviation) I -180° ~ aVF -90°

Reading Heart Rate and Rhythm

The rhythm is the RR interval and is also called the heart rate. If this appears constant, it is called a regular rhythm, otherwise, it is called arrhythmia. Looking at the overall rhythm or interval in a 12-lead ECG is the first thing to do. There are many ways to measure heart rate, but the simplest and most convenient method is a small square calculation in which 1,500 is divided by the number of small squares between the first R and second R wave [Fig. 3.30].

There are 14 small squares between the first R wave and the second R wave shown in [Fig. 3.30], so this would be calculated as {1,500/14 = 107 bpm}. The second method calculates the number of 5 mm boxes between two QRS waves by applying 300-150-100-75-60-50 [Fig. 3.31]. The heart rate shown in the figure corresponds to 60 bpm. However, recent ECG devices automatically calculate heart rate, so heart rate can easily be obtained.

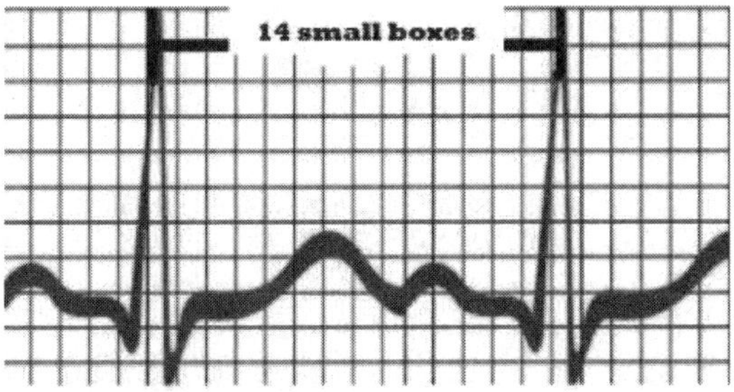

Fig. 3.30 ***Small rectangular calculation method***

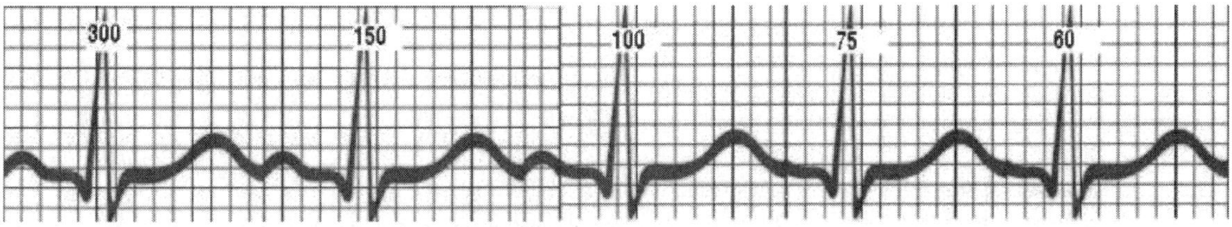

Fig. 3.31 ***Triplicated method***

Reading P Waves

- P waves are regular and point upward in limb lead Ⅱ.
- There is one P wave in front of one QRS complex (1:1).
- The shape of P waves are the same on the same lead.
- P waves point upward in leads I, II, and V_6.
- In lead Ⅱ, the height of a P wave is less than 2.5 ㎜ and the width is less than 0.12 seconds (3 small squares).

Reading PR Interval

- The interval starts from the beginning of the P wave to the beginning of the QRS complex.
- The interval is constant in the same lead, 0.12 to 0.20 seconds (3-5 small squares).
- It should be regular and continuous throughout the entire ECG.
- If the PR interval does not appear constant, an atrioventricular block may be suspected.

Reading QRS Complex

- The QRS width is less than 0.09 seconds or less than 0.12 seconds.
- The maximum height of the QRS complex in a lead is 5 mm or more.
- The R wave height in V_5 or V_6 is less than 27 mm.
- {R wave height of V_5} + {S wave depth of V_1}, should be less than 35 mm (7 large squares). Or
- {R wave height of V_6} + {S wave depth of V_2}, should be less than 35 mm (7 large squares).
- If the width is too wide, blocks in the left bundle or right bundle may be suspected.

Reading Q Waves

- The depth of Q waves should be less than 25% of the R wave (RQ ratio) and less than 0.04 seconds in width.
- Significant Q waves may indicate myocardial damage and aneurysms.

Table 3.15 *Changes in ST segment*

ST segment elevation	ST segment normalization	ST segment depression
· Appears in resting ECG. · As the heart rate increases, it can return to the isoelectric line. 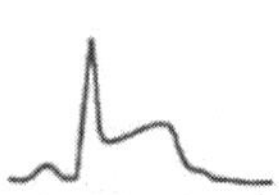 ST elevation (≥ 1mm) 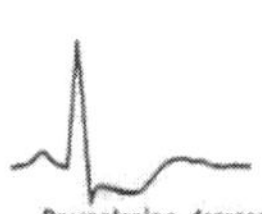 Downsloping depression (≥ 1mm)	· CAD patients have T wave inversion and ST segment depression on resting ECG, but may return to normal during exercise. · Normalization of the ST segment is interpreted as the ST segment elevation. 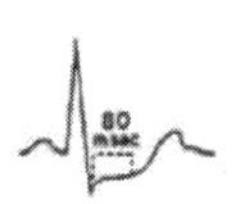 Horizontal ST depression (≥ 1mm for 80 msec) 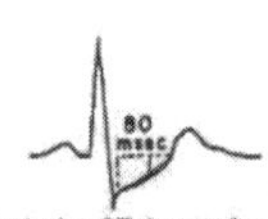 Upsloping ST depression (≥1.5mm at 80 msec)	· Exercise-induced myocardial ischemia · A ST segment depression of 1 mm or more from the isoelectric line was positive within 0.08 seconds from J point. · In ST segment depression, downsloping and horizontal type are more likely to have myocardial ischemia, and upsloping and adduction types are less likely. · The ST segment depression is independent of the ischemic area and the involved coronary artery. However, when the ST depression appears in multiple leads, myocardial ischemia is severe. · In patients with left or right bundle brunch block, ST segment changes indicate myocardial ischemia. · ST segment changes in V_1, V_2, and V_3 are meaningless, and ST changes in V_4, V_5, and V_6 indicate myocardial ischemia.

Reading ST Segments

- ST segments are in line with the isoelectric line, but there is a possibility of a decrease in 1 mm or less, or a rise in 2 ㎜ or less.
- The ST segment is affected by resting ECG and drugs.
- Changes in ST segments are shown in [Table 3.15].

Reading T Waves

- T waves point upward in leads I, II and V_6.
- Usually it is possible to shown downward or upward in V_1 and V_2.

Reading U Waves

- The height is less than 25% of T wave and is the largest in V_2~V_4.
- Almost none.

Reading QT Intervals

- The interval starts from the beginning of the QRS complex to the end of the T wave.
- QT intervals are normal when they are less than 0.42~0.43 seconds.

The waves, intervals, and segments of the ECG described so far are shown in [Fig. 3.32].

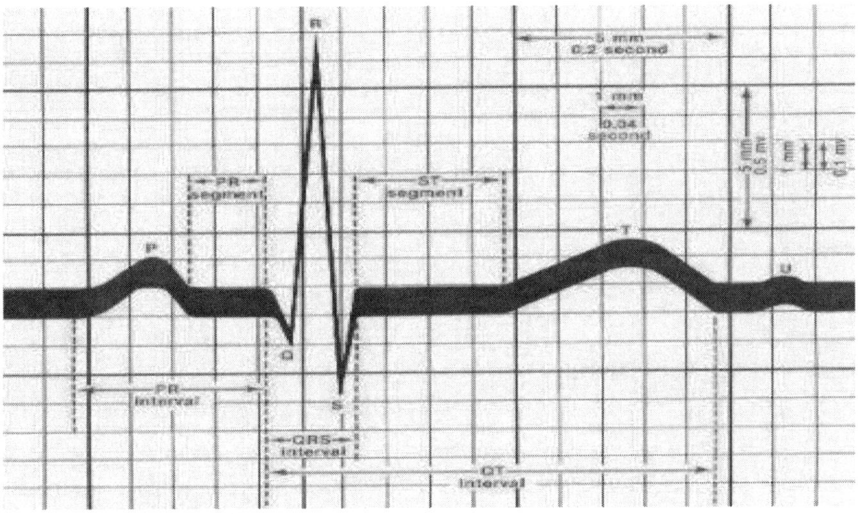

Fig. 3.32 ***Electrocardiographic wave, interval, segment***

Interpretation of Abnormal ECG

Arrhythmia

Arrhythmia is an abnormality of the conduction system with a regular or irregular heart rate. The heart rate may be normal, fast, or slow. Arrhythmia is symptomless and does not cause any disability, so treatment is not necessary. However, first aid treatment should be performed in the case of dizziness or syncope. Arrhythmia can be divided into sinus tachycardia, sinus arrhythmia, atrial tachycardia, atrial flutter, atrial fibrillation, premature ventricular contraction, ventricular tachycardia, and ventricular fibrillation. Specific details and waveforms are shown below.

■ *Sinus Tachycardia*

. Regularity: Regular
. Speed: 100 ~ 160 bpm when resting
. P wave: upward, P : QRS = 1 : 1
. PRI: 0.12-0.20 sec (constant)
. QRS: < 0.12 sec

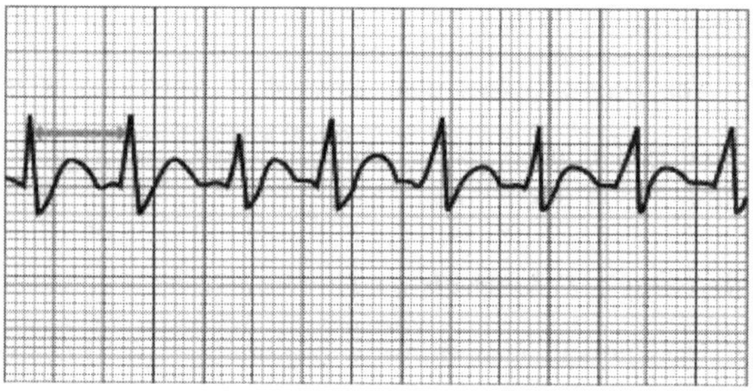

■ *Sinus Arrhythmia*

. Regularity: Irregular
. Speed: 50 ~ 100 bpm
. P wave: upward, P : QRS = 1 : 1
. PRI: 0.12-0.20 sec (constant)
. QRS: < 0.12 sec

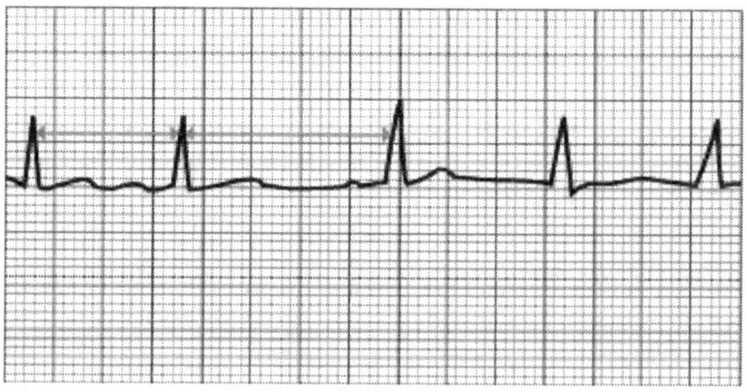

■ *Atrial Fibrillation*

. Cause: overwork / drinking alcohol
. Regularity: irregular
. Speed: > 350 bpm (atrium) +
. P wave: Not shown
. PRI: Not measurable
. QRS: < 0.12 sec
. mitral valvular disease/ ischemic heart disease/ hyperthyroidism

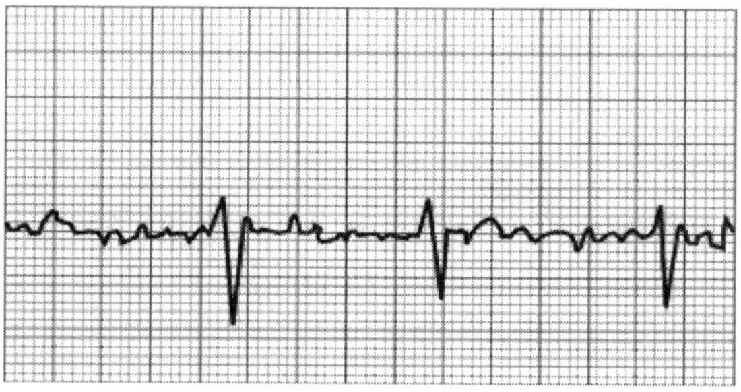

■ *Premature Ventricular Contraction (PVC)*

. Regularity: Regular or irregular
. QRS: > 0.12 seconds faster than normal speed.
. Sporadic (1 PVC / min), multiple (5 PVC / min)
. Bigeminy (1 normal + 1 PVC), trigeminy (2 normal + 1 PVC)
. Ischemic heart disease/ myocarditis/ hypertensive heart disease/ heart failure/ hyperthyroidism

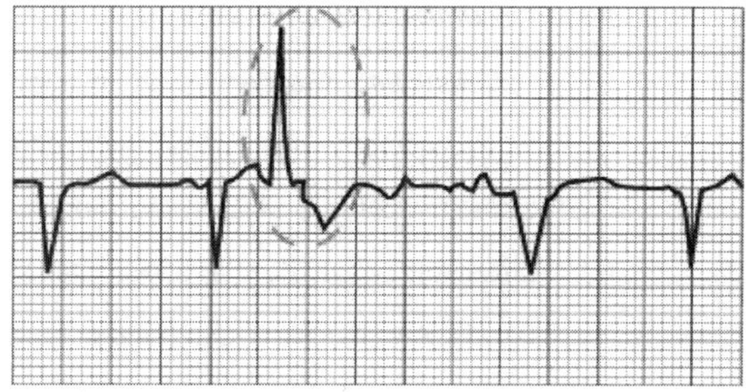

■ *Atrial Tachycardia*

. Regularity: Regular
. Speed: 150 ~ 250 bpm
. P wave: It disappears by T waves.
(P: QRS = 1:1, sometimes 2:1)
. PRI: 0.12-0.20 sec (constant)
. QRS: < 0.12 sec

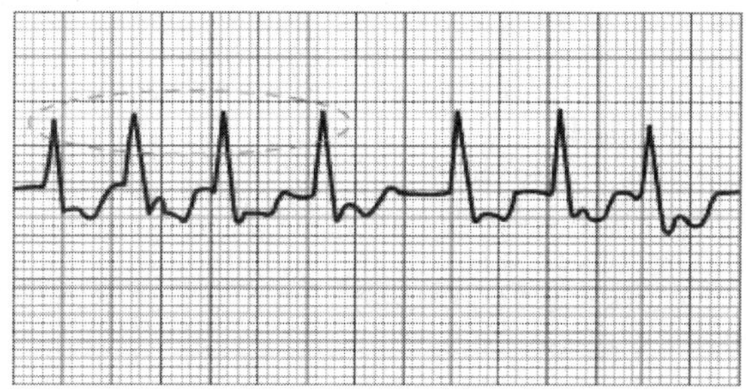

■ *Atrial Flutter*

. Regularity: Regular
. Speed: 250 ~ 350 bpm (atrium)
. P wave: small, sharp, rapid fluctuations (shape of a saw blade) (P: QRS = 3:1 or 4:1)
. PRI: Not measurable
. QRS: < 0.12 sec

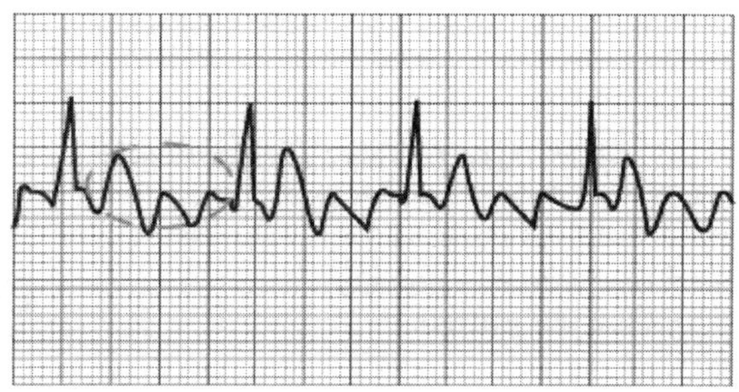

■ *Ventricular Tachycardia*

. Regularity: Regular
. Speed: 150 ~ 163 bpm
. P wave: Not shown
. PRI: Not measurable
. QRS: 0.16 sec
. Severe end-stage heart disease/ mitral valve prolapse/ shock, etc.

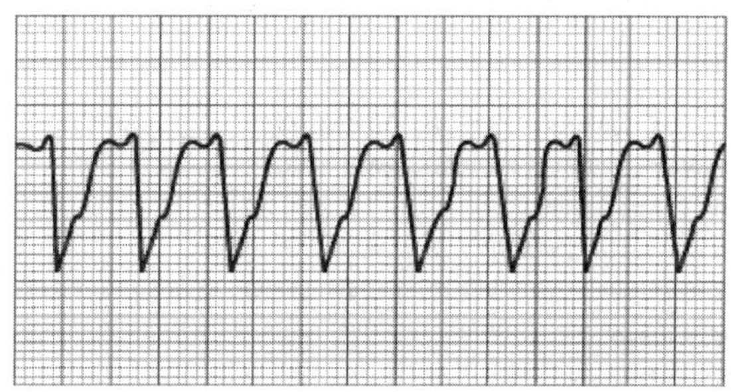

■ *Ventricular Fibrillation*

. Regularity: Irregular
. Speed: 150 ~ 300 bpm
. Coarse ventricular fibrillation
. Suspension and first aid
. End stage heart disease/ acute myocardial infarction/ shock/ hypokalemia or hyperkalemia/ hypocalcemia or hypercalcemia/ hypoxia/ drug addiction

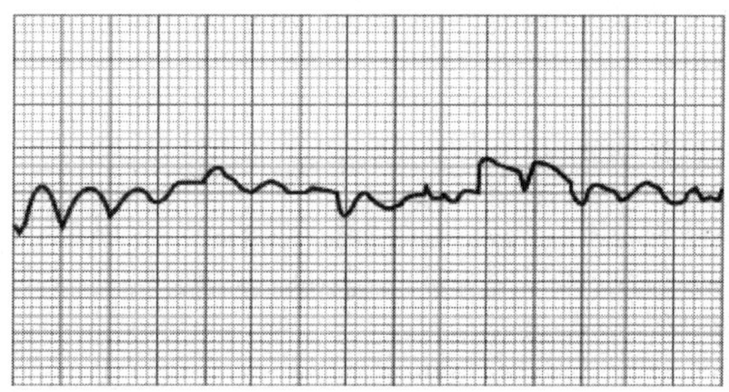

Conduction Disorders

Conduction disorders occur in normal people and most cases are congenital in children. It is generally associated with coronary heart disease, hypertension, aortic stenosis, cardiomyopathy, and drug addiction (especially digitalis). Types of conduction disturbances can be classified into 1° AV blocks, 2° AV blocks (Mobitz I and Mobitz II), 3° AV blocks, right bundle blocks, and left bundle blocks. The specific details of each type and the waveforms are as follows.

■ *1° AV Blocks*

. Cause: Elderly / vagus nerve ↑
. Regularity: Sinus rhythm / incomplete block
. Speed: Normal sinus speed
. P wave: Sinus (including medication)
. PRI: > 0.20 sec (constant)
. QRS: < 0.12 sec
. Myocardial infarction/ ischemic heart disease/ hypertensive heart disease/ rheumatoid heart disease

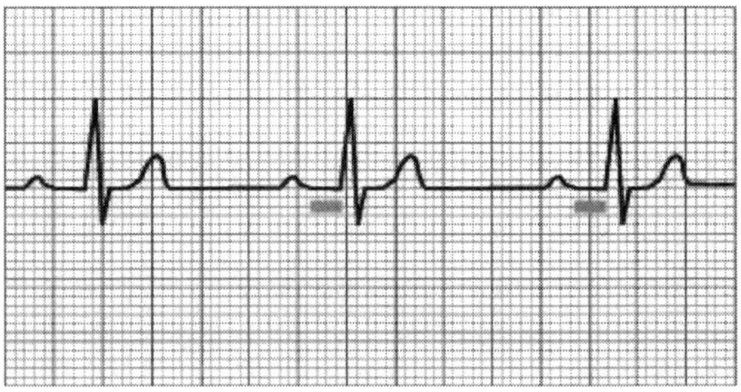

■ *2° AV Blocks (Type I, Mobitz I, Wenchebach)*

. Regularity: sinus rhythm / incomplete blocks
. Speed: Normal sinus velocity, bradycardia, tachycardia
. P wave: sinus (occasionally blocked)
. PRI: One more after graduation
. QRS: < 0.12 sec
. Same with 1°AV blocks including myocarditis or cardiomyopathy

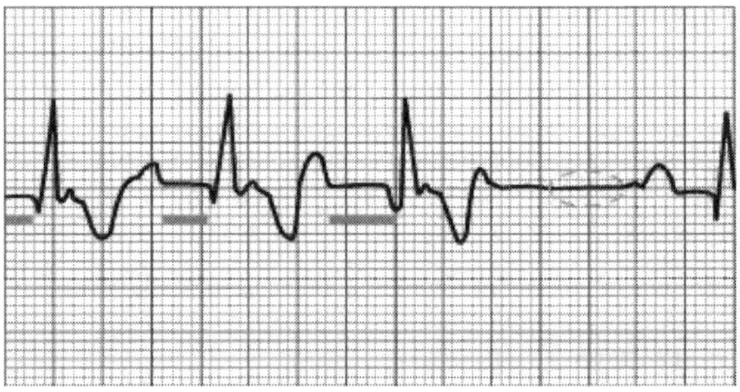

■ *2° AV Blocks (Type II, Mobitz II)*

. Regularity: Sinus rhythm / incomplete blocks
. Rate: Normal rhythm
. P wave: Sinus (blocked P wave increase) / P: QRS = 2: 1 Or 3: 1
. PRI: Constant
. QRS: < 0.12 sec
. Heart disease/ taking medication/ not shown to normal people.

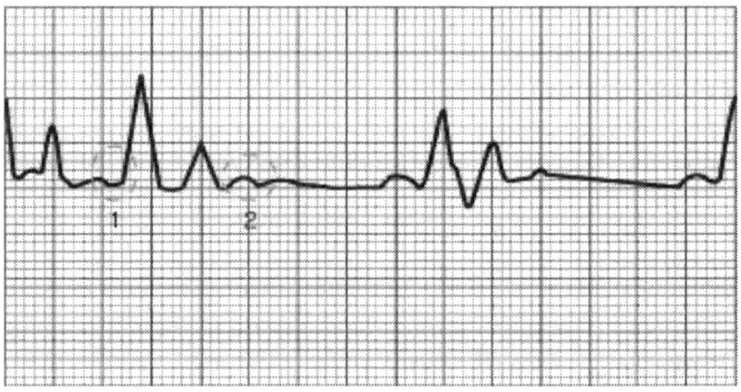

■ *3° AV Blocks*

. Regularity: Sinus rhythm disappears
. Speed: Normal sinus speed, bradycardia, tachycardia
. P wave: Sinus (40 ~ 50 bpm) / independent of QRS
. PRI: Not measurable
. QRS: nodal < 0.12 sec, ventricular > 0.12 sec
. Arrhythmia is not caught by palpation.

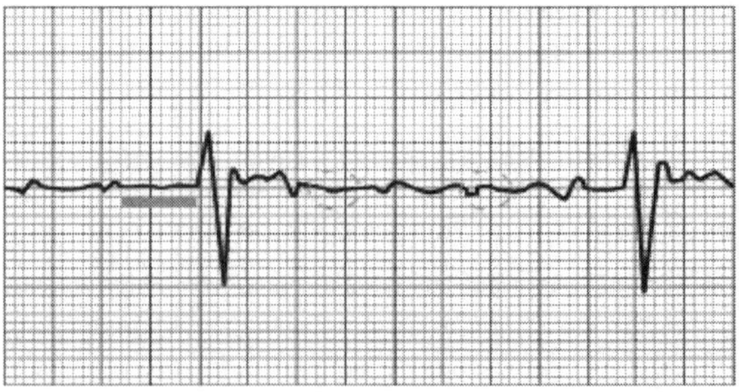

■ ***Right Bundle Branch Blocks***

. V1 to QRS (≥ 0.12 sec): complete
. V1 to QRS (0.1 ~ 0.12 sec): incomplete
. The appearance of rSR, rSRs in V_1 and V_2.
. In general, S waves are wide in lead I and V_6.
. Chronic coronary artery/ hypertensive heart disease/ acute heart failure/ pericarditis/ myocarditis

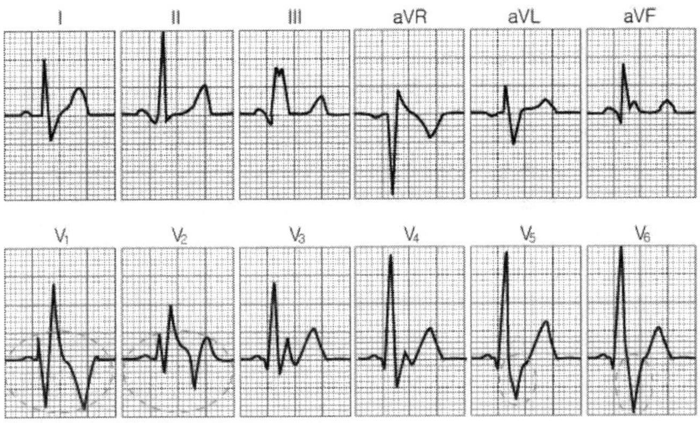

■ ***Left Bundle Branch Blocks***

. Cause: Predominantly in the elderly
. V_1 to QS (≥ 0.12 sec): complete
. V_1 to QS (0.1 to 0.12 sec): incomplete
. Wide QRS wave (≥ 0.12 sec) sinus rhythm.
. ST decreases in V_5 and V6.
. ST increases in V_1, V_2 (T increase).
. Ischemic heart disease/ hypertensive heart disease/ aortic stenosis/ rheumatic disease/ heart failure/ pericarditis/ myocarditis

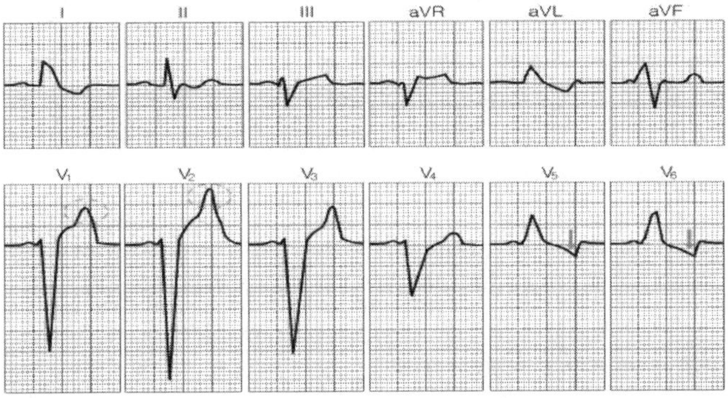

Cardiomegaly

Cardiomegaly is an abnormally thickened state of either or both of the atrial wall and the ventricular wall. It is caused by excessive pressure of blood flow into the heart. The term enlargement can also be used with the same meaning.

■ ***Left Atrial Hypertrophy***

. P-wave width of 0.12 sec or longer in leads I and II
. Wide and depressed P waves (mitral P).
. Mitral stenosis/ cardiac insufficiency/ left ventricular hypertrophy
. P mitrale formation

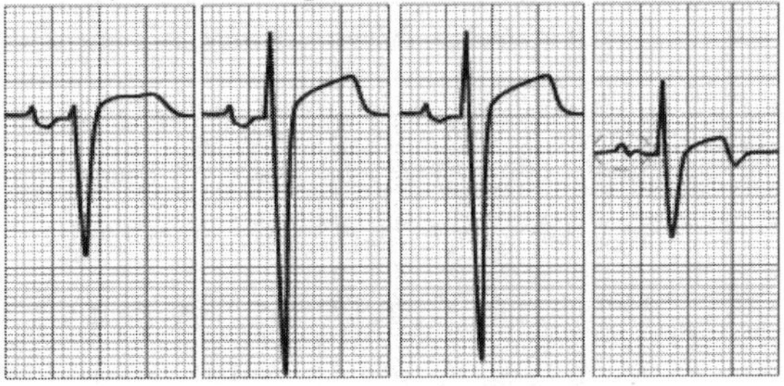

■ ***Right Atrial Hypertrophy***

. A height of more than 2.5 ㎜ in leads II, III, aVF.

. Large, pointed P waves

. In V_1, P waves appear similar to the above.

. Tricuspid stenosis/ obstruction/ right ventricle hypertrophy/ COPD

. P pulmonale formation

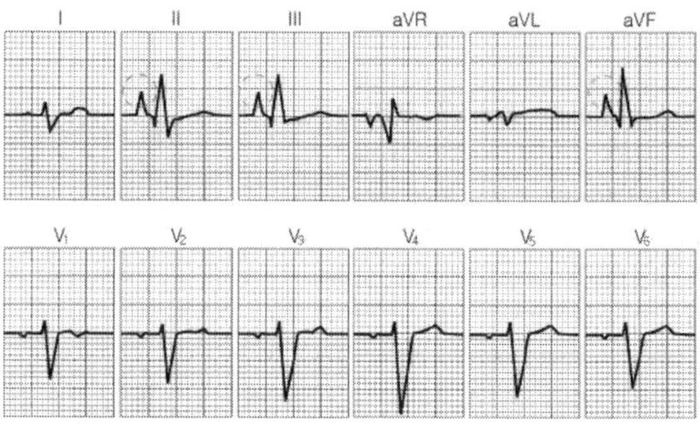

■ ***Right Ventricular Hypertrophy***

. Right axis deviation > 90°

. The ratio of R / S wave in V_1 is > 1.0 sec

. ST depression / T inversion in V_1, V_2, V_3.

. Chronic cor pulmonale/ primary pulmonary hypertension/ pulmonary valve stenosis/ COPD

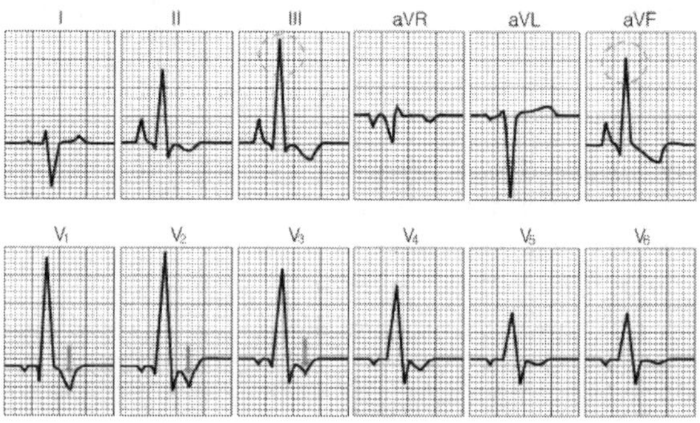

■ ***Left Ventricular Hypertrophy***

. Left axis deviation >-15°

. R wave of all limb leads > 15 ㎜

. V_5 (R) + V_2 (S) = > 35 ㎜

. A negative P wave depth of 0.04 or more in V_1

. Hypertension/ aortic valve disease/ cardiomyopathy/ mitral valve/ cardiac insufficiency/ ventricular septal defect

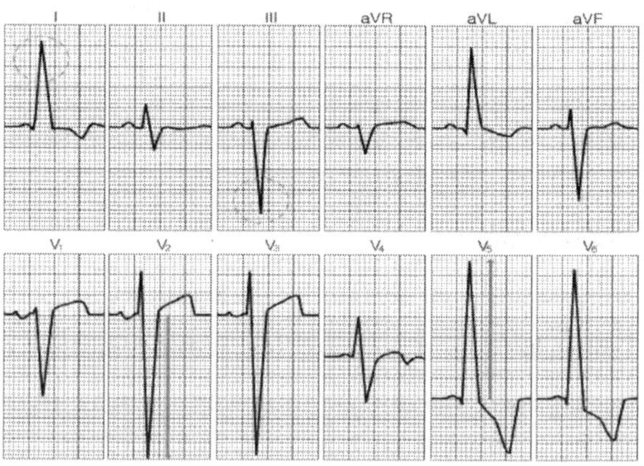

Myocardial Ischemia and Myocardial Infarction

Myocardial ischemia is a temporary and reversible decrease in blood flow to the myocardium. The most common cause is atherosclerosis of the coronary arteries, but it is reported as left ventricular hypertrophy, aortic stenosis, pulmonary arterial hypertension, and anemia. When there is chest pain due to myocardial ischemia, it is clinically referred to as angina, and is widely referred to as angina.[46] However, if this condition deteriorates and blood supply to the myocardium is cut off and insufficient, necrosis of the myocardium may develop and progress to myocardial infarction. The cause of myocardial infarction is the same as myocardial ischemia. It is also caused by the complete closure of the coronary artery. However, it is caused by the incomplete closure if the blood supply to the myocardium suddenly decreases. However, even with the complete closure of the coronary arteries, myocardial infarction does not occur if the collateral circulation is well developed.

■ *Myocardial Ischemia*

. ST segment depression: ≥ 1 ㎜ (3 ㎜)

. ST segment elevation: ≥ 1 ㎜ (severe myocardial ischemia)

. R wave: In the case of severe myocardial ischemia, the left ventricular volume increases due to exercise or the R wave becomes larger due to conduction disorders.

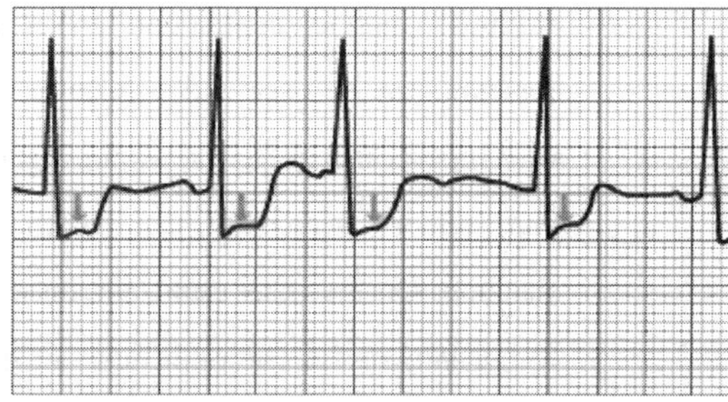

■ *Myocardial Infarction*

. Significant Q wave: ≥ 0.04 sec (QR ratio ≥ 25%)

. ST segment elevation: It is upward in the lead of the myocardial infarction area, and downward in the opposite lead.

. T wave inversion: K^+ is leaked into the extracellular fluid in the injured myocardium.

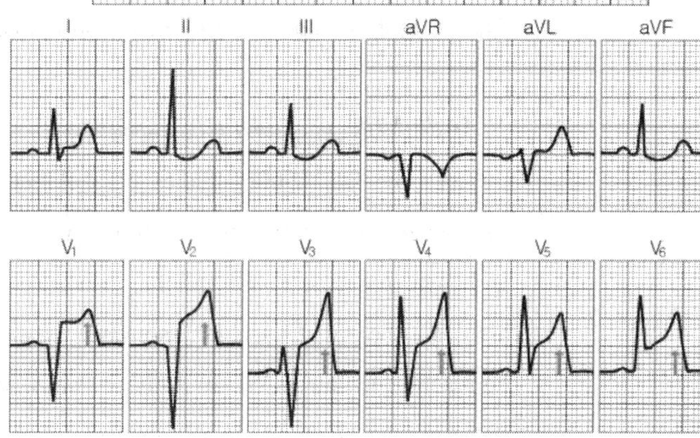

Musculoarticular Function Test

Musculoarticular function test is stable and reliable because it uses isokinetic equipment,[14,48-50] which is speed-centered rather than weight-centered. In other words, the stability is secured by examining the main muscle-joint region before the physical examination, and it can be used as the data of the rehabilitation treatment when the abnormal musculoskeletal joint is found [Fig. 3.33].

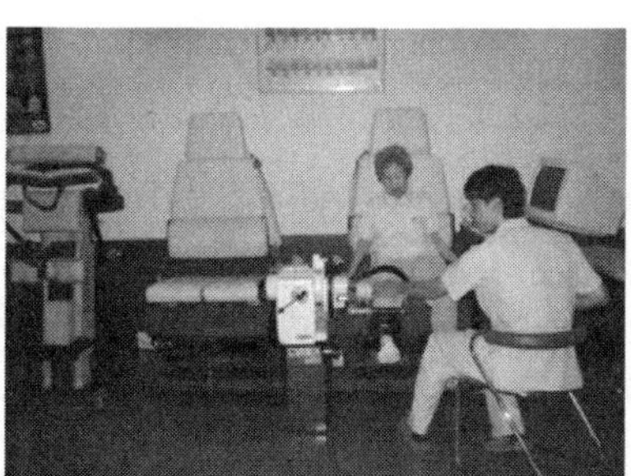

- Epidemiological changes in the musculoskeletal system and the control of pain / fatigue[43]
- Induce maximal contraction of entire ROM without influence of inertia
- Take advantage of tension on muscle length
- Record and observe results every time you repeat the exercise
- Minimize pain and use in patients with myocardial injury
- Automatic speed control helps to restore function

Fig. 3.33 ***Musculoarticular function test***

The advantages of isokinetic equipment are as follows. First, it can be used on severe patients with musculoskeletal abnormalities by automatically adjusting the mechanical changes of the musculoskeletal system during exercise, pain, and fatigue. Second, it avoids the inertia or acceleration that occurs during isotonic exercise and induces maximal muscle contraction throughout the entire ROM. Third, the length-tension function can be used independently. Fourth, the results can be recorded every time the user repeats the exercises within a stable ROM. Fifth, it can help patients with spasticity and tremors overcome pain. Sixth, speed can be adjusted to help the recovery of function. On the other hand, the disadvantages are: expensive equipment, a lack of skilled technicians in the clinic, difficult to move, lengthy time period for inspection and repairs. The contents of specific isokinetic musculoarticular function tests are as follows.

Availability of Isokinetic Equipment

Since the late 1960s, studies on isokinetic exercise have provided important data on musculoarticular function. Recently, its effectiveness has been proved by adopting isokinetic movements for general resistance movements not only in clinical settings, but also in the field. Unlike isotropic motion, isokinetic motion can induce muscle contraction in the ROM. In addition, since the speed of motion is constant, it measures the resistance exerted by the subject (speed change motion). Isotonic exercise induces muscle contraction with weight, which commonly causes injury. However, isokinetic exercise induces muscle contraction using speed, so the risk of injury is low. In addition, there is an advantage in effectively providing a load to the target muscle because it minimizes changes in gravity, exercise posture, and arm length during muscle contraction.

Characteristics of Isokinetic Training

Isokinetic equipment can perform precise muscular functional testing at various angular velocities, help in rehabilitation, and provide strength training to parts that require strength. For example, the difference in bilateral muscular functions at low speeds (less than 60°/sec) is mainly attributed to "deficit of muscle strength" and the difference in bilateral muscular functions at high speeds (over 180°/sec) is mainly attributed to "deficit of power or muscular endurance". Considering this, the program can be set for rehabilitation treatment.

On the other hand, isotonic exercises do not meet the speed requirements required for sports activities because they are done through weight-centered testing and training methods. Isokinetic exercise can stimulate various muscle fibers because it induces exercise at various speeds, even if it does not meet the speed of normal sports activities. In addition, high-speed loading in isokinetic exercise can strengthen the muscles while minimizing swelling and pain because it can reduce the pressure on the joints. In addition, even if the patient suddenly stops or reduces muscle contraction due to pain during testing or training, it is evaluated as clinically safe because resistance by speed is immediately reduced and does not exceed the amount of force given. This stability is of greater significance as Davies reported on the alleviation of pain and improvement in joint lubrication during isokinetic submaximal training.[15]

Principles of Isokinetic Testing and Training

For accurate and reliable measurement and training, it is desirable to use a "standardized protocol" that has been longitudinally studied and developed by many researchers. In particular, isokinetic testing is not a problem for healthy people with no symptoms, but it is important for patients with subjective symptoms or problems specific to the musculoskeletal system or cardiovascular system to seek consent from a physician before testing. Refer to the following for information regarding the restrictions of isokinetic testing. In addition, the following items must be considered before isokinetic testing or exercise.[11]

Patient Education

As with any test, isokinetic testing is a very new sensory type of testing for the general people. Therefore, it is advisable to inform patients about the concept of isokinetic exercise for reliable and valid examinations. Specifically, the isokinetic dynamometer is performed at a preset angular velocity, and the resistance is constant. However, the patient should be told that the maximal ability is recorded only if the patient contracts as strongly and quickly as possible. Since the active isokinetic dynamometer has been developed, it can be tested and trained in various forms such as the eccentric contraction protocol, as well as the ramp protocol. Therefore, it is necessary to inform them about the kind of testing or training that will be performed. On the other hand, it is important to select a set of warm-ups for different test speeds for adjustment and stability for isokinetic tests. In general, most experts recommend performing three or four submaximal exercises in preparation for each isokinetic test.

Posture Fixation and Joint Adjustment

Place the subject on the dynamometer before the test and fix the target muscle group to ensure stability and accuracy. In particular, other limbs and the torso, excluding the target muscle group to be examined, are fastened with strips to prevent them from being mobilized. For example, the waist and chest of a subject are strapped down in a knee test. Also, when the upper leg muscle group is examined, the leg is suspended from the floor so that only the upper extremity is examined.

However, the above-described postural fixation methods are not clinically significant compared to cases without using such methods. Therefore, it is recommended to emphasize stability over accuracy when examining patients or elderly people who lack balance. On the other hand, it is important to know the anatomical postures of the human body at all times to fix the muscle group to be tested. For example, it is advisable to adjust the joints according to the basic manual with consideration of flexion and extension in the sagittal plane, abduction and adduction in the coronal plane, and rotation in the transverse plane.

Gravity Correction

All objects are affected by Earth's gravity. When the human muscular function is accelerated by gravity, torque is increased, while in the opposite situation, torque is decreased. Therefore, to measure only muscular function, the effect of gravity should be minimized. One of the greatest advantages of isokinetic muscular function testing is the ability to correct for gravity, which makes it easier to understand the differences in measuring the quadriceps[10] and hamstring muscle groups[11]. For example, if the test is performed without correcting for gravity, the muscle strength of the quadriceps varies from a minimum of 4% to a maximum of 43%, and the hamstring difference is between 15% and 510%. In addition, it is difficult to determine the ratio of relative muscular function due to weight when gravity correction is performed incorrectly. Therefore, correcting for gravity is recommended for muscle groups that can be increased in strength or resistance by gravity.

---

10) Quadricep muscle: A group of four muscles consisting of rectus femoris, vastus lateralis, vastus medialis, and vastus intermedius.

11) Hamstrings muscle: A group of muscles consisting of semitendiosus, long headed bicep femoris, short headed bicep femoris, and semimembranosus.

Overshoot Phenomenon

The resistance mechanism of isokinetic exercise is to obtain the maximum value by accelerating the target limb at the predetermined angular velocity. However, when suddenly increasing the force in the muscle contraction process, a temporary torque curve appears, which is called "overshoot or spike" phenomenon. These temporary and artificial spikes cause confusion in assessing the subject's true maximum contraction ability. Therefore, many researchers and engineers have adopted the "damp", "ramp" or "preload" approach to overcome this problem to prevent overshoot. More recently, "isoaccleration software" has been developed to prevent acceleration or deceleration that may occur during resistance movement.

Confusing Factors in Isokinetic Tests

The maximal ability of the muscle to generate force is exerted when the 'muscle-tendon unit' is not injured and receives normal nerve stimulation from the nervous system with the absence of pain. Therefore, in some cases, submaximal isokinetic training is recommended to the human body area where the site of the neuromuscular defect present. However, if the subject is suffering from pain at the time of examination, it is not easy to accurately assess the deficit factor of each variable such as torque, workload, or power in a single muscle group. Examples are presented in [Fig. 3.34] and [Fig. 3.35].

[Fig. 3.34] shows the result of isokinetic testing of both the uninjured[12)] and injured side[13)] of the knees of a patient with anterior cruciate ligament (ACL) tear in the lower right limb. In this picture, it can be visually confirmed that the extensor graph of the pain-free and healthy knee joint (LT or Left) is much higher than that of the injured side (RT or Right). In other words, the graph on the injured side is small and does not exhibit peak torque. This point is referred to as the "weakest point" and generally, pain is most intense at this point. [Fig. 3.35] shows the point of pain and the weakest point in the knees of chondromalacia patients.

It is difficult to accurately assess and evaluate patients with musculoarticular injury with isokinetic testing. However, even if there are many confusing factors in assessing these musculoskeletal patients, if the muscular function is restored through active rehabilitation for several weeks, the pain and the weakest point will be reduced and the confusion factor will be reduced. For example, it was found that there were initially confusion factors in the muscular functions of the patients presented in [Fig. 3.36] and

---

12) Uninvolved side or Uninjured side: Healthy limbs without injury or pain.

13) Involved side or Injured side: Injuries or painful limbs.

[Fig. 3.37], but the factors were excluded after 12 and 18 weeks of rehabilitation treatment, respectively. Paradoxically, the initial confusing factor serves as a parameter for treatment or as a definitive therapeutic goal.

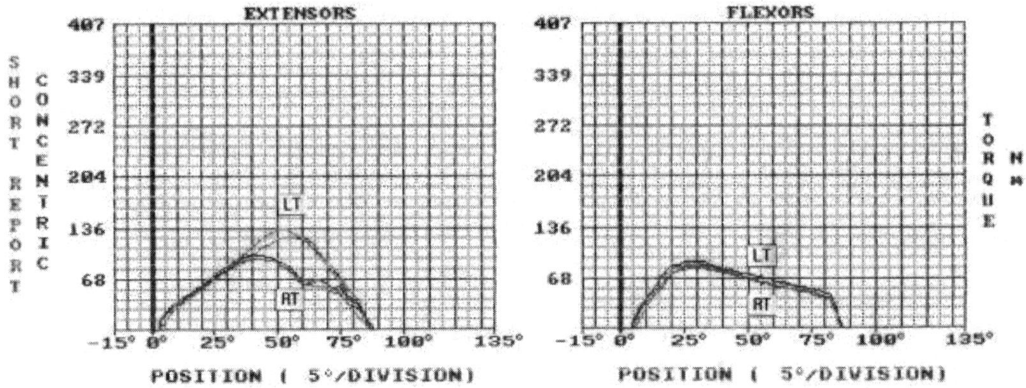

Fig. 3.34 ***Weakest point in RT knee extensor of ACL injured patient***

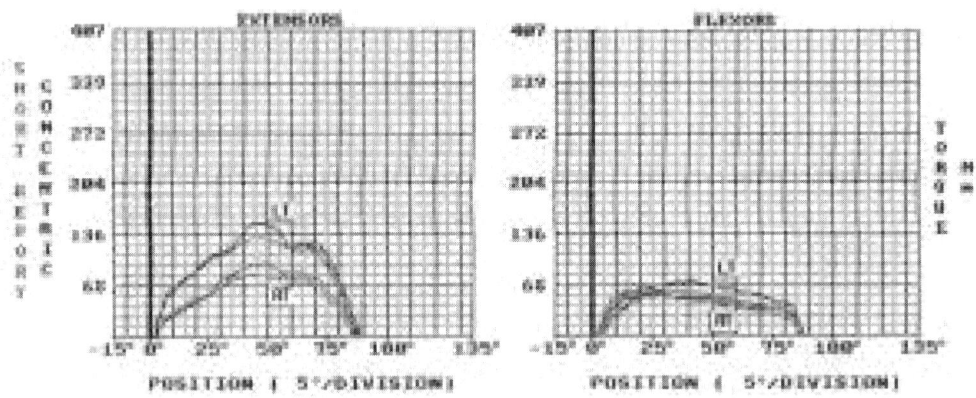

Fig. 3.35 ***Weakest point in RT knee extensor and flexor of chondromalacia patient***

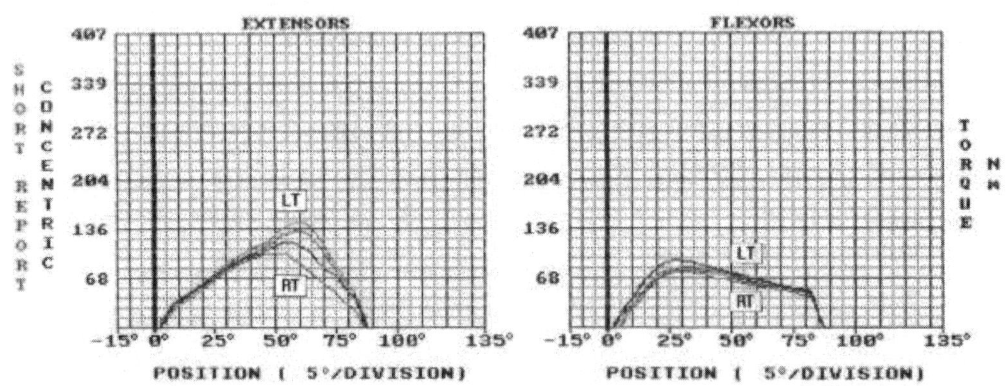

Fig. 3.36 ***Weakest point disappeared in RT knee extensor of ACL injured patient***

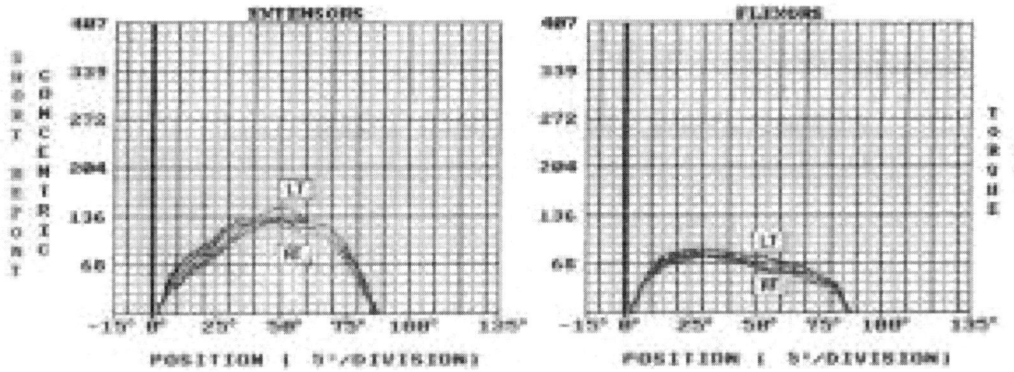

Fig. 3.37 ***Weakest point disappeared in RT knee extensor and flexor of chondromalacia patient***

Testing Protocol

There are many protocols for isokinetic testing. Commonly, these protocols are configured to measure variables such as torque, workload, and power, but most importantly, the testing protocol should be stable and reliable. The details are as follows and the summary is as shown in [Table 3.16].

Table 3.16 ***Recommended protocol for isokinetic testing***

1. Inspection and palpation of the musculoskeletal system	9. Maximum test at low speed (repeat 4 ~ 6 times)
2. Typical stretching and warm-up	10. Rest (30 seconds ~ 1 minute)
3. Patient fixation considering stability	11. Maximum test at high speed (repeat 4 ~ 6 times)
4. Joint adjustment to the motor shaft of the dynamometer	12. Rest (30 seconds ~ 1 minute)
5. Conceptual explanation of isokinetic exercise	13. Endurance tests (usually 24 to 50 times) with many repetitions
6. Gravity compensation for specific joints	14. Other limb test
7. Warm-up (3 times submaximal, 3 times maximum repeat)	15. Records and archives of tests for re-measurement
8. Rest (30 seconds ~ 1 minute)	16. Explanation of the results to the patient

Warm-Up

As with any exercise or test, warm-up through submaximal exercise and maximal exercise is absolutely necessary before isokinetic testing. In order to perform a stable and effective test, three submaximal and three maximal exercises have been reported to be necessary for warming up. Furthermore, it has been reported that after performing warm-up, reliable peak torque, workload, and power can be obtained in 'knee flexion / extension test', 'shoulder flexion / extension test', and 'internal rotation / external rotation test'. It is important to perform a warm-up before the test. However, for more stable and efficient testing, one or two days of adaptive training before the actual testing can be one way to increase the reliability of isokinetic testing.

Rest Time

The isokinetic testing protocol must provide a certain amount of break time between the number of iterations and the speed of the test. Previous studies have shown that having a pre-test rest time provides a significant difference in the outcome, producing a significant amount of isokinetic strength and providing a higher level of reliability. However, the amount of rest time provided should be adjusted differently depending on the type and characteristic of the test. In other words, a sufficient time to recover after 4 maximal repetitions is 30 seconds to 1 minute of rest, whereas 25 to 30 repetitions of an endurance type test requires at least one minute or more of rest. It is also important to provide rest time by distinguishing the characteristics of the subjects (i.e., athletes, non-athletes, or patients).[52]

Testing Speed

The speed of isokinetic testing should be varied at low speeds (less than 60°/sec), medium speeds (60~180°/sec), and high speeds (more than 180 °/sec) in order to closely observe motor unit recruitment patterns and the muscle fiber ratio of one muscle or muscle group. In fact, isokinetic resistance is most likely a new experience for everyone, so it is recommended to start the first test at a low speed. This is because testing at low speeds facilitates learning capabilities and subjects with limited experience with isokinetic equipment have low reliability when high-speed tests precede low-speed tests.

On the other hand, it is a mistaken idea that high-speed isokinetic movements are similar to the movement speeds of athletes. The average rotational torque of the shoulder during the acceleration phase of a professional baseball pitcher is 6,180°/sec, and the highest is 9,198°/sec. These peak angular velocities are about 18 times faster than the fastest test speed of isokinetic equipment (550°/sec).[14] However, even if the isokinetic equipment does not measure the athlete's actual performance, the nerve components needed for athletic function and recruitment patterns of muscle fibers (e.g., the angle of peak torque and acceleration time) can be measured. Therefore, it contributes greatly to rehabilitation and exercise programs.

Number of Repetitions

The number of repetition of the isokinetic test must be constant to obtain the maximum value of force and torque regardless of angular velocity. Studies show that peak torque is typically achieved during the second to sixth rounds of muscle contraction. However, recent studies report that a larger peak torque can be obtained when the isokinetic test is repeated three to five times. In fact, the peak torque is not output at the initial time when the muscle is not contracted at all, that is, when the energy is sufficient, and even after the execution of many repetition times. Therefore, the technique of obtaining peak torque within a certain number of repetitions is very important. Therefore, many isokinetic equipment manufacturers have developed their own unique software, but the measurement method using the visual overlay technique seems to be more useful. In other words, this technique shows a graph of each overlapping number of repetitions to stimulate psychological incentives to outperform previous iterations. Some scholars based on these techniques report that a range of 3 to 5 repetitions is a reasonable range for reaching peak torque.

Encouragement

Verbal encouragement results in a variety of outcomes depending on whether or not they are implemented. In other words, depending on the kind of measurement testing, it must be decided whether it is more effective to increase motivation with a loud or soft voice. In general, however, it seems more effective to stimulate psychological motivation by using a loud voice.

Visual Feedback

All isokinetic power devices display the torque curves of the subjects in numerical or pictorial form. These visual feedbacks lead to active maximum muscle contraction during isokinetic testing. It has been reported that the peak torque of the quadriceps and hamstring muscle group was about 12% different from the angular velocity of 15°/sec when visual feedback was given to subjects. However, this was the result at low speeds, and there is some controversy when performing an isokinetic test at high speeds. The results of the test after applying visual feedback at 180°/sec and 300°/sec suggest that there is no significant difference in each variable. However, most researchers have found that the subjects did not have enough time for the central nervous system to see or process visual feedback at high speeds. In addition, visual feedback in the isokinetic test, whether at high speeds or low speeds, was an important means of inducing high overload.

Table 3.17 ***Isokinetic test protocols***

	1set	2set	3set	4set	5set		1set	2set	3set	4set	5set
Knee extension / flexion						**Ankle plantarflexion / dorsiflexion (knee flexion posture)**					
Angular velocity(°/s)	60	180	300			Angular velocity(°/s)	60	180	180		
Repetitions	4	4	30			Repetitions	3	20	20		
Rest(sec)	20	20	1			Rest(sec)	20	90	1		
Angular velocity(°/s)	60	180	240			Angular velocity(°/s)	30	120	180		
Repetitions	3	3	20			Repetitions	3	3	20		
Rest(sec)	20	20	1			Rest(sec)	20	20	1		
Knee joint tibial axis internal / external rotation						**Ankle inversion / eversion**					
Angular velocity(°/s)	60	120				Angular velocity(°/s)	60	150			
Repetitions	4	4				Repetitions	3	15			
Rest(sec)	20	1				Rest(sec)	20	1			
Angular velocity(°/s)	30	120	180			Angular velocity(°/s)	30	120	30		
Repetitions	3	3	20			Repetitions	3	4	3		
Rest(sec)	20	20	1			Rest(sec)	20	20	1		
Ankle plantarflexion / dorsiflexion (extended knee posture)						**Shoulder abduction / adduction**					
Angular velocity(°/s)	60	180	180			Angular velocity(°/s)	120	300			
Repetitions	3	20	20			Repetitions	4	20			
Rest(sec)	20	90	1			Rest(sec)	20	1			
Angular velocity(°/s)	30	120	30			Angular velocity(°/s)	60	180	240		
Repetitions	3	3	20			Repetitions	3	3	20		
Rest(sec)	20	20	1			Rest(sec)	20	20	1		
Shoulder extension / flexion						**Shoulder internal / external rotation (correction posture)**					
Angular velocity(°/s)	120	300	300			Angular velocity(°/s)	60	120	180		
Repetitions	4	20	20			Repetitions	3	4	20		
Rest(sec)	20	90	1			Rest(sec)	20	20	1		
Angular velocity(°/s)	60	180	240			Angular velocity(°/s)	60	180	240		
Repetitions	3	3	3			Repetitions	3	3	25		
Rest(sec)	20	20	1			Rest(sec)	20	20	1		
Shoulder horizontal abduction / adduction						**Antebrachial muscle pronation/ supination**					
Angular velocity(°/s)	60	180				Angular velocity(°/s)	30	150			
Repetitions	3	4				Repetitions	4	15			
Rest(sec)	20	1				Rest(sec)	20	1			
Angular velocity(°/s)	60	180	240			Angular velocity(°/s)	60	150	150		
Repetitions	3	3	20			Repetitions	4	15	15		
Rest(sec)	20	20	1			Rest(sec)	20	90	1		

	1set	2set	3set	4set	5set		1set	2set	3set	4set	5set
Shoulder internal / external rotation (90° abduction posture)						**Shoulder internal / external rotation (90° flexion posture)**					
Angular velocity(°/s)	60	120	180			Angular velocity(°/s)	60	120	180		
Repetitions	3	4	20			Repetitions	3	4	20		
Rest(sec)	20	20	1			Rest(sec)	20	20	1		
Angular velocity(°/s)	60	180	240			Angular velocity(°/s)	60	180	240		
Repetitions	3	3	25			Repetitions	3	3	25		
Rest(sec)	20	20	1			Rest(sec)	20	20	1		
Wrist extension / flexion						**Elbow extension / flexion**					
Angular velocity(°/s)	30	60	120	120		Angular velocity(°/s)	60	180	240	240	
Repetitions	3	3	15	15		Repetitions	3	4	20	20	
Rest(sec)	20	20	20	1		Rest(sec)	20	20	90	1	
Angular velocity(°/s)	30	120	180			Angular velocity(°/s)	60	180	240		
Repetitions	3	3	20			Repetitions	3	3	25		
Rest(sec)	20	20	1			Rest(sec)	20	20	1		
Wrist radial / ulnar deviation						**Lumbar extension / flexion**					
Angular velocity(°/s)	30	60	120			Angular velocity(°/s)	30	60	90	60	
Repetitions	3	3	15			Repetitions	4	4	4	4	
Rest(sec)	20	20	1			Rest(sec)	30	30	30	1	
Angular velocity(°/s)	30	120	180			Angular velocity(°/s)	30	60	90	120	150
Repetitions	3	3	20			Repetitions	4	4	4	4	20
Rest(sec)	20	20	1			Rest(sec)	30	30	30	30	1
Hip flexion / extension						**Hip abduction / adduction**					
Angular velocity(°/s)	30	60	120			Angular velocity(°/s)	60	120	150		
Repetitions	3	4	15			Repetitions	3	4	4		
Rest(sec)	20	20	1			Rest(sec)	20	20	1		
Angular velocity(°/s)	30	120	180			Angular velocity(°/s)	30	120	150		
Repetitions	3	3	20			Repetitions	3	4	15		
Rest(sec)	20	20	1			Rest(sec)	20	20	1		

Ultimately, the protocols for isokinetic testing vary widely. However, as described above, it is recommended to configure the protocol by appropriately applying the principles of warm-up, rest time, testing speed, the number of repetitions, encouragement, and visual feedback after the stability and reliability of the subjects are secured. [Table 3.16] summarizes these principles, and [Table 3.17] gives examples of clinically recommended protocols.

Caution and Contraindication

Several factors influence the selection of the test protocol. These factors include the muscle group required for the test, the progress of the rehabilitation program, and the physical condition and age of the patient or athlete. For example, in patients with habitual shoulder dislocation requiring surgery, maximal lateral rotation test should be excluded, and isokinetic exercise and testing should be performed within a limited ROM. Patients with cardiovascular problems due to aging or inactivity should be careful during isokinetic testing or exercise. This is because low-speed or high-speed isokinetic exercise of the trunk and limbs may have an adverse effect on the cardiovascular system. Particularly, isokinetic exercise at low speed is similar to resistance exercise in isometric form, resulting in 'Valsalva maneuver'14), which increases intrathoracic pressure and intraabdominal pressure. The maximum isokinetic resistance exercise should be contraindicated in patients with cardiorespiratory conditions because Valsalva maneuvers may cause life-threatening consequences in severe cases.[47] However, it is advisable to be aware of 'absolute contraindications' and 'relative contraindications' as in [Table 3.18], since some patients may be given isokinetic tests even with contraindications.

In [Table 3.18], some tests are possible for patients with relative contraindications. The test starts at a medium speed and then slowly progresses to a high speed. However, in some cases, the test speed starts at a high speed and then proceeds to a low speed. Patients with spasticity or flaccidity due to neurological problems cannot perform accurate muscle function tests and exercises. Patients with spastic symptoms may perform certain types of isokinetic testing or exercise at medium or high speeds. However, in the case of flaccidity patients, it is difficult to induce muscle contraction because the nerves are not dominant in the affected muscle.

Table 3.18 ***Contraindications in isokinetic tests***

Absolute contraindication	Relative contraindication
▪ Soft tissue healing constraints	▪ Mild to moderate pain
▪ Severe pain	▪ Limited ROM
▪ Excessively limited ROM	▪ Effusion or synovitis
▪ Severe joint effusion	▪ Subacute sprains
▪ Unstable joint	▪ Chronic 3rd degree sprain
▪ Acute strain	▪ Pregnancy

14) Valsalva maneuver: A phenomenon developed by hypertensive response triggered by increased intrathoracic pressure caused by stopping respiration during muscle contraction.

Selection of a Training Protocol

When selecting an isokinetic training protocol, consideration should be given to the time and speed of the exercise, the ROM of the joint to be trained, and the length-tension relationship of the muscle group to be trained. Each of these components can be defined by the characteristics of the musculoskeletal injuries.

Training Time

As a result of comparing the 6-second high repetition with the 30-second low repetition for knee joint extension exercise, it has been reported that lactic acid increased in the muscles after only 30 seconds of exercise.[13] This suggests that only a single component among the ATP-PC involved enzyme, the glycolysis involved enzyme, and the Krebs-cycle involved enzyme was increased, even though repeated motions over 6 seconds and 30 seconds showed the same total work. In other words, the stimulus needed to increase intramuscular enzyme activity is more closely related to the time spent in a single training session than the total work obtained by repeatedly performing a short training cycle.

Therefore, it seems advisable to construct the isokinetic training time using time rather than repetition or frequency. Because isokinetic training is performed at a predefined fixed angular velocity, slow motion in a given ROM requires more time than fast motion. For example, in the case of a knee joint exercise, it takes 30 seconds to perform 30 repetitions at a speed of 90°/sec in a 90° range, while it takes 15 seconds to perform 30 repetitions at a speed of 180°/sec in the same angular velocity range.

Velocity Spectrum Exercise

Rehabilitation protocols often use a range of angular velocities called "velocity spectrum exercises". There have been reports of positive results using the velocity spectrum training protocol, but the physiological mechanisms are still unclear. The derivation of positive results is based on differences in muscle fibers and muscle recruitment patterns in skeletal muscle.

In general, human muscle fibers are classified as Type I (slow-twitch muscle fiber, ST) and Type Ⅱ (fat-twitch muscle fibers, FT) with various subcategories. ST fibers have low threshold levels, low conduction velocities, and long contraction times. On the other hand, FT fibers have high conduction velocities, high threshold levels, and short contraction times.[21] The mobilization of these fibers varies according to the given tension. In fact, ST fibers are mobilized ahead of FT fibers because they are mobilized at low threshold levels. Based on these physiological characteristics, low-velocity isokinetic exercises mainly use ST fibers, whereas high-velocity isokinetic exercises mainly use FT fibers. In other words, the maximum force output for isokinetic muscle contraction is the maximum levels of ST and FT fibers that are independently mobilized. However, according to studies, the recruitment patterns of the two fibers are supported simultaneously rather than independently with the velocity of movement. Therefore, in isokinetic training, velocity spectrum exercise can be said to develop both types of muscle fibers.

ROM and Length-Tension Relationship

Isokinetic training should, if possible, consist of the entire ROM to optimize the contraction-coupling process of actin and myosin within the sarcomere. However, if there is a problem with the joint, it is difficult to develop the overall musculoarticular function because the ROM is limited. Therefore, in these cases, it is recommended to perform isokinetic training only within the joint angles where the pain is weak or absent. For example, in an isokinetic knee joint exercise, the force of the patella femur joint is 5.1 times greater than the weight at a given flexion angle (60-80°). On the other hand, when the angle (0-30°) is small, the force is extremely reduced. Therefore, it is necessary to induce isokinetic motion in a narrow range and to exercise in the entire ROM.

In order to establish the isokinetic training protocol with the selection of the ROM, special attention should be paid to the length-tension relationship of the muscle group to which the load is applied. Particularly, it is preferable that such a relation is derived from imitating the activity of the subject during daily life or physical activity in which the action is performed. For example, training in the development of a rotator cuff of a baseball pitcher is more effective at a 90° abducted position, which is similar to the position when pitching. Using another example, muscle training for the quadriceps for a runner that is performed only in the sitting position is difficult to develop the hip strength needed for running. Therefore, training in a prone position or a lying position is more effective.

Submaximal Isokinetic Exercise

The most important advantage of the isokinetic resistance exercise is that the maximum load of the muscle group is within the full ROM of the joint. However, if maximal contraction is not achieved (e.g., an injury to the neuromuscular or skeletal muscle system occurs and the maximum contraction is not possible), the submaximal exercise of the affected side is performed considering the peak torque ratio of the unaffected side.

Overall, the isokinetic training protocol can provide a rehabilitation program for patients who need rehabilitation and a muscle function development program for athletes who need muscle function reinforcement training. However, it is more important to build clinical experience because this part is difficult to understand theoretically. Even if it is a process of accumulating experience, it is important to study [Table 3.19] and continue researching 'program standardization work'.

Table 3.19 ***Recommended protocol for isokinetic exercise***

1. Used for observation of musculoskeletal system 2. Stretching and warm-up before exercise 3. Apply an ideal fixation position similar to the patient's activity pattern and set up the equipment in consideration of the muscle length-tension. 4. Joint adjustment to the motor shaft of the dynamometer 5. Perform submaximal warm-up to know the speed of movement 6. Perform workout at low speed (about 30 seconds) 7. Rest	8. Perform warm-up and workout at medium speed (about 30 seconds) 9. Rest 10. Perform warm-up and workout at high speed (about 30 seconds) 11. Repeat workout at other muscle groups 12. Common stretching and cool-down 13. 20 minutes of ice applied to the affected joint or muscle group

※ Precautions : Isokinetic exercise protocols should include both concentric and eccentric muscle contraction. If the eccentric contraction type is not applicable, an eccentric contraction type should be performed by performing isotonic exercises or free weights.

Effects of Isokinetic Training

Isokinetic training offers many benefits to most patients and athletes, as mentioned in the introduction. However, isokinetic equipment has built-in continuous passive motion (CPM) and isometric and isotropic protocols. In addition, it can be used for muscle contraction training based solely on velocity.

Many previous studies have yielded positive results on the effects of isokinetic training. Particularly, athletes with musculoarticular injuries have been reported to improve peak torque, workload, and power when performing maximal afferent isokinetic training for weeks or months.[13,27,42] One study showed that an 8-week rehabilitation exercise for rugby athletes who incurred grade Ⅱ injuries in posterior cruciate ligaments resulted in improved pain perception on the injured knee every week after rehabilitation exercise.[28] At the end of the study, the maximal ROM was reduced by up to 68%, and the ROM of the joints was improved by 20% compared with that before treatment. Particularly, the peak torque of the quadriceps muscles and the peak torque per body weight were increased by 86% and 85%, respectively, and the peak torque of the hamstring and peak torque per body weight were increased by 74% and 76%, respectively. In addition to the peak torque, the improvement in knee ankle function was also found to be very favorable for average power, total work, and acceleration time. In addition, a study comparing the lower extremities of the patients and normal people reported that there was a significant difference in the pre-training quadriceps muscles. However, after the training, the function of the knee joint was highly developed and it was able to overcome the posterior instability of the knee joint.[6,56] Moreover, the results of a isokinetic muscle strength test, electromyogram, and gait analysis of professional soccer players with chronic posterior cruciate ligament defects in the right knee showed that when the right quadriceps muscles were rehabilitated, walking speed was much faster on the left side and symptoms disappeared.[10] In addition to studies on the knee, positive results have been reported in patients with injuries to the shoulder due to excessive use and in patients with injuries to the ankle joints such as soccer players, dancers, and marathon runners.[1,20,60,61]

Interestingly, however, there are studies that increased muscle strength by isokinetic training does not cause changes in muscle cross-sectional areas or hypertrophy[42], but actually improves muscle function due to increased anaerobic metabolic ability, increased enzyme of the TCA-cycle, and improved ability to mobilize exercise units.[13] In other words, isokinetic training only results in the enzymatic or neurological development of muscle cells. According to some researchers, isokinetic training does not cause hypertrophy for a number of reasons, among which the lack of 'eccentric muscle contraction’ is the most prominent.[50,55] However, other researchers have suggested that isokinetic training can cause hypertrophy, making it impossible to come to a definitive conclusion. Therefore, it is necessary to observe statistical differences between the group with and without eccentric muscle contraction in the future and to observe changes in muscle cross-sectional areas and hypertrophy from isokinetic training.

Interpretation and Evaluation of Isokinetic Testing

The purposes of interpreting and evaluating isokinetic tests are as follows. First, it can predict the degree of injury in a healthy person. Second, it makes it possible to observe patients who have already incurred injuries due to the damage of muscle joints. Third, it provides the necessary preparation for returning to daily life or athletic activity after the exercise program. In order to achieve this process, it is necessary to carefully analyze the ability of the subject to exhibit torque, workload, and power, depending on the instrumental capability of the isokinetic equipment. The details of this are as follows.

Torque

Once muscles contract, they generate force. If this force is measured at the rotation axis of the joint, the moment of force is expressed as torque. The method of measuring the tension generated by the muscles from the rotation axis of an isokinetic dynamometer is to measure these torques. In other words, force is measured by the muscle's ability to generate tension from the resistance pads of a dynamometer, and torque is calculated by the distance from the rotation axis of the joint to the resistance pad. If the forces and torques generated by these muscles can be measured with the full ROM, the measurements may be presented as peak torque or average torque. In other words, peak torque refers to the force generated at the point where the strongest torque is generated in the ROM of the joint during testing, and the average torque refers to the tension generated over the full ROM of joints measured. Therefore, the average torque needs to be standardized for the ROM when comparing before or after both muscle groups. On the other hand, since peak torque occurs in the middle of the measured ROM, standardization is not necessarily required.

Specifically, peak torque is obtained at the highest point of one of the torque curves shown in several isokinetic tests, but the average torque is obtained from the complete waveform of one or several successive isokinetic curves. The advantage of calculating the average torque is that it can prevent the 'artifact' phenomenon that occurs when decelerating the force of the arms or legs involved in the test. Therefore, for accurate examination, it is necessary to confirm whether the ROM between the affected side and the unaffected side is constant. During the rehabilitation program, it is very important to continuously evaluate the ROM and the muscle function of the affected side, especially the average torque value. However, the correlation between peak torque and average torque for torque and force is very high, so both variables reflect the performance of a given muscle group.

Ultimately, peak torque or average torque is a frequent parameter used to assess the ability of the human body to perform an ankle function. However, the shared area of the microprocessor in the isokinetic dynamometer provides an 'angle-specific torque (AST)' that allows the torque to be determined at some point across the ROM [Fig. 3.38].

Work and Power

The isokinetic dynamometer quantifies the force and torque quickly and accurately. If the force and distance of a given muscle contraction are known, the amount of tension produced in the muscle can be obtained. This is called total work. On the other hand, if the amount of time required to calculate work is known, power can also be calculated. Previous studies have shown that the predicted levels of work and power from peak torque produce good results in healthy muscle joints or joints with lesions.[32,34-36,45] In particular, as shown in [Fig. 3.39], the first picture on the left is the uninjured side and the second picture is the injured side. In the case of duplication, it presents another goal of the rehabilitation program because it shows a work deficit as shown in the third figure.

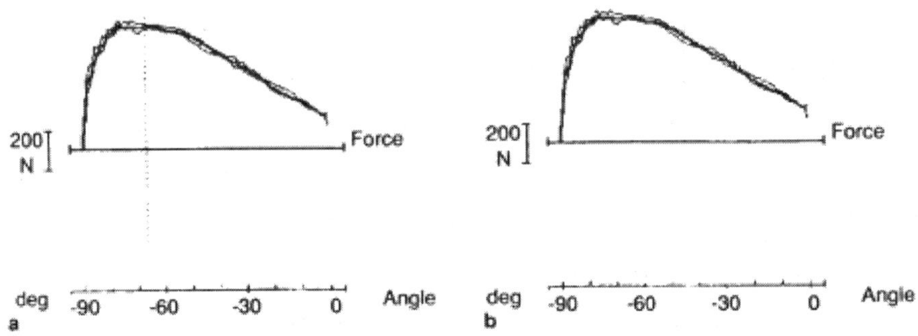

Fig. 3.38 ***Angle-Specific Torque; AST***

A is **a** figure showing a torque value at 60 °, and **b** is a figure showing no specific angle. That is, **a** figure helps to rehabilitate at a certain angle.

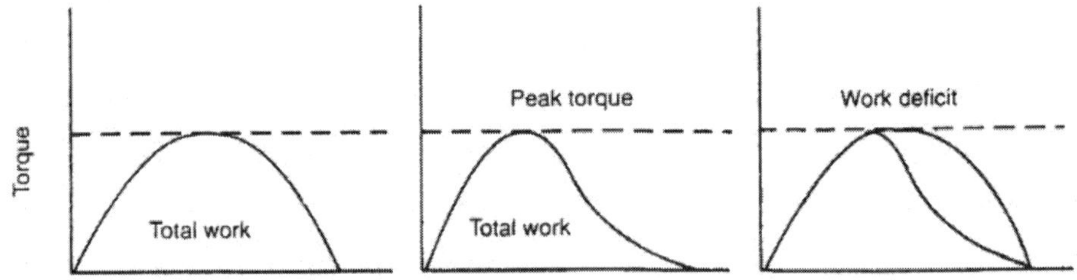

Fig. 3.39 ***Comparison of Total Work***

Endurance Measurement

Endurance refers to the muscle's ability to generate force over a series of isokinetic contractions. In order to measure endurance using isokinetic equipment, the isokinetic dynamometer can calculate the amount of work, so the total work generated from isokinetic contraction represents the endurance ability of the measured muscle groups. It is reported that the work and total work performed during the last 5 of 25 repetitions are as meaningful as measuring the peak torque and estimate the improvement of the endurance ability.[31]

Concentric and Eccentric Contractions

The ability of the muscles to generate tension over part or all of a joint is called 'dynamic contraction'. Muscles produce dynamic tension through two methods: shortening or lengthening. For example, when the direction of movement of the joint is opposite to the direction of gravity and when the muscle tension exceeds the external resistance, the muscle contraction soon becomes a concentric contraction in the form of shortening. On the other hand, if the movement of the joint is in the direction of gravity and the external resistance exceeds the force of the muscle, the muscle contraction soon becomes an eccentric contraction in the form of lengthening. These two types of muscle contractions have long been used in isotonic exercises that are commonly seen today.

In the past, isokinetic equipment was able to only measure concentric contractions. However, since the development of the 'active dynamometer' in the past decade, it has become possible to measure eccentric contractions. In fact, in order to accurately evaluate and interpret isokinetic exercise capacity, it is necessary to understand the relationship between force and velocity in concentric and eccentric contractions. Specifically, concentric muscle contractions are largest when the isokinetic velocity is low and decreases linearly when the test velocity is increased. In other words, the concentric peak torque decreases as the isokinetic test velocity increases from 60 °/sec to 240 °/sec. This phenomenon helps to correctly interpret the relationship between normal muscle groups and interacting muscle groups.

On the other hand, the force-velocity curve formed during eccentric motion is very different from the curve during concentric contraction. In other words, concentric muscle contraction decreases as the test speed increases, whereas eccentric muscle contraction increases as the speed increases. This inconsistency between concentric and eccentric muscular contractions can be explained by the differences in the binding capacity of actin and myosin and the mechanism of neuromuscular inhibition in the Golgi tendon organs, including the muscle spindle in terms of physiological mechanisms.[51,57] In other words, as the angular velocity increases, the torque curve of eccentric muscle contractions, total work, and power are higher than that of concentric contractions because the inhibitory mechanism of the nervous system, which prevents bodily injury, is mobilized.

Normal Torque Curve and Abnormal Torque Curve

The isokinetic equipment creates an analog signal through the dynamometer and displays the activity of the muscle generated by a specific repetitive motion as a curve or a numerical value. Isokinetic resistance adjusts the amount of force generated by a given muscle group. Analyses of the 'muscle length-tension relationship' and 'muscle contraction efficiency' of isokinetic exercises showed the highest torque in the middle area of the full ROM, and lower levels of torque toward the beginning and end [Fig. 3.40]. In other words, the torque curve reflects a change in ability to generate force when one muscle contracts within the ROM.

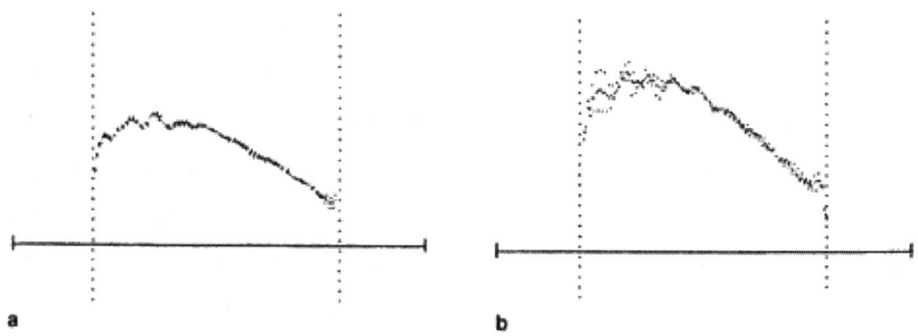

Fig. 3.40 *Concentric(a)/ Eccentric(b) Torque Curve*

Figure b shows the eccentric contraction's curve at 90°/sec at full load. That is, the curve does not start from the baseline.

Some equipment uses a "preload force" to avoid collision of the load in isokinetic testing and to minimize the impact of deceleration. The concept of preload force refers to the amount of pre-set force before the isokinetic contraction begins. The torque curve obtained from the isokinetic test using the preload force [Fig. 3.40b] shows a slight difference compared to the other curve in [Fig. 3.40a].

In fact, the normal, smooth and harmonic isokinetic torque curve has many factors, but among them, it is most important that there is no pain or injury in the muscle group or joint to be examined. The isokinetic dynamometer necessarily reduces the load when the patient is unable to exert strength. It also suggests that pain has been induced. However, pain from muscle-tendon units within the joint that intersects a single muscle group may be accepted as a result of artifacts on the torque curve. However, this flaw can be identified through clinical experience and patient symptoms. For example, as shown in [Fig. 3.36], the isokinetic test results of patients with anterior cruciate ligament injury show two peak torque curves. The mechanism of the first peak torque curve is related to the anterior translation that occurs in the proximal tibia when the quadriceps muscle begins to contract. In the mid-dented area, the temporary reduction in power output is due to pain or dislocation while the second small peak torque curve can be interpreted to potentially overcome the anterior translation of the tibia by other soft tissue structures of the knee. Some clinicians state that it is possible to identify abnormalities in several other joints or muscles through the torque curve obtained from isokinetic testing, especially chondromalacia patella, patella subluxation, and even knee plica syndrome.[29] However, the scientific evidence for this is somewhat lacking, so more research is needed in the future. Regardless, it is important to understand the torque curve formed by the output of muscle torque, work, and power.

Torque Value in Terms of Body Weight

Many studies have reported on the normal absolute muscle values of several muscle groups in athletes from various sports, as well as sedentary people. This information provides the basis for an appropriate peak torque level. However, since the difference in peak torque with respect to body weight is very large, it is necessary to calculate a relative value based on weight. In addition, it is also important to consider the physique, gender, and age of all subjects.[58]

The effect of body weight on the results of the isokinetic test can be easily seen by comparing men and women. The absolute value of peak torque, not considering body weight, is very different between male and female. However, when considering body weight, the difference is not significant. Rather, it can be seen that women have a higher peak torque than men. On the other hand, the relative value of the peak torque by body weight is further reduced between men and women when lean body mass is applied. In other words, if only the absolute value is taken into consideration, the range of error can become larger. Therefore, it is important to calculate the absolute value in order to minimize the difference, but it is also very important to evaluate the relative value in consideration of lean body mass and weight.

Table 3.20 ***Myofunction range of bilateral limbs***

Ratio	Evaluation
± 10% ↓	**Normal**
± 10~20%	**Abnormal possible**
± 20% ↑	**Abnormal**

Ratio of Bilateral Muscle Groups

Comparing and evaluating the bilateral muscle groups of the limbs offers several advantages over evaluating only the muscle group of the unilateral limb. However, for accurate evaluation, test protocols for the right and left sides should be consistent in all situations. In particular, when the ROM of the injured side limb is limited during isokinetic testing, the ROM of the uninjured side must be identified with the injured side so that it does not cause confusion when comparing the average torque or when evaluating the total work.[17] The difference ratio formula for the muscle groups of the bilateral limbs after the completion of the calibration process is as follows.

{(Left - Right) / Right × 100} or {(Right - Left) / Left × 100}

However, patients with muscle-joint injuries generally have a reduced ROM, so that increasing the deficit on the injured side compared to the normal ROM on the other side constitutes a goal of rehabilitation exercise therapy. For example, if the ROM identified on the injured side limb of an ACL injured patient is 90°, the ROM for returning to the normal range (135°) is 45°. It is very important to compare the muscle function of the bilateral limbs. To date, most researchers have the same context in determining 'normal' if the torque range of both limbs is within 10-15%. Specifically, [Table 3.20] shows the range of torque of both limbs.[33] In other words, if the muscle function range of both limbs is less than 10%, it is considered 'normal'. If the range is between 10-20%, it is considered 'abnormal', and when the difference is more than 20%, it is reported as 'abnormal'.

As shown in [Table 3.21], the interpretation should be applied to the general people who do not specialize in sports or athletes who use their limbs in a balanced way. On the other hand, athletes using disproportionate use of both limbs (e.g., tennis players and javelin throwers), are 15% higher in the muscle function of major muscle groups than the other muscle groups. Therefore, in order to calculate the accurate bilateral strength ratio of each athlete, the isokinetic evaluation of many athletes should be given priority.[58]

Table 3.21 ***Knee ipsilateral flexion (F) / extension (E) ratio***

	Authors (year) / Subjects	Gender	Age (yr)	Dominant F/E ratio	Non-dominant F/E ratio
60°/sec	Berg et al. (1985)/ College basketball player	Women	20	63%	67%
	Appen and Duncan (1986)/ College Athletes	Men	18~21	54%	-
90°/sec	Stafford and Grana (1984)/College football player	Men	20	67%	68%
	Chmelar et al. (1988)/ Ballet / Modern Dancer	Women	25	67%	-
120°/sec	Berg et al. (1985)/ College basketball player	Women	20	67%	71%
	Bumie (1987)/ Early childhood gymanst	Women	11	67%	71%
150°/sec	Colliander and Tesch (1989)/ Physically active general	Women Men	27 27	70% 69%	-
180°/sec	Stafford and Grana (1984)/ College football player	Men	20	73%	75%
	Kannus (1988c)/ Patients with chronic ACL failure	Women/ Men	35	78% (uninjured)	88% (injured)
240°/sec	Berg et al. (1985)/ College basketball player	Women	20	76%	79%
	Chmelar et al. (1988)/ Ballet / Modern Dancer	Women	25	90%	-
300°/sec	Stafford and Grana (1984)/ College football player	Men	20	82%	85%
	Appen and Duncan (1986)/ College Athletes	Men	18~21	84%	-

Table 3.22 ***Ankle ipsilateral dorsiflexion (DF) / plantarflexion (PF) and eversion (EV) / inversion (IV) ratios***

	Authors (year) / Subjects	Gender	Age (yr)	Dominant DF/PF ratio	Non-dominant DF/PF ratio
30°/sec				39%	37%
60°/sec				44%	43%
90°/sec	Berg et al. (1985)/ College basketball players	Women	20	49%	46%
120°/sec				54%	54%
150°/sec				60%	59%
Authors (year) / Subjects		**Gender**	**Age (yr)**	**Dominant EV/IV ratio**	**Non-dominant EV/IV ratio**
30°/sec				87%	-
60°/sec	Wong et al. (1984)/ General people	Men	29	90%	-
120°/sec				86%	54%

Table 3.23 ***Trunk flexion (F) / extension (E) ratio***

	Authors (year) / Subjects	Gender	Age (yr)	Trunk F/E ratio
30°/sec	Davies and Gould (1982)/Athletes	Men	21	80%
		Women	20	80%
	Thompson et al. (1985)/The general public	Men	43	93%
		Women	38	97%
60°/sec	Davies and Gould (1982)/Athletes	Men	21	91%
		Women	20	88%
	Thompson et al. (1985)/The general public	Men	43	97%
		Women	38	102%
90°/sec	Davies and Gould (1982)/Athletes	Men	21	99%
		Women	20	98%
	Thompson et al. (1985)/The general public	Men	43	102%
		Women	38	106%
120°/sec	Davies and Gould (1982)/Athletes	Men	21	110%
		Women	20	110%
	Thompson et al. (1985)/The general public	Men	43	105%
		Women	38	105%

Table 3.24 ***Hip ipsilateral flexion (F) / extension (E) and abduction (AB) / adduction (AD) ratios***

	Authors (year) / Subjects	Gender	Age (yr)	Dominant F/E ratio	Non-dominant F/E ratio
30°/sec	Smith et al. (1981)/ Ice hockey player	Men	24	64%	-
180°/sec				59%	-
	Authors (year) / Subjects	**Gender**	**Age (yr)**	**Dominant AB/AD rato**	**Non-dominant AB/AD rato**
30°/sec	Poulmedis (1985)/ Elite soccer player	Men	26	74%	-
60°/sec	Donatelli et al.(1991)/ General public	Women	26	41%	-
		Men	26	48%	

Table 3.25 ***Elbow ipsilateral flexion (F) / extension (E) ratio***

	Authors (year) / Subjects	Gender	Age (ys)	Dominant F/E ratio	Non-dominant F/E ratio
60°/sec	Berg et al. (1985)/ College basketball player	Women	20	90%	86%
180°/sec				104%	92%
240°/sec				104%	90%

Table 3.26 ***Shoulder ipsilateral abduction (AB) / adduction (AD) ratio***

	Authors (year) / Subjects	Gender	Age (ys)	Dominant AB/AD ratio	Non-dominant AB/AD ratio
60°/sec	Connelly Maddux et al. (1989)/ General public	Men	34	66%	65%
		Women	27	61%	66%
90°/sec	Alderink and Kuck (1986)/ Baseball pitcher	Men	18	54%	57%
120°/sec	Alderink and Kuck (1986)/ Baseball pitcher	Men	18	54%	57%
180°/sec	Connelly Maddux et al. (1989)/ General public	Men	34	49%	56%
		Women	27	74%	82%
300°/sec	Alderink and Kuck (1986)/ Baseball pitcher	Men	18	51%	50%

Table 3.27 ***Shoulder ipsilateral external rotation (ER) / internal rotation (IR) ratio***

	Authors (year) / Subjects	Gender	Age (ys)	Dominant ER/IR ratio	Non-dominant ER/IR ratio
60°/sec	Connelly MAddux et al. (1989)/ Normal (90° abduction posture)	Men	34	63%	62%
		Women	26	70%	71%
90°/sec	Alderink and Kuck (1986)/ High school/ college student	Men	18	66%	70%
120°/sec	Alderink and Kuck (1986)/ High school/ college student	Men	18	68%	72%
180°/sec	Cook et al. (1987)/ College baseball pitcher, same age non-exerciser	Men	18~25	70%	81%
		Men	18~25	83%	78%
300°/sec	Cook et al. (1987)/ College baseball pitcher, same age non-exerciser	Men	18~25	70%	81%
		Men	18~25	87%	79%

Table 3.28 ***Shoulder ipsilateral flexion (F) / extension (E) ratio***

	Authors (year) / Subjects	Gender	Age (ys)	Dominant F/E ratio	Non-dominant F/E ratio
60°/sec	Berg et al. (1985)/ Basketball players	Women	18~22	77%	81%
90°/sec	Alderink and Kuck (1986)/ Baseball players	Men	18	52%	55%
120°/sec	Berg et al. (1985)/ Basketball players	Women	18~22	80%	79%
180°/sec	Cook et al. (1987)/ Baseball players	Men	18~25	74%	81%
300°/sec	Cook et al. (1987)/ Baseball players	Men	18~25	70%	71%

Ratio of Ipsilateral Muscle Groups

The muscles of the trunk and limb joints work simultaneously and interactively to produce a smooth, identical motion. The agonist is responsible for the movement of the joint desired by the muscle group, and the antagonist is responsible for the opposite joint activity.[48-50,58] For example, the quadriceps muscle group is an agonist and the hamstring acts as an antagonist during knee extensions. Conversely, when knee flexion occurs, the hamstring acts as the agonist and the quadriceps muscles act as the antagonist. Therefore, the ratio of the ipsilateral muscle group calculated by the formula is as follows.

{Antagonist / Agonist × 100}

On the other hand, it is important for the instructor to understand the properties of the agonist and the antagonist regarding a joint and pursue a balanced development. This is because injuries can easily occur in a region with excessive imbalances in the ratio of the ipsilateral muscle group.[25,44] It is reported that when the ipsilateral flexion/extension ratio is less than 50%, that is, when the hamstring muscle function is less than ½ of the quadriceps muscles, an injury may occur.[40] Likewise, if the ipsilateral flexion/extension ratio of the knee joint is less than 75%, injuries to the knee joint may occur.[19]

However, the ipsilateral flexion/extension ratio of the knee reported above is somewhat different from the results of studies performed by different researchers. In addition, the ratios in other joints, other than the knee joint, are different. Furthermore, there are differences in the isokinetic angular velocity of athletes. Therefore, it is recommended to consider each of the joints with reference to [Table 3.21] and [Table 3.28].

Returning to the Field

The performance of muscle function is limited by several factors. In particular, muscle-tendon injuries such as strain, tearing, and tendinitis further limit the muscle's ability to generate forces. In addition, immobilization due to injuries of the joints or surrounding muscles may result in joint laxity and atrophy of the muscles leading to inadequate transfer from the nervous system to the muscles. Isokinetic training is used as an appropriate rehabilitation tool for the damage of these neuromuscular joint systems and is useful for determining when to safely return to daily activity.[58]

In particular, the level of isokinetic test results is a very important item in evaluating the injured side (ipsilateral flexion/extension ratio) with the goal of rehabilitating musculoskeletal injuries (achieving more than 90% of uninjured side limbs). In addition, flexibility, proprioceptive state, functional ability, and psychological status are secondary to returning to daily life.[59,60]

Physical Fitness Test

To prescribe exercise according to the individual's health condition and physical fitness, muscular strength factors (grip, back, and leg strength), respiratory circulatory ability (cardiopulmonary endurance), and the nervous system function (balance, agility, flexibility, and coordination should be measured. The factors of physical fitness can be divided into health-related and skill-related fitness factors as shown below.

Health-related Components of Physical Fitness	Skill-related Components of Physical Fitness
Flexibility	Power
Cardiorespiratory endurance	Speed
Muscular strength	Agility
Muscular endurance	Balance
Body composition	Coordination

Test Method and Evaluation of Flexibility

The "distance method" measures by length, the "angle method" measures by angle, and "exponential method" which measures by ratio. Generally, the distance method is easy to measure and is widely used. The distance method includes the 'sit & reach flexion test' and the 'back extension test' method, but the former is used for safety.

Sit & Reach Flexion Test Method

A sit and reach box with a ruler that measures 25 ㎝ up and 40 ㎝ down is used. First, a subject get both talus bones together and attach the feet to the examination table with both legs about 5 ㎝ apart. After taking a deep breath, breathe out and bend forward to position the fingertips as far as possible [Fig. 3.41].

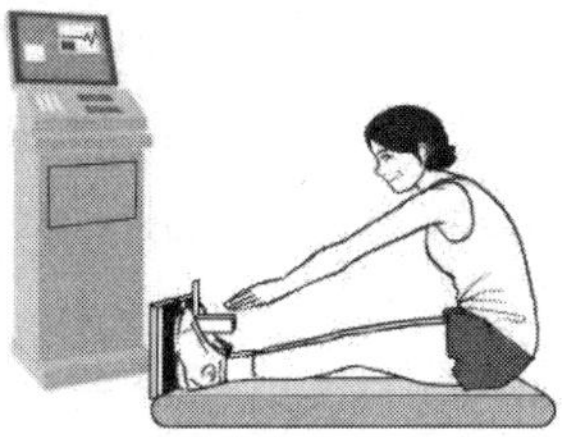

※ Test Tips and Precautions

- Gather both fingertips and put feet on the measuring instrument.
- When you bend your body, do not give back reaction.
- Try to put your head between your arms when you bend your torso forward.
- Do not bend your knees and let the meter slide with both hands while breathing out.
- The bending posture is stopped by stopping for about 2 seconds.
- Record the highest value after two measurements [Table 3.29].

Fig. 3.41 Sit-and-Reach Test

Table 3.29 ***Sit-and-Reach Evaluation***

Unit : cm

	Percentile	Age(years)									
		20~29		30~39		40~49		50~59		60~69	
		Men	Women	Men	Women	Men	Women	Men	Women	Men	Women
Very good	90	42	43	40	42	37	40	38	40	35	37
Good	80	38	40	37	39	34	37	32	37	30	34
	70	36	38	34	37	30	35	29	35	26	31
Average	60	33	36	32	35	28	33	27	32	24	30
	50	31	34	29	33	25	31	25	30	22	28
	40	29	32	27	31	23	29	22	29	18	26
Low	30	26	29	24	28	20	26	18	26	16	24
	20	23	26	21	25	16	24	15	23	14	23
Very low	10	18	22	17	21	12	19	12	19	11	18

※ If the reference of the measurement unit is set to 26 cm, then the point is zero, and if it is set to 23 cm, the point is zero. That is, if a 20-year-old man records 40 cm, the actual length extended from the toe is 14 cm.

Cardiopulmonary Endurance Test Method and Evaluation

Cardiopulmonary endurance is best measured in the clinic through GXT. The evaluation variable generally uses the $\dot{V}O_2max$ [Table 3.30]. In general, the $\dot{V}O_2max$ is determined by the amount of oxygen ingested per body weight (mℓ/kg/min). The GXT for measuring the $\dot{V}O_2max$ is done with a treadmill, but a cycle ergometer is used for patients who are uncomfortable with walking, and an arm ergometer is used for patients with paraplegia. In addition to the $\dot{V}O_2max$ obtained in the laboratory, cardiorespiratory

Table 3.30 ***Maximum Oxygen Uptake Evaluation***

Unit : ml/kg/min

	Percentile	Age(years)									
		20~29		30~39		40~49		50~59		60 or more	
		Men	Women	Men	Women	Men	Women	Men	Women	Men	Women
Very good	90	51.4	44.2	50.4	41.0	48.2	39.5	45.3	35.2	42.5	35.2
Good	80	48.2	41.0	46.8	38.6	44.1	36.3	41.0	32.3	38.1	31.2
	70	46.8	38.1	44.6	36.7	41.8	33.8	38.5	30.9	35.3	29.4
Average	60	44.2	36.7	42.4	34.6	39.9	32.3	36.7	29.4	33.6	27.2
	50	42.5	35.2	41.0	33.8	38.1	30.9	35.2	28.2	31.8	25.8
	40	41.0	33.8	38.9	32.3	36.7	29.5	33.8	26.9	30.2	24.5
Low	30	39.5	32.3	37.4	30.5	35.1	28.3	32.3	25.5	28.7	23.8
	20	37.1	30.6	35.4	28.7	33.0	26.5	30.2	24.3	26.5	22.8
Very low	10	34.5	28.4	32.5	26.5	30.9	25.1	28.0	22.3	23.1	20.8

※ Regardless of age and gender, if the maximum oxygen uptake is below 20, the mortality rate from CAD increases rapidly(Blair et al., 1989).

endurance can be assessed by time and distance which are measurable on a track. The advantage of the former test is that it can be analyzed accurately, but the disadvantages include the fact that it is time-consuming, expensive, and lacking experts. On the other hand, the advantage of the latter is that it can be carried out collectively so that it takes less time and costs less. The disadvantage is that seasonal and environmental impacts can lead to inaccurate data. Therefore, this section presents cardiovascular endurance as the $\dot{V}O_2max$ obtained in the laboratory [Appendix B].

Muscle Strength Measurement and Evaluation

Measurement of muscle strength includes measurement of static strength and measurement of dynamic strength. Static muscle strength measures the subject's maximum isometric strength, including grip strength, back strength [Fig. 3.42], and leg strength [Fig. 3.43]. On the other hand, dynamic muscle strength measures the subject's maximum isotonic muscle strength, using bench press and leg press.

Measurement of Static Strength

The method of measuring static strength is as follows. The evaluation grade can be evaluated by separately classifying grip strength, back strength, and leg strength as shown in [Table 3.31]. The total score is the absolute static strength, and the absolute value divided by body weight is the relative static strength.

Grip Strength Test Method

A smedley-type dynamometer is used to measure the maximum strength of the upper limb by the coordination of the four fingers and the thumb. Muscles related to grip strength are the flexor digitorum and flexor carpi, which measure the static strength of the forearm.

Back Strength Test Method

The back muscles of the upper, lower and lumbar muscles are measured while holding the hand grips attached to the back dynamometer with both hands and stretching the back [Fig. 3.42, Table 3.31].

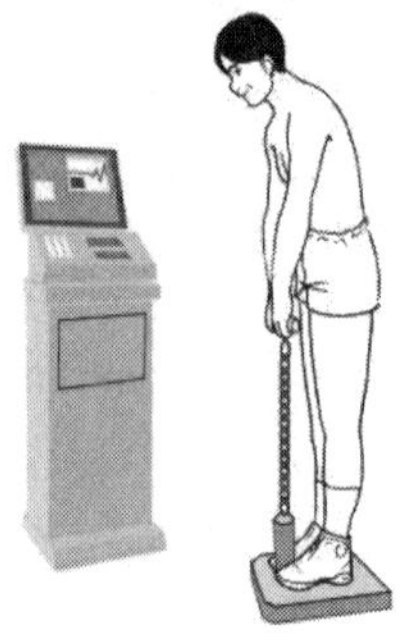

※ Test Tips and Precautions

- Adjust the length of the handle so that the upper body is bent by 30° on the back muscle strength tester.
- Be sure to hold the handle with a pronated grip.
- Practice rehearsal lightly.
- Keep the torso straight and slowly pull up the handle so that it will give you maximum strength in about 10 seconds.
- Take a rest for 1 min, then perform this test and record the highest value.
- Be careful not to bend your arms or knees, or to move your body to the back.

Fig. 3.42 Back muscle strength test

Table 3.31 Static strength evaluation by leg press

Unit : kg

	Evaluation grade †	Left grip	Right grip	Back strength	Leg strength	Total score: Absolute value	Total score: Relative value ‡
Men	Very good	≥68	≥70	≥209	≥241	≥587	≥7.50
	Good	56~67	62~69	177~208	214~240	508~586	7.10~7.49
	Average	43~55	48~61	126~176	160~213	375~507	5.21~7.09
	Low	39~42	41~47	91~125	137~159	307~374	4.81~5.20
	Very low	≤38	≤40	≤90	≤136	≤306	≤4.80
Women	Very good	≥37	≥41	≥111	≥136	≥324	≥5.50
	Good	34~36	38~40	98~110	114~135	282~323	4.80~5.49
	Average	22~33	25~37	52~97	66~113	164~281	2.90~4.79
	Low	18~21	22~24	39~51	49~65	117~163	2.10~2.89
	Very low	≤17	≤21	≤38	≤48	≤116	≤2.09

†: Evaluation grade adjustment: For subjects older than 50, score 10% lower.

‡: Relative value refers to the absolute value converted into body weight.

Leg Strength Test Method

The leg dynamometer can be used in combination with the back dynamometer. It is the difference from the back strength test that the muscles of the lower leg are measured while holding the attached handle with both hands and spreading the legs.

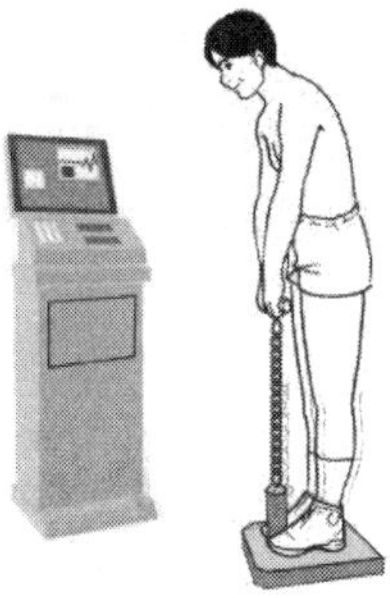

※ ***Test Tips and Precautions***

- Adjust the length of the knob so that the knee will bend about 130-140 degrees on the platform.
- Be sure to hold the handle with a pronated grip.
- Do not use lumbar muscle strength.
- Practice the rehearsal twice to pull up the handle with only leg strength.
- Slowly pull up the handle to give the maximum power in 10 seconds.
- Take a rest for 1 minute, then perform this test and record the highest value.

Fig. 3.43 Leg strength test

Measurement of Dynamic Strength

The method of measuring dynamic muscle strength is as follows. The evaluation grade is shown in [Table 3.32] for bench press and [Table 3.33] for leg press.[18] The dynamic muscle strength can be evaluated by measuring the 1RM that can be lifted or pushed to its maximum.

Bench Press Measurement

In the past, the bench press in which the subject lied down was mainly used. Currently, it is recommended to perform the bench press in a sitting position for stability. The bench press measures dynamic muscle strength of related muscle groups, including the pectoralis [Fig. 3.44].

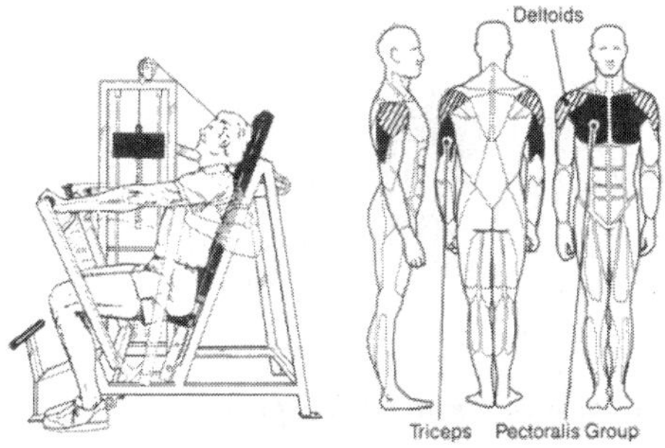

Fig. 3.10 Dynamic strength measurement by bench press

※ ***Test Tips and Precautions***

- Adjust the height of the saddle so that the knob height of the bench press is on your chest.
- When pushing the handle, check that the height of the elbow is pushed from the chest line.
- Perform a light warm-up 5 to 10 reps at a weight corresponding to 40-60% of the maximum predicted value before 1RM measurement.
- After 1 minute of rest, lightly stretch and lift 3-5 reps for 60-80% of the maximum predicted value.
- When the load increases to some extent, it takes about 2-3 minutes of rest in the middle.
- Repeat until you have lifted up to 1 reps, increasing the weight on the bench by 5 to 10 pounds (lbs).
- Once 1RM is determined, the weight is divided by its pound weight and converted.
- The evaluation by bench press is shown in [Table 3.32].

Table 3.32 ***Dynamic strength evaluation by bench press***

		Age (years)				
		20~29	30~39	40~49	50~59	60 or more
Men	Very good	≥1.26	≥1.08	≥0.97	≥0.86	≥0.78
	Good	1.17~1.25	1.01~1.07	0.91~0.96	0.81~0.85	0.74~0.77
	Average	0.97~1.16	0.86~1.00	0.78~0.90	0.70~0.80	0.64~0.73
	Low	0.88~0.96	0.79~0.85	0.72~0.77	0.65~0.69	0.60~0.63
	Very low	≤0.87	≤0.78	≤0.71	≤0.64	≤0.59
Women	Very good	≥0.78	≥0.66	≥0.61	≥0.54	≥0.55
	Good	0.72~0.77	0.62~0.65	0.57~0.60	0.51~0.53	0.51~0.54
	Average	0.59~0.71	0.53~0.61	0.48~0.56	0.43~0.50	0.41~0.50
	Low	0.53~0.58	0.49~0.52	0.44~0.47	0.40~0.42	0.37~0.40
	Very low	≤0.52	≤0.48	≤0.43	≤0.39	≤0.36

※ If a 35-year-old man with 70 kg raised the bench press by 200 lbs, this person's dynamic strength corresponds to "very good" because {(70 kg × 2.2) = 154 lbs} → {(200 lbs ÷ 154 lbs) = 1.29}.

Leg Press Measurement

In the past, leg presses used a squat motion to lift the weight on the shoulders. In recent years, the semi-seated type is recommended in which the subject sits in a reclined position and performs the leg press. The leg press is a measure of the dynamic strength of a group of related muscles, including the gluteals [Fig. 3.45].

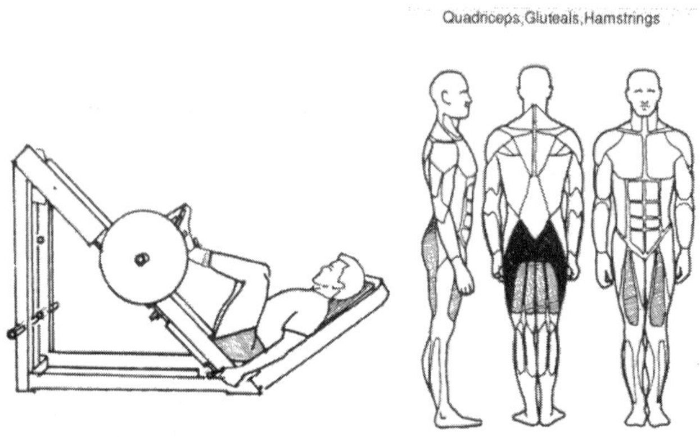

Fig. 3.45 ***Dynamic strength measurement by leg press***

※ Test Tips and Precautions

- Adjust the height of the bar so that the angle of the knee is bent 90 to 110 degrees.
- When pushing the bar, make sure that the knee does not move outward or inward.
- 1RM measurement is performed by the same method as bench press.
- Evaluation by leg press is shown in [Table 3.33].

Table 3.33 ***Dynamic strength evaluation by leg press***

		Age (years)				
		20~29	30~39	40~49	50~59	60 or more
Men	Very good	≥2.08	≥1.88	≥1.76	≥1.66	≥1.56
	Good	2.00~2.07	1.80~1.87	1.70~1.75	1.60~1.65	1.50~1.55
	Average	1.83~1.99	1.63~1.79	1.56~1.69	1.46~1.59	1.37~1.49
	Low	1.65~1.82	1.55~1.62	1.50~1.55	1.40~1.45	1.31~1.36
	Very low	≤1.64	≤1.54	≤1.49	≤1.39	≤1.30
Women	Very good	≥1.63	≥1.42	≥1.32	≥1.26	≥1.15
	Good	1.54~1.62	1.35~1.41	1.26~1.31	1.13~1.25	1.08~1.14
	Average	1.35~1.53	1.20~1.34	1.12~1.25	0.99~1.12	0.92~1.07
	Low	1.26~1.34	1.13~1.19	1.06~1.11	0.86~0.98	0.85~0.91
	Very low	≤1.25	≤1.12	≤1.05	≤0.85	≤0.84

Muscle Endurance Measurement and Evaluation

In the measurement and evaluation of muscle endurance, there are field type tests such as pull-ups, dips, and sit-ups using their own weight, and dynamic muscle endurance tests which use seven kinds of instruments. Dynamic muscle endurance tests measure muscle endurance using barbells, dumbbells, weights, and other training devices as a load without complicated measuring devices.

Field Type Tests

Field tests that can be used for endurance testing include pull-ups, flexed-arm-hang, curl-ups, and push-ups. However, this chapter describes sit-ups and push-ups that can be performed indoors.

Curl-Ups

Curl-ups measure the endurance of the abdominal muscles as shown in [Fig. 3.46]. Although there is a lack of scientific data to date, it is believed that weak endurance of abdominal muscles may cause lower back pain.[26]

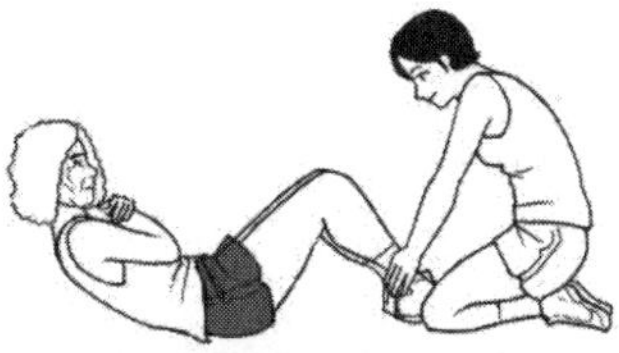

Fig. 3.46 ***Curl-Ups***

※ *Test Tips and Precautions*

- Lie on the mat with your feet spread about 30 ㎝ wide.
- The assistant can hold his ankle with both arms, or mount the foot where it can be fixed.
- The knees bend at an angle of 90°, and both hands cross at the chest.
- Bend your upper body forward with the start signal and let your elbow touch your knee.
- The moment when both elbows touch the knee and the back touches the floor is regarded as one time.
- Record the total repetitions for 1 minute [Table 3.34].

Table 3.34 ***Evaluation of curl-ups***

Unit : reps

	Percentile	Age (years)									
		20~29		30~39		40~49		50~59		60~69	
		Men	Women	Men	Women	Men	Women	Men	Women	Men	Women
Very good	90	75	70	75	55	75	50	74	48	53	50
Good	80	56	45	69	43	75	42	60	30	33	30
	70	41	37	46	34	67	33	45	23	26	24
Average	60	31	32	36	28	51	28	35	16	19	19
	50	27	27	31	21	39	25	27	9	16	13
	40	24	21	26	15	31	20	23	2	9	9
Low	30	20	17	19	12	26	14	19	0	6	3
	20	13	12	13	0	21	5	13	0	0	0
Very low	10	4	5	0	0	13	0	0	0	0	0

※ If abdominal muscle strength is weak, it is likely to cause back pain (LBP) (Jackson et al., 1998).

Push-Ups

Push-ups are suitable for men, as shown in [Fig. 3.47a, b], where a large force is required of the upper body. However, this can be modified for women by bending the knees.

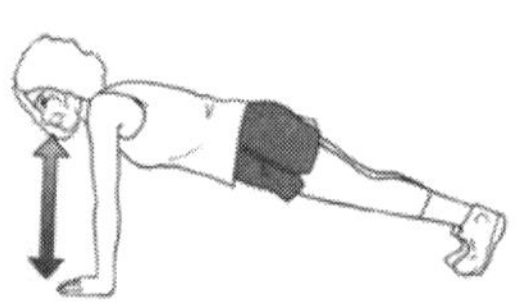

Fig. 3.47a ***Men's Push-Ups***

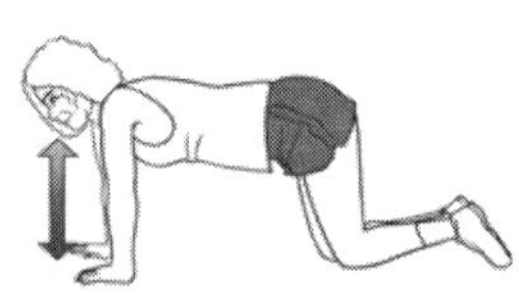

Fig. 3.47b ***Women's Push-Ups***

※ Test Tips and Precautions

- Take a prone position with both arms perpendicular to the torso.
- In the case of a woman, she bends both knees and acts like a man.
- Bend your arms with the start signal and hold your chest until it touches the floor.
- The state that returned to the initial posture is counted once.
- Record the maximum number of reps [Table 3.35].

Table 3.35 ***Evaluation of push-ups***

Unit : reps

	Percentile	Age (years)									
		20~29		30~39		40~49		50~59		60~69	
		Men	Women	Men	Women	Men	Women	Men	Women	Men	Women
Very good	90	41	32	32	31	25	28	24	23	24	25
Good	80	34	26	27	24	21	22	17	17	16	15
	70	30	22	24	21	19	18	14	13	11	12
Average	60	27	20	21	17	16	14	11	10	10	10
	50	24	16	19	14	13	12	10	9	9	6
	40	21	14	16	12	12	10	9	5	7	4
Low	30	18	11	14	10	10	7	7	3	6	2
	20	16	9	11	7	8	4	5	1	4	-
Very low	10	11	5	8	4	5	2	4	-	2	-

※ If muscle endurance is weak, ability to recover from fatigue in everyday life is very poor.

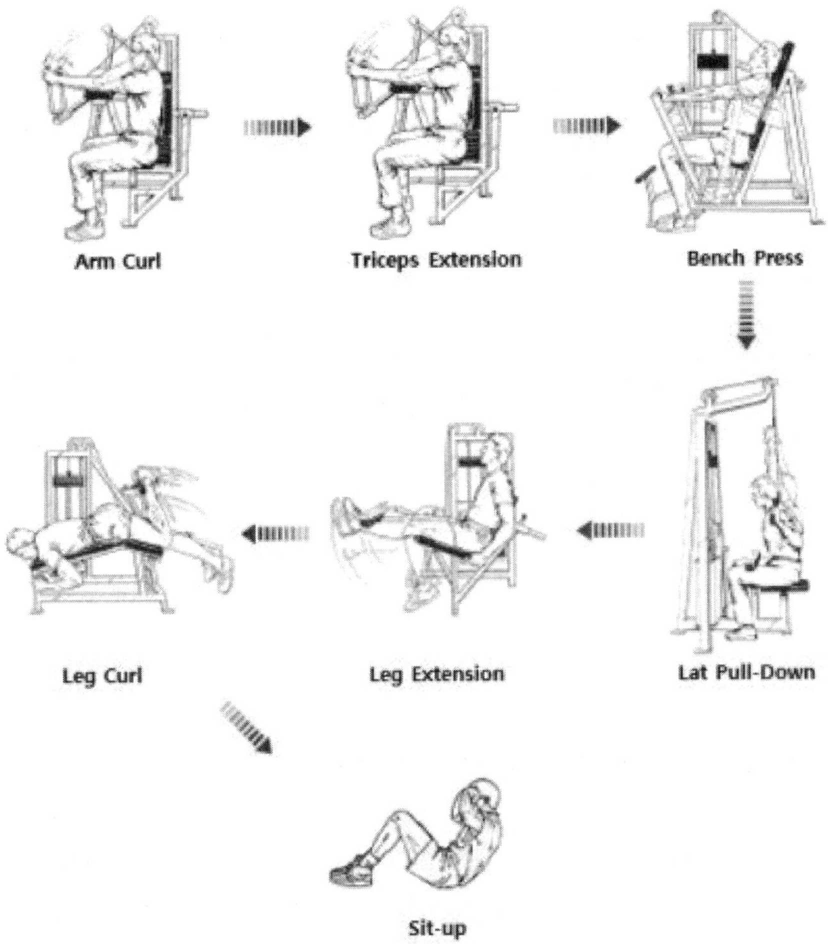

Fig. 3.48 ***Seven dynamic endurance tests***

※ Test Tips and Precautions

- Dynamic endurance can be evaluated by recording as many repetitions as possible using 1RM or body weight.
- When using weight equipment, set 70% of 1RM and evaluate whether you can lift up to 15 reps.
- Multiply the number of repetitions from six weighting devices by the index for body weight.
- The sit-up is evaluated by the number of reps it has been performed for one minute.
- The total number of reps is added to evaluate muscle endurance in six steps [Table 3.36].

Dynamic Muscle Endurance Tests

As shown in [Fig. 3.48], this test, which is performed indoors, consists of arm curl, triceps extension, bench press, lateral pull down, leg extension, leg curl, and sit-up. It is evaluated by the total score. For dynamic muscle endurance evaluation, set 70% of 1RM and measure how much weight can be lifted. The order is as follows. If someone has successfully completed 15 repetitions from the arm curl to the leg curl, multiply that index by 15 times. For men, the number of repetitions 15 × index 0.33 = 4.95 for arm curl, 4.95 for triceps extensions, the 9.9 for bench press, 9.9 for lateral pull-downs, 7.5 for leg extensions, and 4.95 for leg curls. If all of these points are combined, it will total 42.15 points. If the person performs sit-ups 50 times in 1 minute, it total 92.15 points and belong to the "highest grade".

Table 3.36 ***Evaluation of dynamic endurance test***

Unit: Times

	Index*			Evaluation		
	Men	Women		Repetitions(15)	Total number of reps	Rating
① Arm curl	0.33	0.25	=	________	91~105	Utmost
② Triceps extension	0.33	0.33	=	________	77~90	Very good
③ Bench press	0.66	0.50	=	________	63~76	Good
④ Lateral pull down	0.66	0.50	=	________	49~62	Average
⑤ Leg extension	0.50	0.50	=	________	35~48	Low
⑥ Leg curl	0.33	0.33	=	________	<35	Very low

* The index is based on 250 male and female college students.[24]

Body Composition Measurement and Evaluation

In addition to the bioelectrical impedance method described above, the body composition test can also calculate the body fat percentage using body mass index (BMI), waist-to-hip ratio (WHR), skin fold, bone scan, and computer tomography (CT).

Body Mass Index

BMI is calculated as body weight/height squared [kg/m^2]. In the case of athletes, the body is used to distinguish between light, moderate, and heavyweight categories, but is used to predict obesity in the general population [Table 3.37].

Table 3.37 ***BMI Category***

BMI(kg/m^2)	Category	Recommended Treatment
< 18.5	Underweight	
18.5~24.9	Normal	
25.0~29.9	Overweight	
≥ 30.0	Obesity	
30.0~34.9	1 degree obesity	Diet + Exercise
35.0~39.9	2 degree obesity	Diet + Exercise + Medication
≥ 40.0	3 degrees (pathological) obesity	Diet + Exercise + Medication + Surgery

Waist-to-Hip Ratio

The WHR is a simple and highly reliable way to determine the degree of obesity in the abdomen. The approximate normal range is 0.80-0.95 for men and 0.70-0.85 for women. This method can also be used to estimate the risk of chronic diseases [Table 3.38].

Table 3.38 ***Chronic disease risk assessment by WHR***

	Age (years)	Chronic disease risk rate			
		Low	Normal	High	Very high
Men	20~29	0.83 ⇩	0.83~0.88	0.89~0.94	0.94 ⇧
	30~39	0.84 ⇩	0.84~0.91	0.92~0.96	0.96 ⇧
	40~49	0.88 ⇩	0.88~0.95	0.96~1.00	1.00 ⇧
	50~59	0.90 ⇩	0.90~0.96	0.97~1.02	1.02 ⇧
	60~69	0.91 ⇩	0.91~0.98	0.99~1.03	1.03 ⇧
Women	20~29	0.71 ⇩	0.71~0.77	0.78~0.82	0.82 ⇧
	30~39	0.72 ⇩	0.72~0.78	0.79~0.84	0.84 ⇧
	40~49	0.73 ⇩	0.73~0.79	0.80~0.87	0.87 ⇧
	50~59	0.74 ⇩	0.74~0.81	0.82~0.88	0.88 ⇧
	60~69	0.75 ⇩	0.76~0.83	0.84~0.90	0.90 ⇧

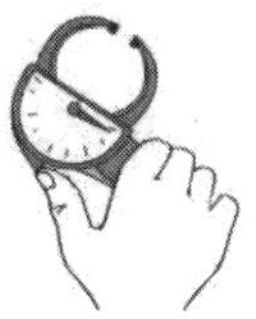

Caliper

※ *Test Tips and Precautions*

- Measurements should be made at the site of primary use by the subject.
- Hold skin with a thumb and a forefinger.
- Measure the thickness of the skin with a caliper. The unit is mm.
- The measurement is carried out three times until the intermediate value is obtained.
- At this time, it is confirmed that the error is 2 ㎜ or less.

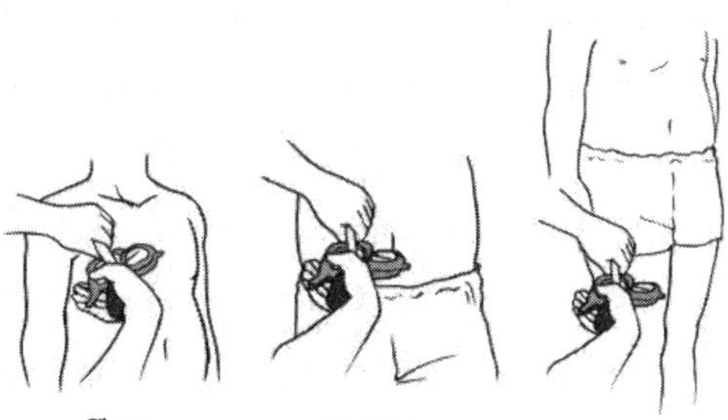

Chest Abdomen Thigh

※ *Test Sites and Tips*

- Chest: Pick up about half a point between the axillary line and the nipple.
- Abdomen: Pick up vertically about 2 ㎝ away from the belly button.
- Thigh: Measure between the knee and the femur vertically.

※ *Calculation Formula*

- Body density, BD = {1.10938−0.0008267 (×3 Site sum)}+{0.0000016(×3 Site sum)×2}−0.0002574 (×Age)
- Fat % = (457÷BD)−414.2

Fig. 3.49 ***Body fat measurement area and calculation formula of man***

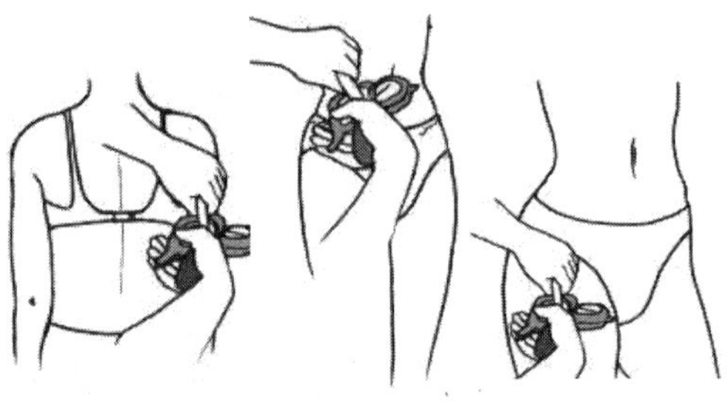

※ Test Sites and Tips

- Triceps: Pick up the midpoint between the shoulders and elbows vertically.
- Suprailiac: Pick up the upper part of the suprailiac pointed diagonally in a natural flow.
- Thigh: Measure between the knee and the femur vertically.

※ Calculation Formula

- Body density (BD) = {1.099421− 0.0009929 (×3 site sum}+{0.0000023(×3 site sum)×2}−0.0001392 (×Age)
- Fat % = (495÷BD)−450

Fig. 3.50 ***Body fat measurement area and calculation formula of woman***

Skin Fold

When calculating fat weight using the skin fold method, fat mass is subtracted from body weight. Lean body mass includes muscles, bones, organs, and moisture of the body. On the other hand, fat is a necessary substance in the human body. Excess fat can reduce performance and increase the prevalence of chronic diseases. Conversely, if the amount of fat is too low (5-7% of younger men and 11-13% of women), it also has a detrimental effect on health. In other words, it is very important to maintain an adequate amount of fat. The proper amount of body fat known to date is 10-20% for men and 18-25% for women. On the other hand, men are judged to be overweight if their body fat mass is 20.1-25% and obese if over 25.1%. On the other hand, women are judged to be overweight if their body fat mass is 25.1-29.9% and obese if over 30% [Fig. 3.49, 3.50].

Bone Scan

Bone scan was originally developed to measure bone mineral density and related variables such as calcium content and bone mineral content, but body composition can also be measured [Fig. 3.51]. The instrument is characterized by high accuracy and sensitivity, low test times, and dual energy X-ray bone densitometer (DPX-L, 1992) using dual energy X-ray absorptiometry with low radiation exposure. On the other hand, unlike previous scans that used to measure bone density, a bone scan can perform a whole body scan to output the bone density and body composition of each patient. However, it is advisable to have the same investigator operate the machine in order to minimize errors in measurement.

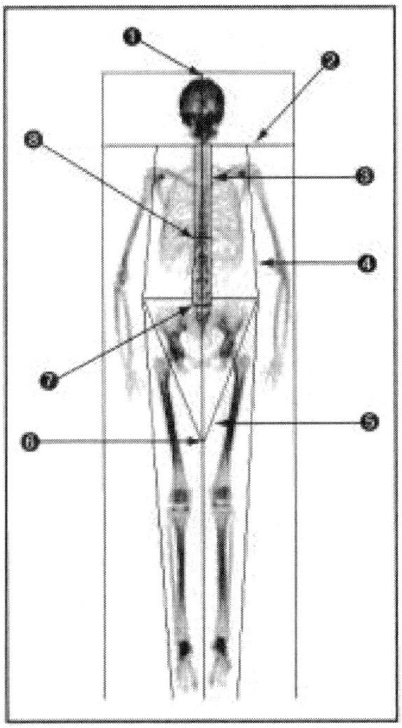

Fig. 3.51 ***Bone Scan***

Computer Tomography

Computer Tomography (CT) is a device for viewing the internal structure of the human body. It is made by complementing the shortcoming of X-rays by only showing bone tissue. This inspection technique has the function of visualizing the structure and tissue state of the body and the advantage of dividing the various tissues in the body vertically or horizontally. In recent years, magnetic resonance imaging (MRI) is being used due to its superior image quality. However, the high costs of an MRI to simply analyze the body composition is burdensome, so the use of CT is high. In particular, CT has been recommended for patients with a BMI greater than 30 kg/m^2 to correctly detect abdominal obesity [Fig. 3.52]. Abdominal CT is a test that generally measures the area of visceral fat and subcutaneous fat. The test site is sliced transversally around the lumbar spine 4-5 (umbilicus). The area of visceral fat and subcutaneous fat should be specified using the cursor. The mitigation range is approximate -190 to -30 Hounsfield units. [Fig. 3.53] shows an example of the result of an abdominal CT scan.

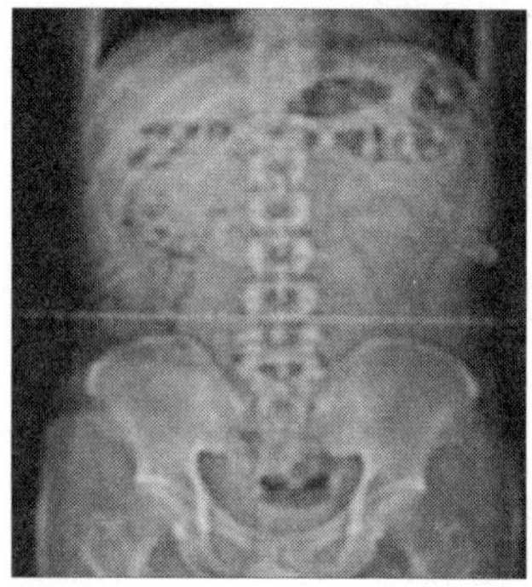

Fig. 3.52 ***Reference point of abdominal CT***

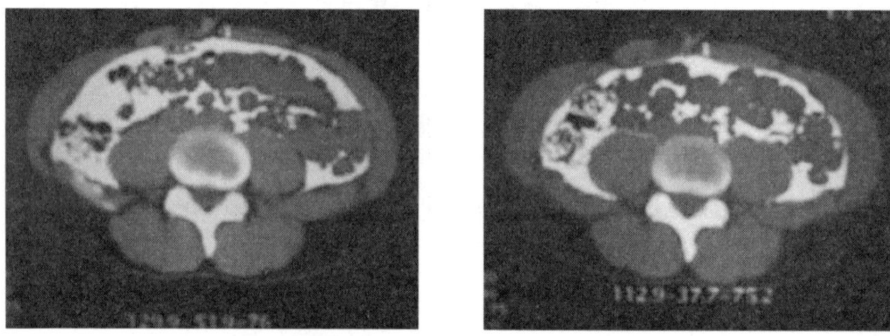

Abdominal site before exercise　　Abdominal site after exercise

Fig. 3.53 ***Results of abdominal CT Scan***

Agility Measurement and Evaluation

Agility is the ability to respond to certain stimuli. In other words, it is the ability to change direction and speed quickly without losing balance. It is based on muscle strength, muscular endurance, power, balance, and flexibility. Agility training is most effective when repeating the required actions accurately and quickly. The tests include the 10m shuttle run, zigzag run, burpee test, reaction time test, and side-step test. This section, however, introduces the side-step and reaction time tests.

Side Step

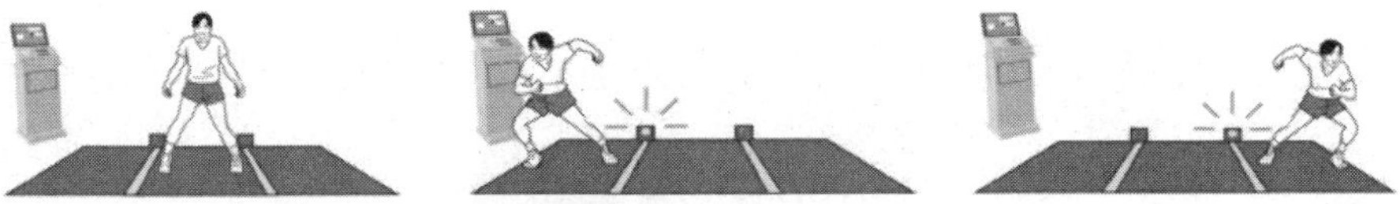

Fig. 3.54 Side Step Test

※ Test Tips and Precautions

- Draw three lines at an interval of 1.2 m for men, 1 m for women.
- Centered around the center line, stand with both feet in shoulder width.
- With the start, one foot goes over the right line, and then back to the center line and over the left line [Fig. 3.54].
- Encourage to do as much as possible.
- The total number of times performed for 30 seconds is measured and evaluated [Table 3.39].

Table 3.39 Evaluation of side step

Unit : reps

	Age (years)									
	Less than 20s		20~29		30~39		40~49		50s or more	
	Men	Women	Men	Women	Men	Women	Men	Women	Men	Women
Very good	≥46	≥40	≥45	≥40	≥45	≥38	≥41	≥36	≥35	≥31
Good	42~45	37~39	42~44	37~39	41~44	34~37	38~40	32~35	33~34	27~30
Average	38~41	33~36	38~41	33~36	37~40	27~33	35~37	27~31	30~32	20~26
Low	34~37	30~32	32~37	29~32	32~36	22~26	31~34	20~26	26~29	15~19
Very low	≤33	≤29	≤31	≤28	≤31	≤21	≤30	≤19	≤25	≤14

Reaction Time

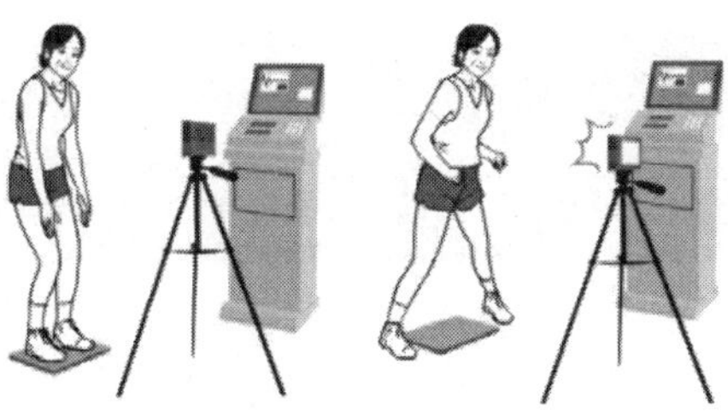

Fig. 3.55 Reaction Time

※ Test Tips and Precautions

- Set the time to "0" using the home switch before measuring.
- The ready position before the reaction is light bent knees.
- Let the subject stand on the reaction plate and quickly get out of the reaction plate as soon as he recognizes the stimulus [Fig. 3.55].
- The shorter the reaction time, the better the agility.
- As a response signal, auditory or visual stimuli can be used without notice [Table 3.40].

Table 3.40 ***Evaluation of reaction time***

Unit : msec

	Age (years)									
	20~29		30~39		40~49		50~59		60~69	
	Men	Women	Men	Women	Men	Women	Men	Women	Men	Women
Very good	≥305	≥386	≥321	≥389	≥322	≥370	≥341	≥400	≥373	≥442
Good	356~306	443~387	380~322	454~390	395~323	454~371	422~342	483~401	463~374	531~443
Average	423~357	512~444	456~381	538~455	490~396	562~455	527~423	592~484	579~464	646~532
Low	475~424	567~516	514~457	602~539	563~491	645~563	608~528	676~593	668~580	735~647
Very low	≤476	≤568	≤515	≤603	≤564	≤646	≤609	≤677	≤669	≤736

※ There is a study in Japan that the better the whole-body reaction time, the longer the life span.

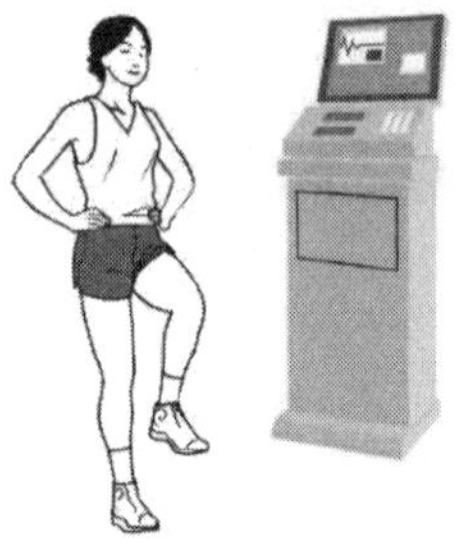

Fig. 3.56 ***Stand on one-leg with eyes closed test***

※ *Test Tips and Precautions*

- The subject puts both arms on the waist and takes a ready stance.
- With the start signal, slowly raise one foot and close eyes. And maintain a stable posture.
- The subject is considered to have terminated when his leg is lowered to the ground or his arm is lowered.
- Three times until completion, record the best measurements.
- [Table 3.41] for evaluation.

Table 3.41 ***Evaluation of stand on one-leg with eyes closed test***

Unit : sec

	Age (years)									
	20~29		30~39		40~49		50~59		60~69	
	Men	Women	Men	Women	Men	Women	Men	Women	Men	Women
Very good	≥216	≥213	≥157	≥157	≥110	≥110	≥75	≥75	≥45	≥50
Good	141~215	139~212	102~156	102~156	72~109	72~109	50~74	50~74	34~44	34~49
Average	44~140	43~138	31~101	31~101	21~71	22~71	16~49	16~49	12~33	12~33
Low	20~43	20~42	16~30	16~30	12~20	12~21	8~15	8~15	4~11	4~11
Very low	19≤	≤19	≤15	≤15	≤11	≤11	≤7	≤7	≤3	≤3

※ Elderly people with reduced balance are at increased risk for falling, and many die.

Balance Measurement and Evaluation

Balance refers to the ability to maintain the body's center of gravity in a static or dynamic state. If there is a high degree of balance, it results in fewer falls and less dizziness. It is very important in terms of stability as balance involves the ability to control the body's automatic and feedback control mechanisms. The most common balance test is standing on one leg with eyes closed [Fig. 3.56].

Coordination Measurement and Evaluation

Coordination is the ability to perform complex motion techniques accurately, which can be measured using three bars. The coordination test involves holding 24-inch-long bars in each hand, balancing the third bar of the same length between them, launching the center bar into the air in a half-turn, and catching it. There is a way of catching the center bar by rotating it around in the air [Table 3.42].

※ *Test Tips and Precautions*

- Practice several times before the test.
- When ready, perform a half turn five times.
- In this case, the score is added one point for every half turn.
- The way to do one turn is the same as turning one half turn, but the score is added two points for each success [Table 3.42].

Table 3.42 ***Evaluation of turning a stick***

Unit: reps

	Men	Women
Very good	14~15	13~15
Good	11~13	10~12
Average	5~10	4~9
Low	3~4	2~3
Very low	≤2	≤1

Power Measurement and Evaluation

Power refers to the amount of work done per unit of time and the ability to exert an explosive force in as short a time as possible. In other words, power is the ability to exert force quickly, which depends on the combination of force and speed (power = muscle power × speed). Therefore, in order to increase power, it is necessary to increase muscle strength or muscle speed. In the case of human muscles, the greater the force, the slower the speed, and the smaller the force, the faster the speed. Because of these characteristics, the greatest power is produced when 30% of maximum muscle strength is performed. In other words, since power is the ability to exert force based on muscle strength, training for power improvement should be based on muscle strength training. Therefore, it is effective to train the motions required for sports with lower loads at a high speed.

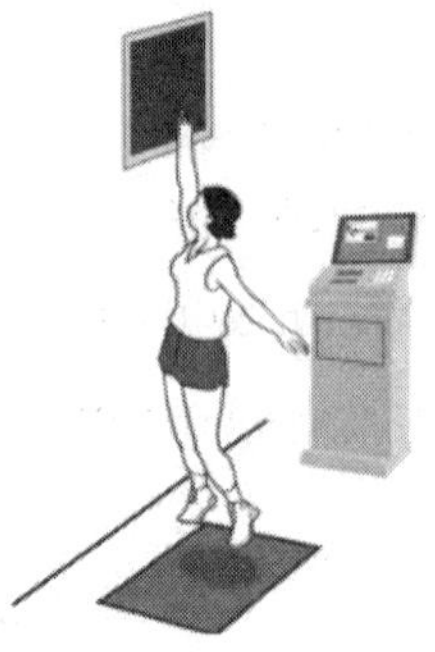

Fig. 3.57 ***Sargent Jump***

※ Test Tips and Precautions

- Gather the legs on the straight line and stand on the side toward the measuring plate [Fig. 3.57].
- Adjust the measuring plate by fully spreading a main side hand and lifting it up.
- Keep the fingertips under the plate.
- Fix the position of the adjusted measuring plate.
- Jump as high as possible and lightly hit the plate with the fingertips.
- Two measurements are made and the average value is evaluated [Table 3.43].

Power measurements include the standing high-jump, standing broad-jump, Margaria Kalmen test, 50 m running, Wingate test, and Lewis Nomogram method. This section introduces only the standing high jump [Fig. 3.57].

Table 3.43 ***Evaluation of sargent jump***

Unit : cm

	Age(years)									
	20~29		30~39		40~49		50~59		60~69	
	Men	Women	Men	Women	Men	Women	Men	Women	Men	Women
Very good	≥67	≥44	≥61	≥40	≥55	≥36	≥49	≥31	≥43	≥26
Good	61~66	40~43	55~60	35~39	49~54	31~35	43~48	27~30	37~42	22~25
Average	52~60	33~39	46~54	28~34	41~48	25~30	35~42	21~26	30~36	16~21
Low	46~51	28~32	40~45	24~27	35~40	21~24	30~34	17~20	24~29	12~15
Very low	45≤	≤27	≤39	≤23	≤34	≤20	≤29	≤16	≤23	≤11

※ If you have good power, you have good athleticism and easy to lead a powerful game.

Speed Measurement and Evaluation

Speed can be defined as the ability to speed up movement. To perform a speed run test, it is necessary to have enough space to run, a precise stopwatch, and a whistle [Fig. 3.58].

※ ***Test Tips and Precautions***

- This test is conducted mainly for young people under 40 years old.
- The starting line and nine lines are displayed in 10 yards (0.9m) [Fig. 3.58].
- The subject is 1 or 2 yards behind the start line and runs as soon as possible with the start.
- Press the stopwatch when passing the start line.
- After the stopwatch is turned on, blow the whistle exactly 3 seconds later.
- The inspector correctly displays the whistle position.
- The score shall be the distance that arrived after 3 seconds. The test is carried out twice, and the farthest distance is used as the score [Table 3.44].

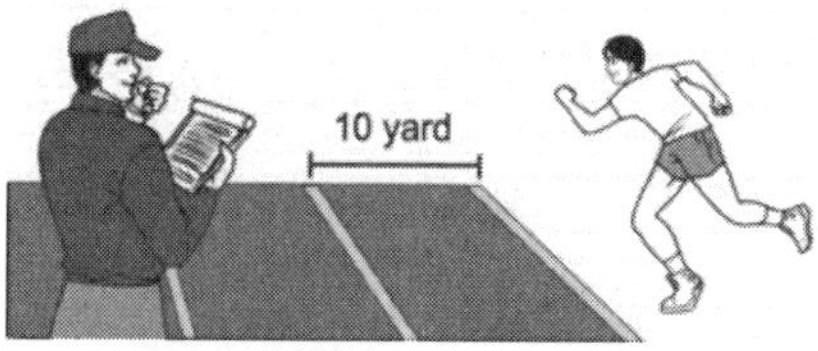

Fig. 3.58 ***Speed Running***

Table 3.44 ***Speed running evaluation***

Unit : yard

	Men	Women
Very good	24~26	22~26
Good	22~23	20~21
Average	18~21	16~19
Low	16~17	14~15
Very low	≤15	≤13

❖ Study Questions

1. 1. The term exercise prescription was invented by Dr. (*Igao Michio*) of Japan, Dr. (*Horman*) of Germany in 1960s.

2. The term "clinical" refers to the case of an experiment, rehabilitation, treatment or surgery on a person at a (*hospital*) or a research institute.

3. The principle of exercise prescription is as follows: the (*specific*) principle that only the muscles and related elements are changed when exercising, the (*overload*) principle that the physical element is developed only when the load is higher than the daily load, the (*progressive*) principle that it should increase the load and time deliberately, the (*individualized*) principle that each individual's gender, age, family history, exercise history, and physical fitness level should be considered, and the (*diverse*) principle that it should increase interest and maximize exercise participation.

4. This principle of exercise prescription is somewhat different from the specific principle. It is the (*neural crossover*) principle that one limb develops to some extent when the other limb exercises. This is called the (*cross-transfer*) effect.

5. The changes of the human body, which is increased by exercise, is restored when you take a rest. This principle is called (*reverse*) principle and you should not be rest for at least (*two*) weeks.

6. Functional capacity refers to upper physical factors from eating, dressing, toileting, walking indoors, light housework that are the most basic and (*independent*) activities in daily life. This can be evaluated by MET, and running over walking requires about (*5*) or more METs of functional ability.

7. The reserve oxygen uptake ($\dot{V}O_2R$) formula: the prescribed intensity × {(maximum oxygen uptake) - 3.5} + 3.5.

8. The reserve heart rate (HRR) formula: the prescribed intensity × {(*maximum HR*) - resting HR} + resting HR.

9. If exercise intensity can not be prescribed with oxygen uptake or heart rate, use

(*Ratings of perceived exertion, or RPE*).

10. If there is a problem with the pulmonary function, use the (*Dyspnea scale*) if you can not prescribe exercise intensity with oxygen uptake or heart rate.

11. (*Angina scale*) should be used for patients with angina pectoris or myocardial infarction who can't be prescribed exercise intensity with oxygen uptake or heart rate.

]12. Using the HR Reserve formula, a person with 60-year-old age and a resting heart rate of 80 bpm has a 60% exercise intensity of (*128*) bpm and a 90% exercise intensity of 152 beats per minute.

13. When an obese patient aged 30 and having a resting heart rate of 65 bpm is running at a target heart rate of 160 beats per minute, the exercise intensity is (*77*)% and the RPE is (*16*).

14. To improve cardiopulmonary function in the FITT principle, the ACSM recommends exercise frequency of (*3~5*) days per week, exercise intensity of HRR (*40/50~85*)% and exercise time of (*20~60*) minutes.

15. To improve muscle function in the FITT principle, the ACSM recommends exercise frequency of (*2~3*) days per week, exercise intensity of HRR (*60~80*) % selecting between 8 and 10 items.

16. You want to calculate exercise time with MET. When a person weighing 60 ㎏ had an exercise test, the maximum MET was 13. It is assumed that the person has a high fitness level and can consume 400 ㎉. At this time, when exercise intensity is prescribed at 50%, exercise time is calculated as (*61.54*) minutes.

17. Regardless of the type, exercise should be continued for at least (*12*) weeks to observe an increase in fitness levels.

18. The adult disease is called 'the illness that does not heal' or (*the illness that should be managed for life*).

19. Ideally, the unit of activity should be a (*weekly*) unit in planning the exercise.

20. The annual plan of exercise is recommended for (*4*) weeks of conditioning phase, (*24*) weeks of improvement phase and (*after 24*) weeks of maintenance phase.

21. The warm-up is a pre-workout exercise that should take place for (*10-15*) minutes and include (*flexible*) gymnastics and (*stretching*), or walking in place.

22. The warm-up is to raise the (*rectal*) temperature of 1°C. The sequence of warm-up starts from the ankle far from the heart and progressively reaches the heart. The reason is to prevent (*shock*).

23. When combining aerobic exercise and weight training in workout, (*60*) minutes and (*50*) minutes are recommended, respectively.

24. Cool-down is to reduce the (*rectal*) temperature by 1°C as opposed to warm-up. The order of the cool-down starts from the head close to the heart and progresses gradually to the heart. The reason is to relieve (*fatigue*).

25. The reason for evaluating ACSM preparticipation health screening as (*risk*) factors, (*symptom*) factors, and other factors is to form categories of exercise tests and prescriptions according to each individual's health state risk level.

26. In ACSM exercise qualification test questionnaires, if more than (*2*) items are found in 7 items of the risk factor, they belong to (*moderate*) risk group. Therefore, exercise test should be performed a submaximal test, that is, (*85*)% of the maximum intensity is used as endpoint and exercise is prescribed to consume 200~400 ㎉.

27. In ACSM exercise qualification test questionnaires, if more than (*1*) items are found in 8 items of the symptom factor, they belong to (*high*) risk group. Therefore, exercise test can not be done without the supervision of a doctor, and exercise is prescribed to consume less than 200 ㎉.

28. When the ACSM exercise qualification questionnaire can not classify the patient, a 7-question (*physical activity readiness questionnaire, or PAR-Q*) is used.

29. What is the step to determine whether a precise diagnosis is made during the exercise prescription procedure? (*D*)

A. Counseling
B. Body composition test
C. Muscle function test
D. Medical examination

30. What is the criterion for the need for the precise diagnosis? (*C*)

A. Resting heart rate 100 bpm or more
B. SBP 160 mmHg or more
C. More than 250 mg/dℓ of blood sugar
D. Total cholesterol 260 mg/dℓ or more

31. What is the level at which HDL cholesterol is judged to be "negative" during qualification testing for exercise? (*D*)

A. 35 mg/dℓ or more
B. 40 mg/dℓ or more
C. 50 mg/dℓ or more
D. 60 mg/dℓ or more

32. Which of the following is not a 'low risk level' by ACSM? (*A*)

A. Middle-aged or younger adult and 45 years or younger men / 50 years or younger women
B. No or less than one coronary heart disease risk factor
C. No disease or no symptoms
D. When the maximum exercise test is possible

33. Which of the following is not a 'moderate risk level' by ACSM? (*B, D*)

A. Two or more risk factors for coronary heart disease.
B. Three or more risk factors for coronary heart disease.
C. When submaximal exercise test is required.
D. Less than 200 kcal should be consumed.

34. What is not required to determine liver function during blood tests? (*D*)

A. albumin
B. bilirubin
C. GOT and GPT
D. Cholesterol

35. What is not required to determine kidney function during blood tests? (*C*)

A. Blood Urea Nitrogen
B. Creatine
C. Triglycerides
D. Uric acid

36. What is not the level of blood lipids that increase the risk of heart disease? (*D*)

A. More than 150 ㎎/dℓ of triglycerides

B. Total cholesterol greater than 240 ㎎/dℓ

C. LDL cholesterol more than 160 ㎎/dℓ

D. HDL cholesterol 35 ㎎/dℓ or more

37. Hematocrit is used to diagnose anemia. Which one is the correct level? (*B*)

A. Men 40%, women 45% B. Men 45%, Women 40%

C. Men 45%, women 45% D. Men 40%, Women 40%

38. What is the normal level of white blood cells that diagnose respiratory diseases and stress? (*C*)

A. Average of 5,000 / ㎣ B. Average of 6,000 / ㎣

C. Average of 7,000 / ㎣ D. Average of 8,000 / ㎣

39. When diagnosing diabetes with urine, what is the reference? (*A*)

A.15 ㎎% or less B. 15 ㎎% or more

C. 150 ㎎% or less D. 150 ㎎% or more

40. What is the correct procedure for checking the body composition test? (*B*)

A. Take carbohydrates 4 hours before the test.

B. Stop drinking two days before the test.

C. Have a diuretic taken one week before the test.

D. Holding one's urine 30 minutes before the test.

41. Which of the following is not the purpose of the graded exercise test? (*D*)

A. If there are abnormalities in normal time and need for a test.

B. If there is no abnormality in normal time, but to check for potential illness

C. To predict the risk of cardiopulmonary function during exercise.

D. To predict the risk of cardiopulmonary function after exercise.

42. Who is not the subject of muscle-joint function test? (*C*)

A. Patients with anterior cruciate ligament injury

B. Patients with posterior cruciate ligament injury

C. Knee joint hyperflexion patient

D. Knee joint hyperextension patient

43. What is not an absolute contraindication to the musculoarticular function test?(*C*)

A. Severe pain B. Extremely limited ROM

C. Pregnancy possible to exercise D. Acute contusion of muscle or tendon

44. What is the normal range for the ipsilateral limb of the knee after isokinetic testing? (*C*)

A. 50~60% B. 45~60% C. 50~70% D. 45~65%

45. What is the normal range of the bilateral limb of the knee after isokinetic testing? (*B*)

A. ± 10% or more
B. ± 10% or less
C. ± 20% or more
D. ± 20% or less

46. Which of the elements of fitness do not correspond to health-related fitness? (*D*)

A. Cardiopulmonary endurance
B. Strength and muscle endurance
C. Flexibility
D. Power

47. Which of the elements of fitness do not correspond to skill-related fitness? (*A*)

A. Cardiopulmonary endurance
B. Agility
C. Reaction time
D. Power

48. Which of the following is not 1RM test method and precautions? (*B*)

A. Lift 5-10 reps with 40~60% weight of the maximum predicted value.
B. After 1 minute rest, lift 4-5 reps with 60~80% weight.
C. If the load increases to some extent, take a rest period of 2 to 3 minutes in the middle.
D. Increase the weight by 5-10 pounds and repeat until the subject lift up to 1 RM.

49. What is the type of dynamic muscle endurance test? (*A*)

A. arm curl, triceps extension, bench press, lateral pull down, leg extension, leg curl, sit-up
B. arm curl, triceps extension, leg press, lateral pull down, leg extension, leg curl, sit-up
C. arm curl, cervical extension, bench press, lateral pull down, leg extension, leg curl, sit-up
D. arm curl, triceps extension, bench press, back extension, leg extension, leg curl, sit-up

50. What is the treatment method for class II obesity patients? (*D*)

A. Treat with dieting and exercise therapy.
B. Treat with dieting, exercise and surgical therapy.
C. Treat with exercise and medication.
D. Treat with dieting, exercise, and medication therapy.

51. In a skinfold for determining body fat, what is the measurement area of a woman? (*B*)

A. Chest, Abdomen, Thigh
B. Triceps, Suprailiac, Thigh
C. Chest, Suprailiac, Thigh
D. Triceps, Abdomen, Thigh

52. What is not the kind of agility test? (*D*)

A. 10m shuttle run
B. Zigzag run
C. Reaction time
D. Sargent jump

53. What is wrong about workout? (*B*)

A. Exercise with tennis, bowling, swimming, etc. for people with moderate or more physical fitness.

B. When aerobic exercise and weight-bearing exercise are performed together, 45 minutes for the former and 30 minutes for the latter.

C. When aerobic exercise and weight-bearing exercise are performed together, the former is every day and the latter is every other day.

D. When aerobic exercise and weight-bearing exercise are performed together, gender and age should be considered.

E. When aerobic exercise and weight-bearing exercise are performed together, it is better to consider mobility and physical fitness.

54. What is wrong about the conditioning phase in the annual plan? (*C*)

A. Minimal duration of side effects that may occur during exercise.

B. The adaptation and refinement period of muscles and organs necessary for exercise.

C. Apply 2% lighter intensity and time than the prescribed exercise program.

D. It is good to assign the period to about 4 weeks.

55. What is wrong with the improvement phase in the annual plan? (*B*)

A. Period for maximum exercise effect.

B. Period during which the exercise in the adaptation phase is carried out consistently.

C. A 2% improvement period to fit the prescribed exercise program.

D. It is good to allocate the period to about six months.

56. What is not an arrhythmia on ECG? (*A*)

A. Left bundle branch blocks
B. Atrial fibrillation
C. Atrial tachycardia
D. Ventricular fibrillation

57. Which of the following conduction disorders is characterized by myocardial infarction, ischemic heart disease, hypertensive heart disease, PRI of greater than 0.20 seconds and QRS interval of less than 0.12 seconds in the ECG? (*A*)

A. 1° AV blocks
B. 2° AV blocks
C. 3° AV blocks
D. Right bundle branch blocks

58. Which is characterized by the presence of a large and depressed P wave, a P wave amplitude of 0.12 seconds or longer in the electrocardiographic leads I and II and caused by mitral stenosis, obstruction or left ventricular hypertrophy. (*D*)

A. Left ventricular hypertrophy
B. Right ventricle hypertrophy
C. Right atrial hypertrophy
D. Left atrial hypertrophy

59. What is the arrhythmia that is caused by hypertension, aortic valve disease, cardiomyopathy, or ventricular septum defect and characterized by $V_5(R)$ + $V_2(S)$ ≥ 35㎜? (*A*)

A. Left ventricular hypertrophy
B. Right ventricle hypertrophy
C. Right atrial hypertrophy
D. Left atrial hypertrophy

60. What is the arrhythmia that is caused by end-stage heart disease, acute myocardial infarction, or shock and characterized by very irregular waveforms and velocities of 150~300 bpm? (*B*)

A. Atrial flutter
B. Ventricular fibrillation
C. Atrial Fibrillation
D. Premature ventricular contraction

Chapter 4

Clinical Kinesiology

Goals

- To learn the practice of health-related exercises.
- To understand flexibility exercise methods.
- To understand cardiopulmonary endurance exercise methods.
- To understand muscle strength exercise methods.
- To understand muscular endurance exercise methods.

Flexibility Exercise

If atrophy lasts for a long time due to aging and the pain caused by disease, the connective tissue, which is an inhibitory factor, proliferates and limits the ROM. For example, a right-handed person's left arm is less mobile than the right arm, a farmer's waist is lumbar curvature, and a patient with kidney disease is bent on one side. An exercise that prevents the growth of connective tissues, increases mobility, and improves flexibility, is stretching.

Stretching includes dynamic (or ballistic) stretching using a bounce, static (or passive) stretching to extend the body within the ROM without using any bounce, and proprioceptive neuromuscular facilitation (PNF) combining the both.

Dynamic stretching is used mainly to prevent injuries in athletes. The dynamic recoil of the body to increase the muscles may cause damage to the tendons or ligaments unconsciously. Therefore, the static stretching method of stopping and stretching for 10 seconds at the limit of the ROM is desirable in clinical practice. Ultimately, flexibility exercises are beneficial for all types of training. In particular, it is important to stretch all the joints before exercise. However, when time is lacking, it is preferable to perform only the stretching of the Achilles tendons, calf muscles, hamstrings, back, and trunk. Stretching should be performed immediately after the warm-up or the workout.

Hold-Relax Technique of PNF	*Hold-Relax-Contract Technique of PNF*
• Perform isometric contraction for 8~15 seconds. • Relax for 2~3 seconds. • Perform static stretching for 10~15 seconds. • Relax for 20 seconds. • Repeat the first to fourth actions 3~5 times.	• Perform isometric contraction for 8~15 seconds. • Relax for 2~3 seconds • Isometric contraction of the antagonist is performed again for 7~15 seconds. • Relax for 20 seconds. • Repeat the first to fourth actions 3~5 times.

Proprioceptive Neuromuscular Facilitation

PNF is a stretching method that is performed with partners. The muscle spindle in the muscle contracts the muscle when there is sudden muscle extension, but the tendon spindle on the tendon relaxes the tendon if it contracts excessively. When these two signals work simultaneously, the relaxation signal acts first rather than the contractile signal, and the muscle can be stretched beyond the limit. In other words, the spindle in our muscles and tendons is a protective device that, when overloaded, signals the cerebrum to engage a relaxation mechanism. If the extension and relaxation signals work simultaneously, the relaxation signal overrides the contraction signal, which causes over-relaxation of the muscles. The PNF includes the hold-relax technique and the hold-relax-contract technique.

Static Stretching

Static stretching is performed by first choosing an action that can be done naturally. After that, whole movements should be attempted. Specifically, static stretching gently lengthens the muscles, concentrating consciousness on the stretched muscles and maintaining the state for 10 seconds (maximum 30 seconds). Breathing during the extension of the muscle group should be in the exhalation state [Fig. 4.1].

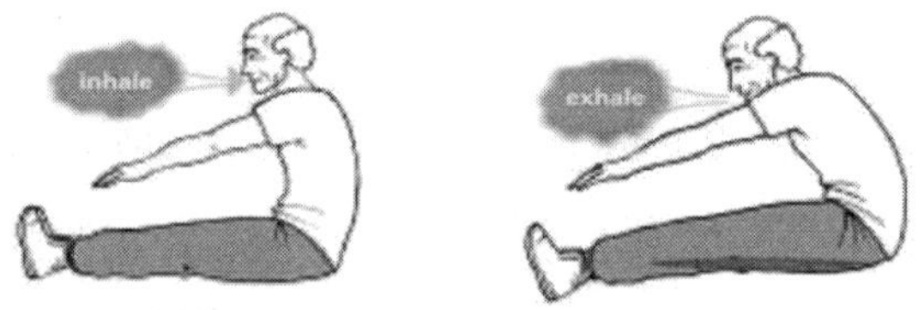

Fig. 4.1 ***Breathing method in static stretching***

When the elderly exercises tightening the thoracic and abdominal cavity, emphasize exhalation more.

If breathing is not natural, or if the subject feels pain or severe discomfort in a stretched muscle group, attempt to stretch it slightly, but maintain the position for 15 seconds. It is also good to repeat the desired action when the activity is over. This stretching should be done twice a day. Moreover, in the case of the elderly, it is desirable to reduce it by 20% compared to the total stretching time of young people. Various methods of stretching that can be performed in a clinic or at home are as follows.

Stretching (1)

※ Considerations : If you train three days a week for 40 minutes a day, flexibility improves and changes your health significantly. In particular, the following stretching is the most basic operation. Stretching at the same time as waking up or before going to bed, you can prevent injuries that can occur in everyday life and sports situations.

Name	Motion	How to Exercise
Whole body stretching	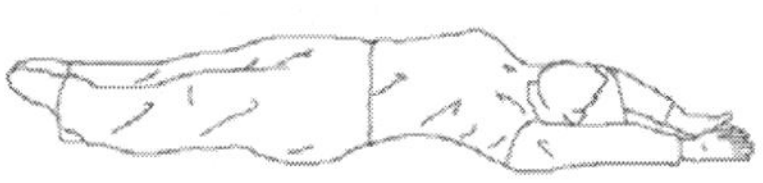	Lie straight on the floor and stretch both arms and feet as much as possible. Keep for 8~10 seconds and increase to 3 sets after it is adapted from the first 2 sets.
Whole body stretching lying sideways	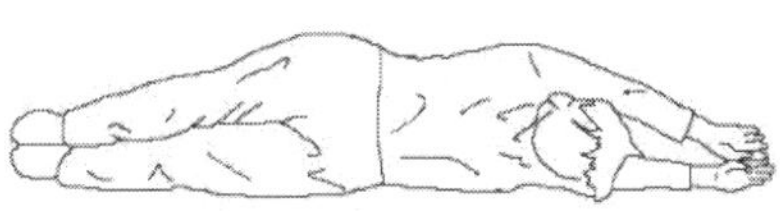	Lie sideways on the floor and stretch arms and feet as much as possible. Keep for 8~10 seconds and increase to 3 sets after it is adapted from the first 2 sets.
Tighten the anus and lift the hips	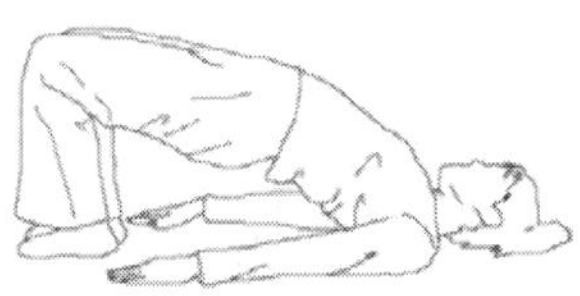	Lie on the floor, tighten the anus, lift the hips as much as possible. Keep for 8~10 seconds and increase to 3 sets after it is adapted from the first 2 sets.
Lift hips and spread one leg	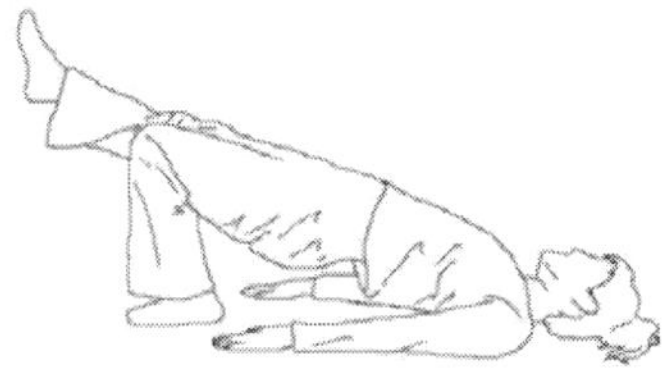	Lie on the floor, fasten your torso with your arms open, and lift one foot. Keep for 8~10 seconds and increase to 3 sets after it is adapted from the first 2 sets.
Abdominal raise	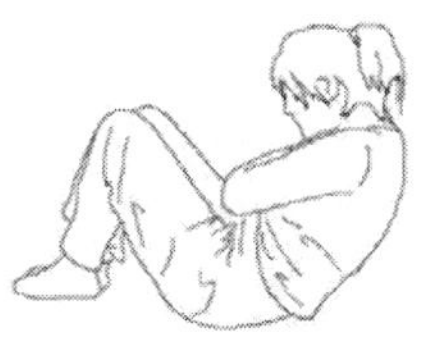	Lie on the floor, put both hands in the chest X-fold, stop at 45 degrees for 10 seconds. Keep for 8~10 seconds and increase to 3 sets after it is adapted from the first 2 sets.
Twist to side	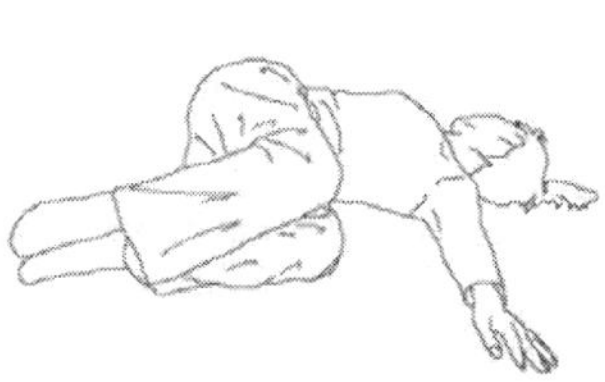	Lay on the floor, open your arms sideways, fold your knees on both sides. Breathe out and lower both knees to the left floor. Point your gaze in the opposite direction to your legs, and attach your elbows, head and shoulders to the floor. Keep for 8~10 seconds and increase to 3 sets after it is adapted from the first 2 sets.

Stretching (2)

※ Considerations : Focus on stretching the muscles of the hands, wrists, arms, shoulders, back, and pelvis. Stretching should begin at low intensity and gradually increase to a point where slight pain is caused.

Name	Motion	How to Exercise
Raise one leg and spread	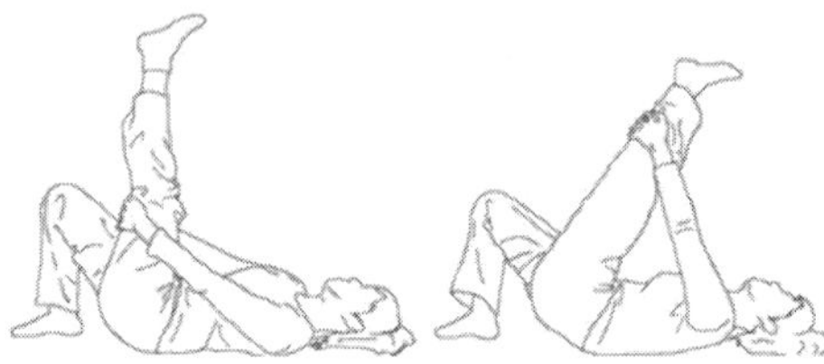	Lie on the floor and fold your knees. Stick your feet close to your hips. Lift your right leg up and hold it with both hands. Breathe out slowly, pulling your knees toward your face. Keep for 8~10 seconds and increase to 3 sets after it is adapted from the first 2 sets.
Pulling the knee to the chest	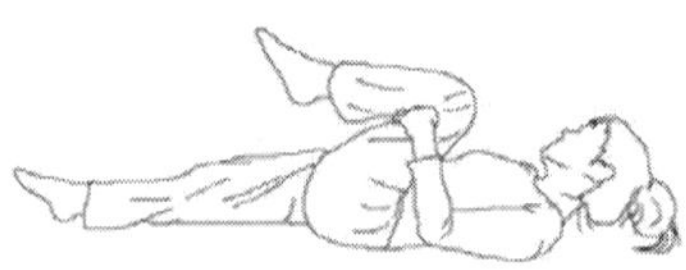	Both hands are interlaced and wrap on the knee. Breathe in and pull your right knee to your chest. Keep for 8~10 seconds and increase to 3 sets after it is adapted from the first 2 sets.
Bend one knee and twist	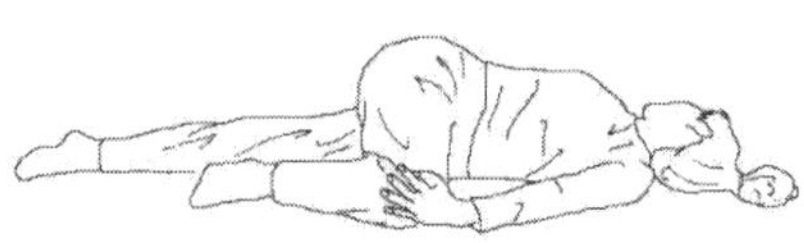	Lay on the floor, stretch both legs, and hold your left knee with your right hand. Breathe out and pull your knees to cross the torso. Keep for 8~10 seconds and increase to 3 sets after it is adapted from the first 2 sets.
Spread one leg and twist	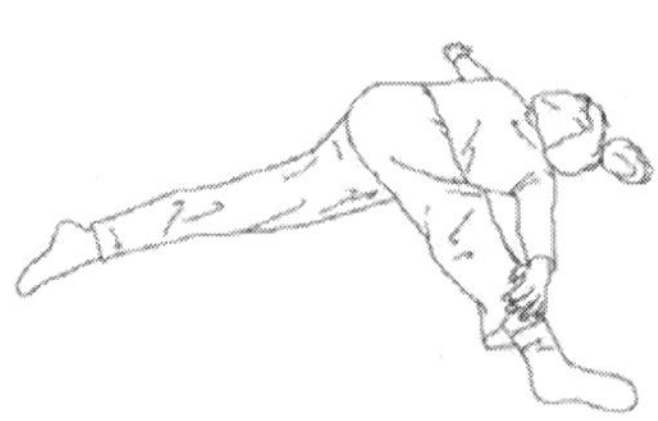	Lie on the floor, open both arms, raise the right leg and straighten the knee. Breathe out and lower your right leg to your left. Keep for 8~10 seconds and increase to 3 sets after it is adapted from the first 2 sets.
Lie down sideways and lift one leg up and down	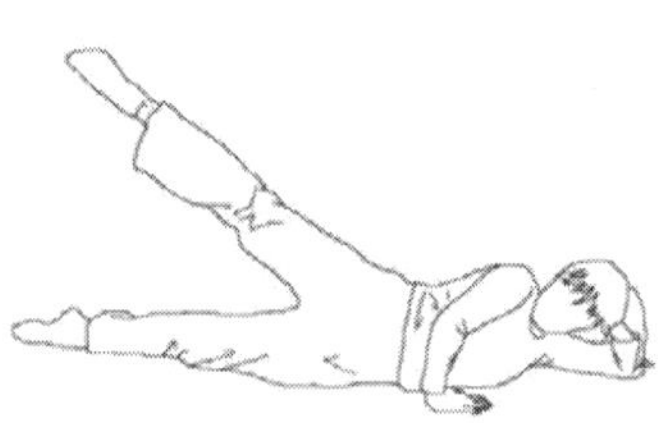	Lie down sideway on the floor and support the head with one hand. Straighten one leg straight up and down, and the other side in the same direction. Keep for 8~10 seconds and increase to 3 sets after it is adapted from the first 2 sets.
Strengthen waist and back muscle (1)	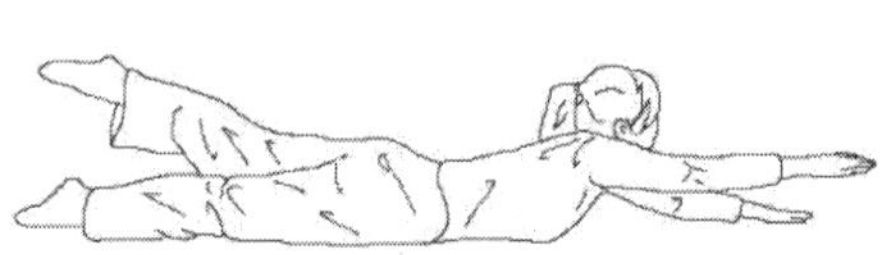	Place abdomen and right arm and left leg on the floor. Straighten left arm and right leg. Keep for 8~10 seconds and increase to 3 sets after it is adapted from the first 2 sets.

Stretching (3)

※ Considerations : Stretching should begin at low intensity and gradually increase to a point where slight pain is caused. If you take more than 30 minutes, the effect of yoga can be expected.

Name	Motion	How to Exercise
Strengthen Waist and Back Muscle (2)	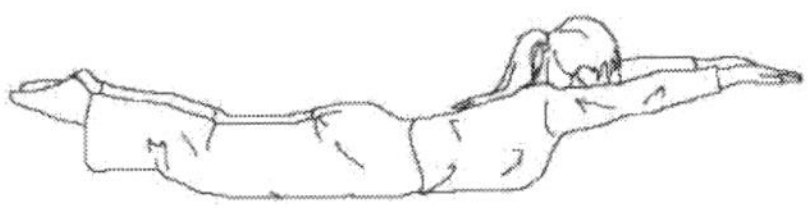	Lie on one's stomach and face to the floor. Spread both arms and legs. Keep for 8~10 seconds and increase to 3 sets after it is adapted from the first 2 sets.
Strengthen Waist and Back Muscle (3)	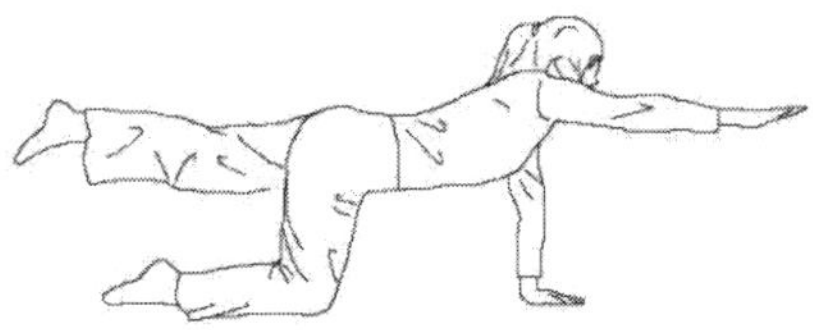	Place your left knee and right palm on the floor. Straighten the right leg and left arm. Keep for 8~10 seconds and increase to 3 sets after it is adapted from the first 2 sets.
Raise Abdomen Up Kneeling on the Floor	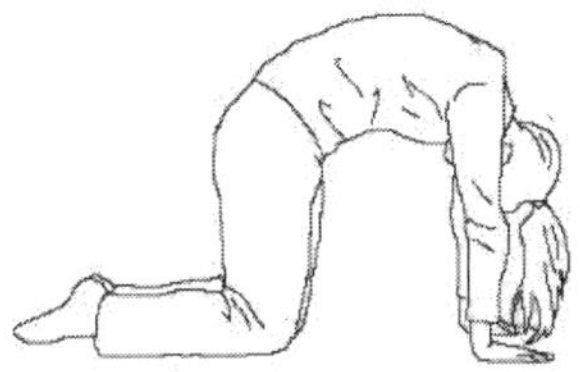	Lay on the floor and spread both hands to shoulder width. Breathe, give strength to the abdomen, and bend the back up. Keep for 8~10 seconds and increase to 3 sets after it is adapted from the first 2 sets.
Put Abdomen Down Kneeling on the Floor	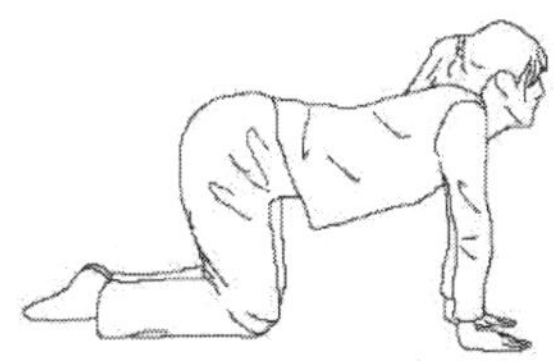	Lay down on the floor in the base posture of four feet and open hands to the shoulder width. Breathe in, give strength to the abdomen, and lower the back. Keep for 8~10 seconds and increase to 3 sets after it is adapted from the first 2 sets.
Shoulder Spread	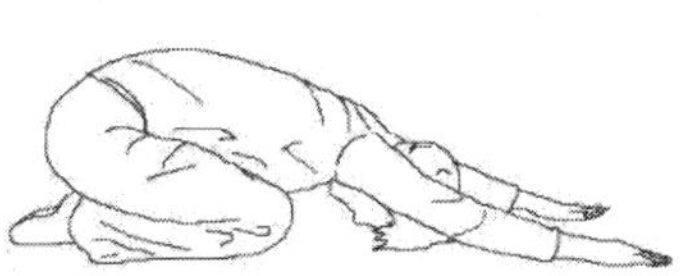	Lay down on the floor in the base posture of four feet and put both arms on the floor. Put your arms on the floor and pull your body back. Keep for 8~10 seconds and increase to 3 sets after it is adapted from the first 2 sets.
Abdomen Extension	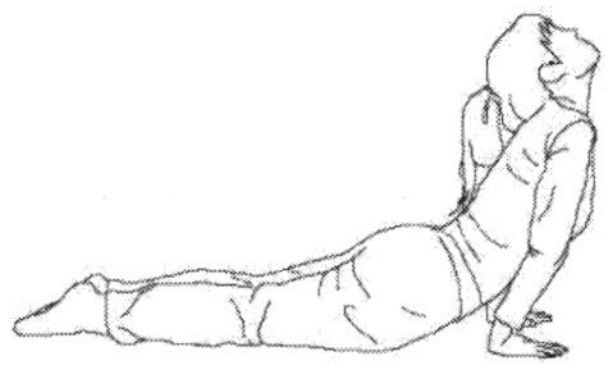	Get down on the floor and have both feet up. Bend your arms, place your fingers forward, put both thighs on the floor, breathe out and pinch your arms. Keep for 8~10 seconds and increase to 3 sets after it is adapted from the first 2 sets.

Stretching (4)

※ Considerations : If you train three days a week for 40 minutes a day, your health and constipation will improve. In particular, if you stretch before and after going to bed in order not to get injured in your life, life can be maximized and injury can be prevented.

Name	Motion	How to Exercise
Sit-ups twisting trunk	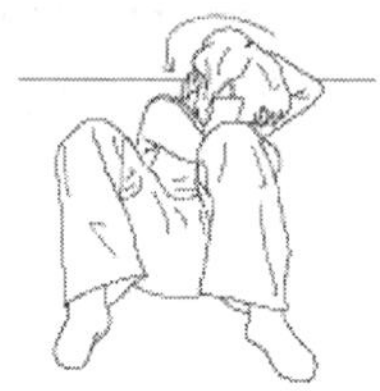	Lay on the floor and put both hands on the head. Take a sit-up posture and come up 45 degrees and stop. Keep for 8~10 seconds and increase to 3 sets after it is adapted from the first 2 sets.
Pelvis spreading	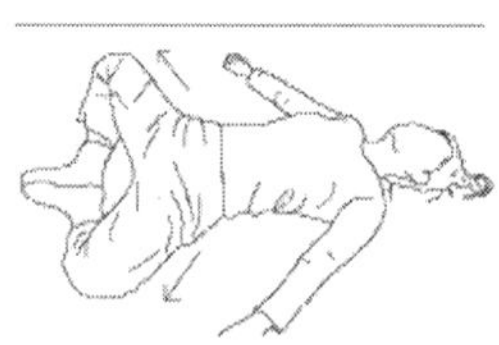	Lie on the floor, bend your knees, collect your legs and pull them towards your hips. Breathe out, spread your knees as wide as possible, and attach them to the floor. Keep for 8~10 seconds and increase to 3 sets after it is adapted from the first 2 sets.
Stretching the pelvis to the side	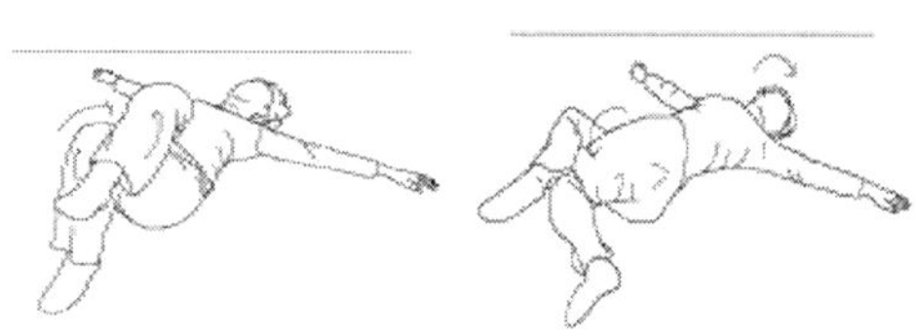	Lift your left leg and put it on your right knee. Pull the left leg and push it toward the right floor. Keep for 8~10 seconds and increase to 3 sets after it is adapted from the first 2 sets.
Bicycling in the air	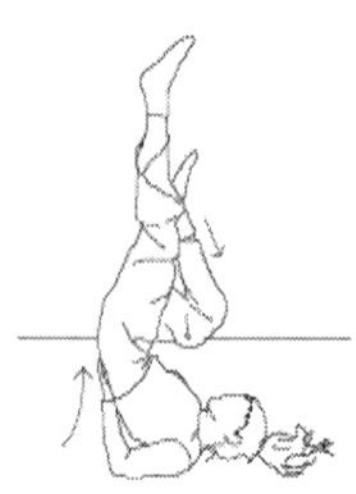	Lie on the floor and put your palm under your waist. Breathing out, push the floor with both hands. And raise knees and lift legs, holding both hands on buttocks. Keep for 8~10 seconds and increase to 3 sets after it is adapted from the first 2 sets.
Knees to chest with gentle rocking	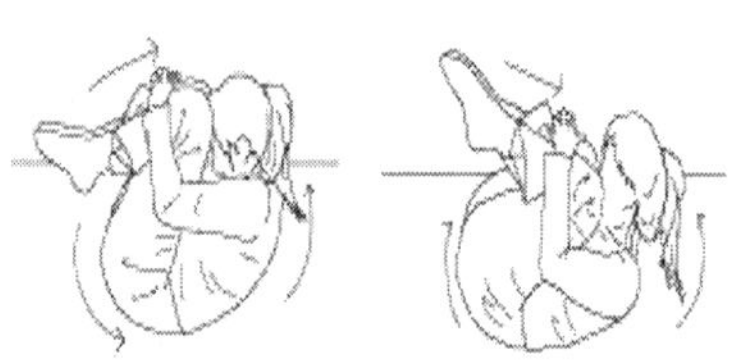	Lie on the floor, bend your knees and pull toward your chest. Grab the back of your knee with both hands. Pull your knees toward your chest and shoulders and raise your hips. Keep for 8~10 seconds and increase to 3 sets after it is adapted from the first 2 sets.
Whole body stretching	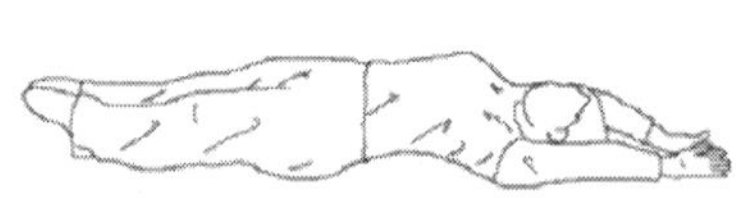	Lie straight on the floor and stretch both arms and feet as much as possible. Keep for 8~10 seconds and increase to 3 sets after it is adapted from the first 2 sets.

Chair stretching (1)

※ Considerations : Chairless gymnastics, which does not take up much space, is a stretch that can be practiced in a small space without special equipment for most people sitting in front of a desk or computer. This stretching is also effective for the elderly and the weak who are not balanced.

Name	Motion	How to Exercise
Rotate ankles	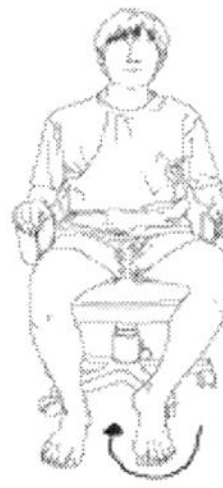	While sitting comfortably on the chair, place both hands lightly on the chair knob or knee, lightly turn the left foot outward, and do the same with the other. Keep for 8~10 seconds and increase to 3 sets after it is adapted from the first 2 sets.
Touch the floor with instep of the foot	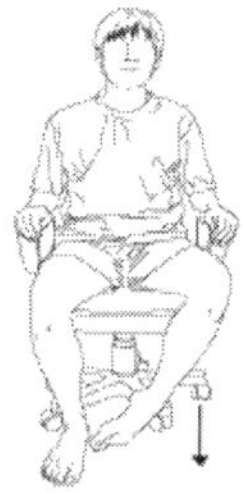	While sitting comfortably in a chair, place both hands lightly on a chair knob or knee, and let your toes touch the floor. It does not give too much force. After the ankle is bent like an bow, the other one is performed in the same way. Keep for 8~10 seconds and increase to 3 sets after it is adapted from the first 2 sets.
Heel lifting	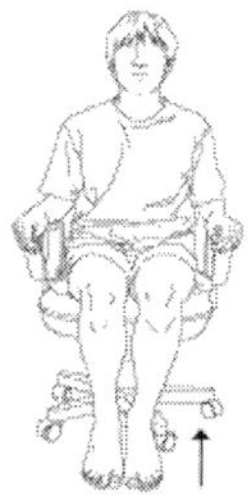	While sitting comfortably on the chair, put both hands lightly on the chair handle or knee, and raise the heel. The other side is carried out in the same way. Keep for 8~10 seconds and increase to 3 sets after it is adapted from the first 2 sets.
Toes lifting	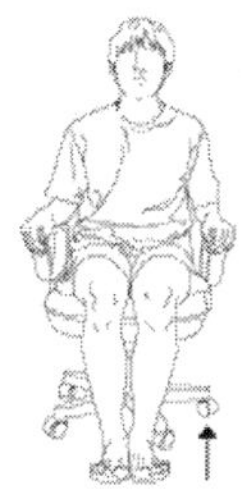	While sitting comfortably in a chair, both hands are lightly placed on a chair knob or knee, and the heel touches the ground on the contrary to the above motion. The other side is carried out in the same way. Keep for 8~10 seconds and increase to 3 sets after it is adapted from the first 2 sets.
Spread one leg	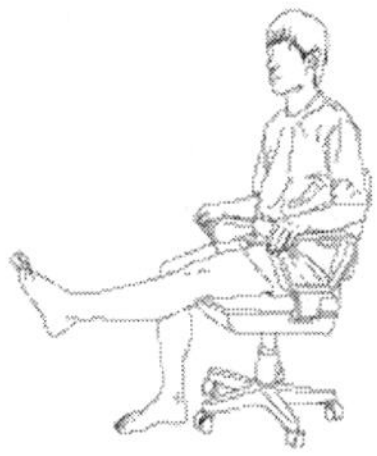	While sitting comfortably in a chair, both hands lightly on the knob of a chair or on the knee, and comfort one foot. At this time, the knees should be fully extended. The other side is carried out in the same way. Keep for 8~10 seconds and increase to 3 sets after it is adapted from the first 2 sets.

Chair stretching (2)

※ Considerations : Chair stretching can increase not only the flexibility of the elderly but also the strength and muscle endurance. However, the stretching operation must be carried out in the exact order so that it is effective in fitness factor development.

Name	Motion	How to Exercise
Raise both legs to make fan-shaped	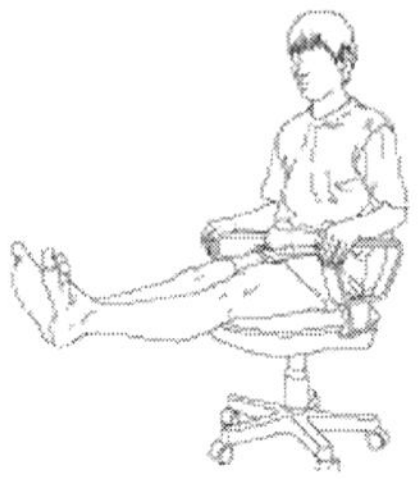	Sit comfortably on your chair and put both hands lightly on your chair knob or knee. After lifting the legs comfortably, make sure that both heels are in contact with each other to form a fan-shaped. Keep for 8~10 seconds and increase to 3 sets after it is adapted from the first 2 sets.
Raise both legs to make triangle-shaped	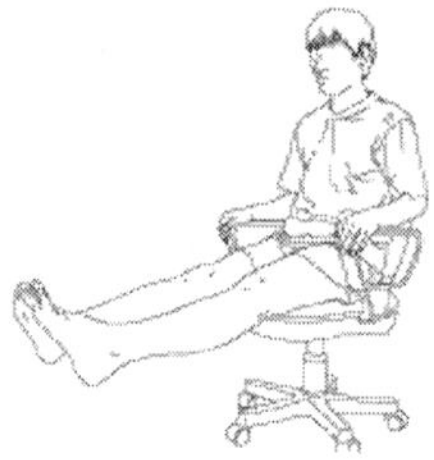	While sitting comfortably in a chair, put both hands lightly on a chair knob or knee, lift both legs comfortably, and make a triangular shape with the toes touching. Keep for 8~10 seconds and increase to 3 sets after it is adapted from the first 2 sets.
Lift one knee	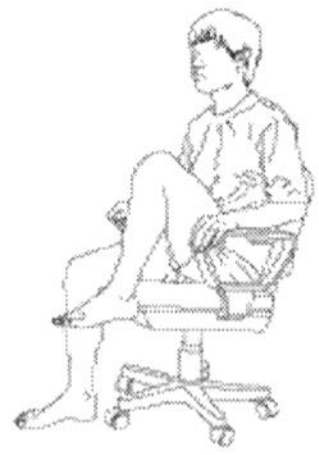	Sitting comfortably on the chair, both hands are placed lightly on the chair knob or knee, and lightly raise one leg to the chest. The other side is carried out in the same way. Keep for 8~10 seconds and increase to 3 sets after it is adapted from the first 2 sets.
Touch the chest with one leg	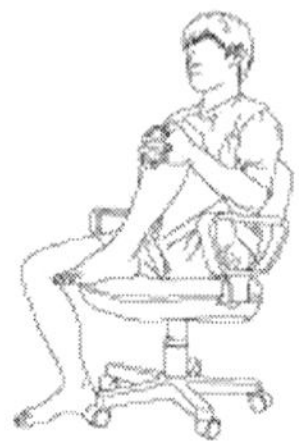	While sitting comfortably on the chair, put both hands lightly, and both hands clasp the pods, grab the knees and pull them to the chest. The other side is carried out in the same way. Keep for 8~10 seconds and increase to 3 sets after it is adapted from the first 2 sets.
Body twist	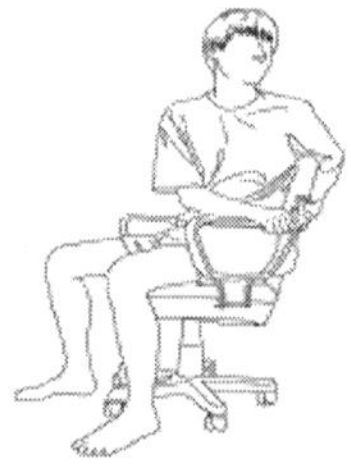	While sitting comfortably in the chair, both hands hold the bar on the chair, then turn the waist. The gaze turns to the direction of turning. The other side is carried out in the same way. Keep for 8~10 seconds and increase to 3 sets after it is adapted from the first 2 sets.

Chair stretching (3)

※ Considerations : Chair stretching increases flexibility, muscular strength and muscle endurance, reducing fatigue and laziness from daily life. It also has the effect of correcting the wrong posture in everyday life.

Name	Motion	How to Exercise
Stretch shoulder forward	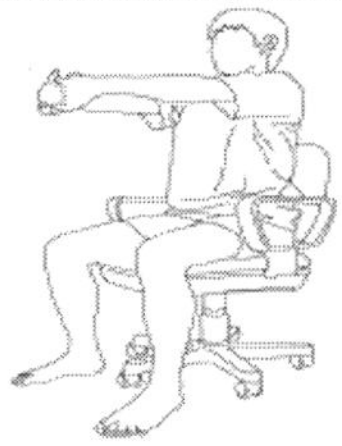	While sitting comfortably in the chair, put both hands in front of the chest, and stretch it forward. Do not lean over your upper body, but keep your back from touching your back. Keep for 8~10 seconds and increase to 3 sets after it is adapted from the first 2 sets.
Stretch shoulder upward	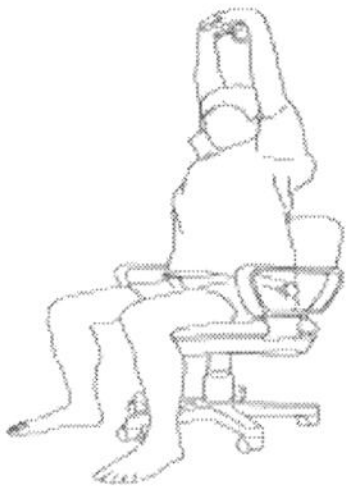	While sitting comfortably in a chair, put both hands in front of the chest, and then stretch it up. Keep your upper body straight, and keep your back from touching your back. Keep for 8~10 seconds and increase to 3 sets after it is adapted from the first 2 sets.
Stretch the side	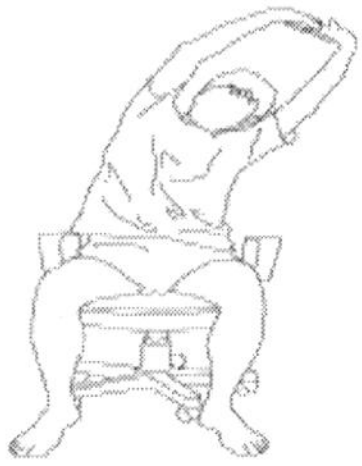	While sitting comfortably in a chair, put both hands in front of the chest, and then stretch it up. Be careful not to bend your arms and slowly bend to one side. The other side is carried out in the same way. Keep for 8~10 seconds and increase to 3 sets after it is adapted from the first 2 sets.
Stretch shoulder sideways	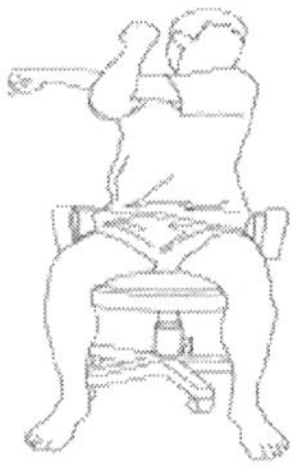	While sitting comfortably on the chair, grab the other elbow with one hand and pull it gently. The gaze moves away from the pulling side. The other side is carried out in the same way. Keep for 8~10 seconds and increase to 3 sets after it is adapted from the first 2 sets.
Stretch shoulder backward	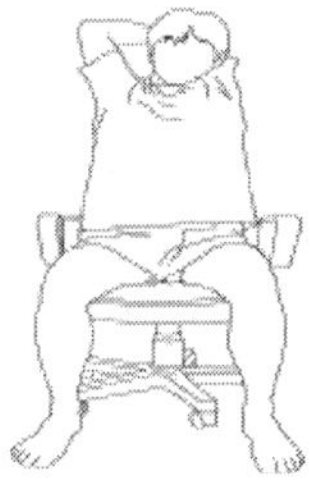	While sitting comfortably on the chair, raise one hand to the shoulder height and hold the elbows with the other hand. The other side is carried out in the same way. Keep for 8~10 seconds and increase to 3 sets after it is adapted from the first 2 sets.

Chair stretching (4)

※ Considerations : Chair stretching increases flexibility, muscular strength and muscle endurance, reducing fatigue and laziness from daily life. It also has the effect of correcting the wrong posture in everyday life.

Name	Motion	How to Exercise
Stretching the palm	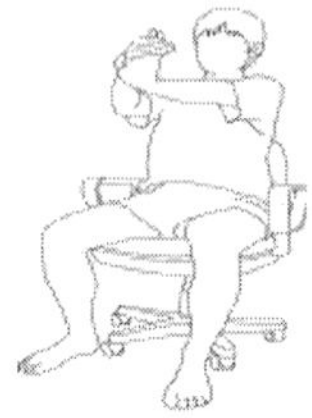	While sitting comfortably in the chair, grab one wrist with the other and pull it to the chest. The other side is carried out in the same way. Keep for 8~10 seconds and increase to 3 sets after it is adapted from the first 2 sets.
Stretching the back of the hand	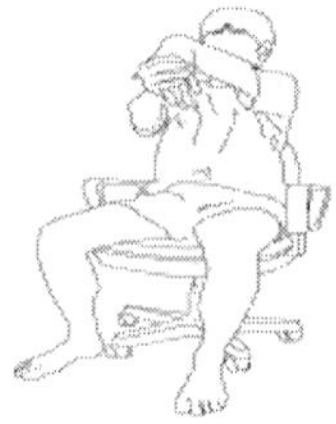	While sitting comfortably in a chair, grab one wrist with the other hand, then push it down and pull it toward your chest. The other side is carried out in the same way. Keep for 8~10 seconds and increase to 3 sets after it is adapted from the first 2 sets.
Pull the head to the left and right	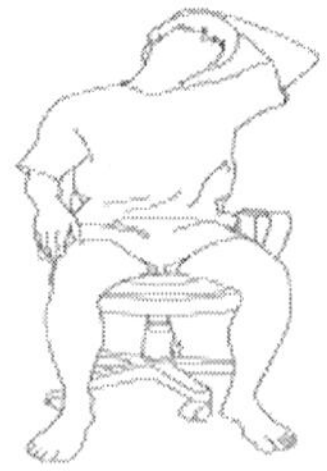	While sitting comfortably on the chair, grab his head with one hand and pull it to the other side. Keep for 8~10 seconds and increase to 3 sets after it is adapted from the first 2 sets.
Pull the head with both hands	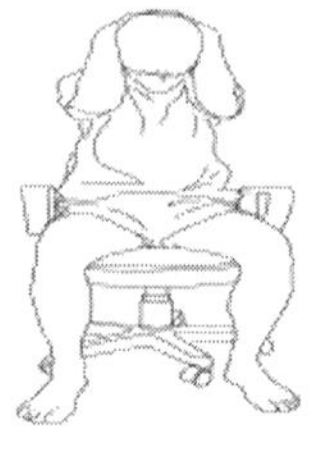	While sitting comfortably in a chair, put both hands in a pod, then push your head with your hand. When you slowly lower your head, let it breathe long. Keep for 8~10 seconds and increase to 3 sets after it is adapted from the first 2 sets.
Push the jaw with both hands	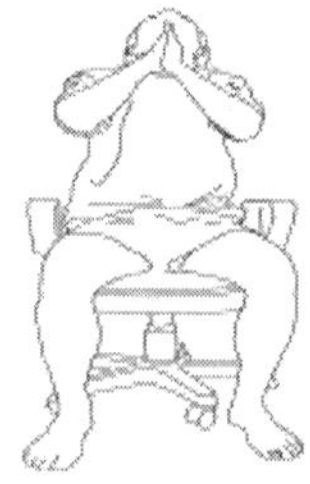	While sitting comfortably in a chair, after both hands are gathered, put both hands on the jaw and push up the head. Keep for 8~10 seconds and increase to 3 sets after it is adapted from the first 2 sets.

Chair stretching (5)

※ Considerations : Chair stretching can increase not only the flexibility of the elderly but also the strength and muscle endurance. In addition, chair gymnastics, which does not take up much space, is a stretching technique that can be performed in a narrow space without special equipment for office workers sitting in front of a desk or a computer, thereby improving obesity as well as constipation.

Name	Motion	How to Exercise
Hand-to-hand pushing and pulling by hand	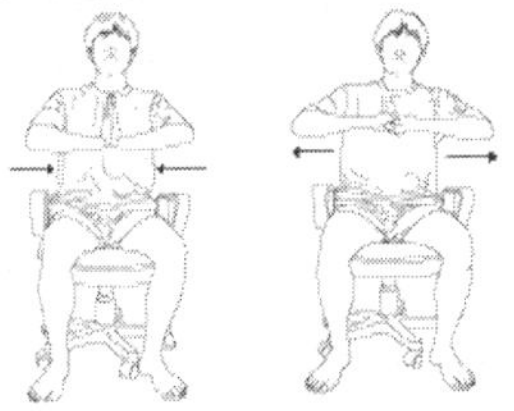	While sitting comfortably on the chair, both hands are gathered in a praying posture, and then the palm is pushed. On the other hand, while holding hands with each other in the opposite direction, pulls out. This is maintained for 8~10 seconds, and after being adapted from the first 2 sets, it is increased to 3 sets.
Turn shoulders in horizontal posture then fold and spread arms upward	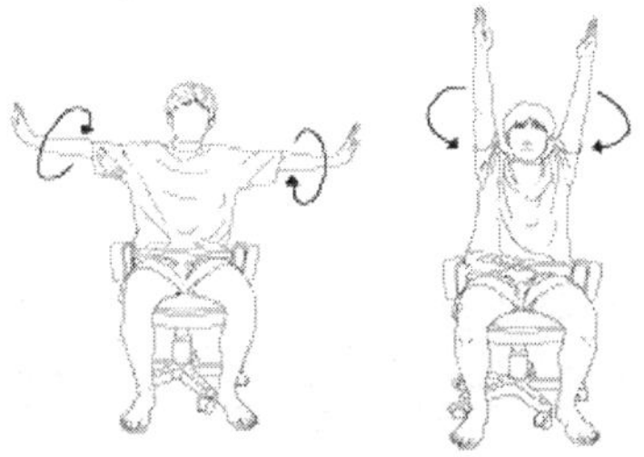	Sit on a chair, raise both hands and turn clockwise. Holding the fists, put the hands up on the shoulder and raise it for 5 seconds. Maintain 8-10 seconds and perform the first 2 to 3 sets. On the other hand, when you are seated, raise your shoulders straight up and onto your head. Repeat 10 times and perform the first 2 to 3 sets.
Folding and unfolding arms	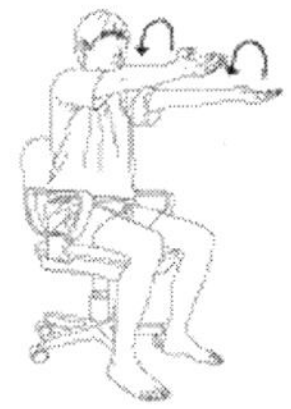	Sit on the chair comfortably and put the hands on the shoulders, unfold the hands forward and repeat. After repeating 10 times and adapting to the first 2 sets, it is increased to 3 sets.
Touch the floor with both hands and cross both legs	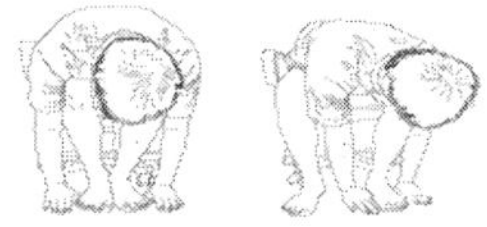	While sitting comfortably in the chair, gather the feet and let both hands touch the floor. Later on, sit on the chair comfortably and reach the floor between the feet. The other side is carried out in the same way. Keep for 8~10 seconds and increase to 3 sets after it is adapted from the first 2 sets.
Tap shoulders	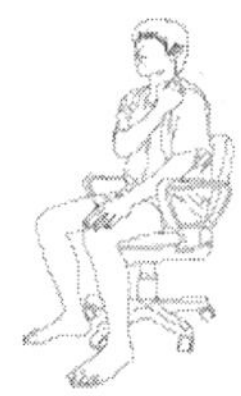	Relax your shoulders in the middle of the stretch while sitting comfortably in the chair. The other side is carried out in the same way. Tap 10 times and repeat according to the situation.
Clap and cool-down with breathing exercise	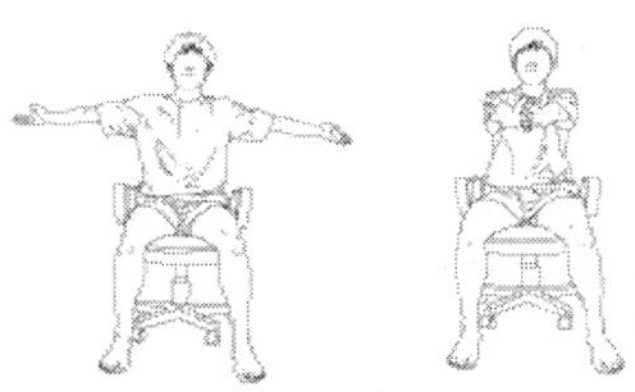	While sitting comfortably in a chair, open both hands and clap to the left and right. After clapping 10 times and adapting to the first two sets, it is increased to three sets. Breathing is performed as the last action. Keep for 8~10 seconds and increase to 3 sets after it is adapted from the first 2 sets.

Cardiopulmonary Endurance Exercise

Cardiopulmonary endurance is the ability to perform whole body movements continuously. This ability is also known as aerobic capacity or endurance because it is closely related to the capacity to supply oxygen to the muscles through the cardiorespiratory system.[3] To improve cardiopulmonary endurance, the ability to provide oxygen through the cardiorespiratory system and the ability to produce energy in muscles using oxygen must develop together. Training to improve cardiopulmonary endurance should be performed in a way that allows the entire body to exercise for a prolonged period of time. Depending on the circumstances, the type of exercise may vary (e.g., continuous or interval exercise). However, the principle of exercising the whole body for long durations must be observed.

Table 4.1 ***Physiological variables according to endurance training***

Variables	General People		Athlete
	Pre	Post	
Heart rate (bpm)			
Resting	74	61	45
Maximal	194	190	185
Stroke volume (㎖/beat)			
Resting	64	82	127
Maximal	122	142	201
Cardiac output (ℓ/min)			
Resting	4.5	4.6	4.4
Maximal	22.3	25.8	34.9
Heart volume (㎖)	750	823	1250
Blood volume (ℓ)	4.8	5.2	6.1
Blood pressure (㎜Hg)			
Resting	120/80	124/78	105/65
Maximal	206/85	202/82	209/69
Ventilatory volume (ℓ/min)			
Resting	7	6	6
Maximal	123	142	201
Respiration rate (reps)			
Resting	14	12	11
Maximal	42	47	59
Tidal volume (ℓ)			
Resting	0.06	0.6	0.6
Maximal	2.8	3.1	3.1

Variables		General People		Athlete
		Pre	Post	
Vital capacity (ℓ)		2.8	3.1	3.1
Residual capacity (ℓ)		5.8	6.1	6.4
Arteriovenous O_2 difference (㎖/100cc)				
Resting		6.1	6.1	6.1
Maximal		14.5	15.2	16.4
Maximal oxygen uptake (㎖/kg/min)		47	55	79
Body weight (㎏)		75	72	62
Body fat percent (%)		16.0	14.9	6.7
Type I fiber ratio (%)		55	55	81
Area of muscle fiber (㎛²)				
Type I		4730	4820	4180
Type IIa		6860	7150	4299
Type IIb		6167	6433	3899
Capillary density				
Number/㎟		290	350	460
Number/muscle fiber		1.2	1.4	3.2
Citrate synthase		28	37	78
Hexokinase		2.4	2.9	4.2
Lactate dehydrogenase		580	654	629
Muscle fibers maximum shortening velocity (muscle length / sec)	Type I	0.86	?	1/10
	Type II	4.85	?	1/74

Factors of Cardiopulmonary Endurance

The most common changes in the human body due to cardiopulmonary endurance training are an increase in $\dot{V}O_2max$ and maximum cardiac output. Moreover, increase in respiratory volume, lower lactate concentration at submaximal exercise intensity, increase in mitochondria and capillary density, and improvement in enzyme activity are common changes in a study in which the results are shown in [Table 4.1].

Physiological adaptation to cardiopulmonary endurance training is closely related to age and gender. Maximum aerobic power decreases with age, and on average, women tend to be lower than men. However, the general physiological response through training is similar. The fundamental difference in the aerobic power between men and women is that women have higher percentages of body fat and lower blood hemoglobin levels than men, while men have larger heart volumes and higher blood flow than women. To examine the physiological effects of endurance training, a study measured physiological variables related to whole body endurance before and after training and compared with the athletes in a group of untrained people who performed endurance training for a short period of 3-6 months.

Types of Exercises to Improve Cardiopulmonary Endurance

The aerobic exercise for cardiopulmonary endurance should be used according to the annual plan. The kinds of exercises performed by clinics include treadmill walking, jogging, running, or indoor cycling, which may cause psychological boredom and fatigue. To avoid these drawbacks, exercise prescribers must apply various forms of cardiovascular endurance exercise. For example, even when walking on a treadmill only, it is necessary to adjust the exercise intensity (speed or slope) intermittently or continuously. However, it is preferable to use these various kinds of exercises for people who are used to a certain degree of exercise or those who have significantly recovered.

Cardiopulmonary endurance exercises include walking, jogging, running, stationary cycling (sitting and standing), arm ergometer, and steppers. There are intermittent exercises (interval training performed by athletes) and continuous training to adjust the exercises.

Intermittent Training

Intermittent training is a method of repetition by distributing incomplete rests between exercises, also called interval training [Fig. 4.2]. This method obtains the benefits of training while preventing the accumulation of fatigue during exercise compared to continuous training. In other words, it is a way to develop the potential ability of the respiratory circulation system by running short distances with incomplete rests in between.

Regarding physiology, intermittent training is a combination of anaerobic exercise and aerobic exercise. It improves the chemical changes in the muscles, leading to improved oxygen debt, cardiac output, and the ability of the ATP-PC system to recover during incomplete resting. As a result, intermittent training enhances the sustainability of exercise.

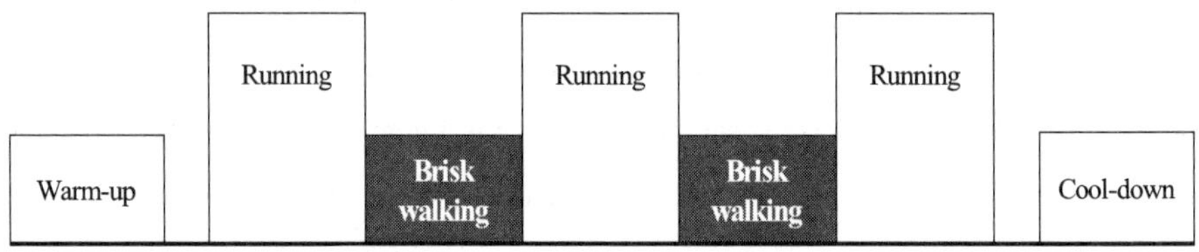

Fig. 4.2 ***Configuration of Interval Training***

Continuous Training

Continuous training is a typical aerobic training method in which a low-intensity exercise is continuously performed for a certain period of time. It can be expected to be effective at 50% of the $\dot{V}O_2max$ or more, and it is essential to continue for 40-60 minutes. This training method has about six types that athletes perform on the field, but low-intensity long distance training seems to be suitable for patients and the general public in clinical settings.

Six Types of Continuous Training of Athletes

① *Low Intensity Long Distance Training* : At 60~80% of maximum heart rate, perform long-distance exercise at low intensity. In the case of athletes, 25~50 ㎞ is divided into two sessions per day. In the off-season, the distance is reduced to 5~6.5 ㎞ to maintain endurance.

② *High Intensity Continuous Training* : At 85~90% of the maximum heart rate, exercise is performed at 1/2 to 3/4 of the distance. Because this method has high exercise intensity, it increases the speed of progression gradually in parallel with fartlek, repetition training. It is a training method that can improve the speed simultaneously during the off-season of the players.

③ *Fartlek Training* : It is a way to enhance speed and endurance by running freely at a constant pace in a coastal road, lawn, or dune environment. This is a training to enjoy the pleasure of play, suitable for middle / long distance running, cross country skiing, cycling, and long distance swimmers. Usually, the exercise time is 30 to 45 minutes.

④ *Speed Continuous Training* : It is a way to run continuously with a speedy and dynamic rest by walking or jogging in the middle. One researcher recommends running 400 m at a speed of 100 m in 20 seconds, and 300 m at a speed of 100 m in 16 seconds, repeating 5 times and resting at 1.5~2 minutes.

⑤ *Repetition Training* : It is a training method to repeatedly perform exercise with all-out intensity or intensity close to all-out and to take a complete rest between exercises several times. The exercise time of the spurt is suitable for 7-8 seconds and speed should be explosive maximum. In the case of running, 30~70 m is recommended, and the rest is 5~10 minutes. If you take more than 10 minutes of rest, the central nervous system will be reduced in the excitability and concentration will be reduced.

⑥ *Highland Training* : It is a training method for improving the cardiopulmonary system by stimulating the oxygen delivery system using the oxygen deficiency state appearing in the high mountain. Highland training can be expected to improve maximal oxygen uptake, increase myoglobin content, increase vascularization, and improve the respiratory system. An altitude of 2,000~3,000 m is appropriate for the training, and the training period is 2~4 weeks.

Amount of Cardiopulmonary Endurance Exercise

Continuous aerobic exercise is appropriate for the initial exercise phase for the development of cardiopulmonary endurance. At this time, exercise intensity is preferably 40~50% of the subject's maximum capacity. It is best to start 10~15 minutes at first, then gradually increase the time to about 45 minutes after two weeks have passed. This phase lasts 4-6 weeks. After that, the improvement phase lasts 16~24 weeks. The intensity is increased to 60~85% and the exercise time is increased by 2~5 minutes every two weeks with a goal of 60 minutes. It is important to calculate the initial exercise time scientifically with MET derived from the GXT results.

When the first exercise begins, it takes about six months. The maintenance phase program is the next step. At this stage, it is also desirable to engage in safe sports activities to prevent boredom and increase interest in exercise. For example, if the subject jogs two to three days a week, a ball game can be played for two days. However, in the early stages when a person with low physical fitness starts to exercise, exercising every other day is useful to prevent damage to the bones and joints and to avoid muscle fatigue. Aerobics, jump-roping, and racquet exercises which are not easy to control intensity are suitable for those who are skilled, and not for beginners.

Cardiopulmonary Endurance Exercise and Energy Expenditure

MET is a term that refers to the calories consumed by body weight per hour and is also expressed as energy consumption. It is also used to calculate the basal metabolic rate (BMR), resting metabolic rate, or exercising metabolic rate. For example, the BMR of an adult male who weighs 70 kilograms is [70 kg × 1 kcal = 70 kcal], and [70 kcal × 24 hours = 1,680 kcal/day]. That is, the BMR of this person is about 1,700 kcal/day. On the other hand, the metabolism of a female is similar to that of an adult male, but the calorie consumption is rather small. The BMR can be calculated by applying 0.9 ㎉/kg/hr. MET is accurately calculated through a GXT and can be used to determine exercise intensity. For example, if a person showed 10 METs after the GXT, it would be regarded as 100%. The lowest intensity of 40~50% would be 4~5 METs, the moderate intensity of 60~70% would be 6~7 METs, and the maximum intensity, 85%, would be 8.5 METs. [Table 4.2] indicates the levels, relative fitness levels, and guidelines for MET.

Table 4.2 ***MET and Functional Ability***

Unit : ㎉/kg/hr

MET	Functional Ability	Expert Participation
1	Resting	
2~3	Walking at 3.2 km/h	
3~4	Walking at 4.8 km/h	
4~5	Walking at 5.6 km/h	Necessary
7~8	Jogging at 8.0 km/h	⇧
8	Jogging at 8.1~9.5 km/h	Expert observation
10	Jogging at 9.6 km/h	⇩
13	Rope skipping at 130 reps/minute	Unnecessary
18	An endurance athlete	
20	A world-class marathon player	

Cardiopulmonary Endurance Exercise and Metabolic Formula

ACSM has developed several formulas to estimate the oxygen consumption during walking, running, stationary cycling, and stair climbing to improve the scientific qualities of exercise.[1] These exercise types are considered to be very accurate because they do not change energy requirements according to age, gender, or exercise techniques. However, body size affects energy demand and should be applied in the metabolic formula. On the other hand, although the metabolic formulas are accurate, it should be recognized that this formula is used for estimating. In other words, it is more accurate to determine oxygen consumption through direct inspection, if possible. However, the reliability of the formulas is very high because of the vast number of researchers and long-term studies. [Table 4.3] shows the metabolic formulas, and [Table 4.4] shows the conversion formula that calculates the calorie consumption per minute and more.[8]

Table 4.3 *Cardiopulmonary endurance metabolism formula*

Items	Formulas	Unit
Walking	$VO_2 = 3.5 + 0.1 \times (Speed) + 1.8 \times (Speed) \times (Slope)$	VO_2 : ml.min^{-1}.kg^{-1}
Running	$VO_2 = 3.5 + 0.2 \times (Speed) + 0.9 \times (Speed) \times (Slope)$	Speed : m . min^{-1}
Cycling	$VO_2 = 7 + 1.8 \times (Workload) / (Weight)$	Workload : kg.m.min^{-1}
Arm cycling	$VO_2 = 3.5 + 3 \times (Workload) / (Weight)$	Step speed : steps.min^{-1}
Stepping	$VO_2 = 3.5 + 0.2 \times (Step\ speed) + 2.4 \times (Step\ speed) \times (Step\ height)$	Step height : m

Table 4.4 *Conversion formula for cardiopulmonary endurance metabolism formula*

Item	Calculation Formula	Item	Calculation Formula
VO_2 (ml.min^{-1}.kg^{-1})	$= \frac{VO_2(\ell.\ min^{-1}) \times 1{,}000}{body\ mass\ (kg)}$	VO_2 (ℓ.min^{-1})	$= \frac{VO_2(ml.min^{-1}.kg^{-1}) \times body\ mass(kg)}{1{,}000}$
VO_2 (ml.min^{-1}.kg^{-1})	$= VO_2\ (MET) \times 3.5$	VO_2 (MET)	$= \frac{VO_2\ (ml.min^{-1}.kg^{-1})}{3.5}$
Calorie# (kcal.min^{-1})	$= VO_2\ (\ell.\ min^{-1}) \times 5$	VO_2 (ℓ.min^{-1})	$= \frac{Calorie\ (kcal.min^{-1})}{5}$
Speed# (m.min^{-1})	$= Speed\ (mph) \times 26.8$	Speed (mph)	$= \frac{Speed\ (m.min^{-1})}{26.8}$
Speed (kph)	$= Speed\ (m.min^{-1}) \times 0.06$	Speed (m.min^{-1})	$= \frac{Speed\ (kph)}{0.06}$
Workload (kg.m.min^{-1})	$= (Power\ W) \times 6$	Power (W)	$= \frac{Workload\ (kg.m.min^{-1})}{6}$
Weight (lbs)	$= Weight\ (kg) \times 2.2$	Weight# (kg)	$= \frac{Weight\ (lbs)}{2.2}$
Height (m)	$= Height\ (inches) \times 0.0254$	Height (inches)	$= \frac{Height\ (m)}{0.0254}$

The metabolic formulas in [Table 4.3] are available for two purposes. First, it allows to calculate the oxygen uptake and thus the energy consumption. It is possible to estimate how many calories were burned during exercise and how much weight loss occurred. Second, it enables to calculate the target workload of the exercise prescription.

Walking

Walking is a type of exercise that can be done anywhere and is recommended for patients, the elderly, as well as obese patients. Walking aims to burn fat by improving distance and duration. It is highly recommended because it is useful for weight control and does not cause the heart strain. When walking, only one foot at a time leaves contact

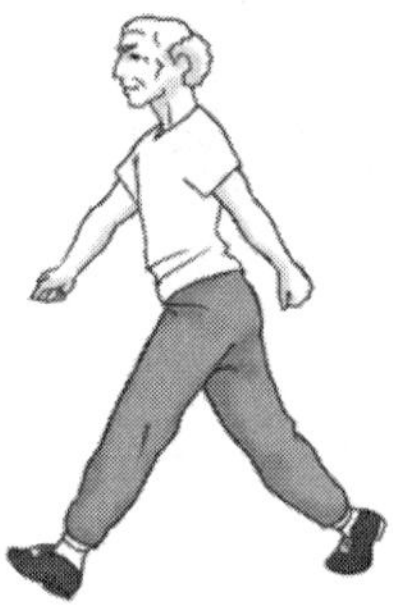

with the ground and there is a period of double-support (both feet on the ground). In contrast, running includes times when both feet are off the ground. Since the center of mass of the sole is on the outer side of both feet, the gait usually tilts to the outside of the foot. Therefore, when walking, the heel should first make contact with the ground and then toward the big toe. Beginners walk 100 m for 65~70 seconds, intermediate walkers for 60~65 seconds, and advanced walkers for 50~65 seconds.

Example Study 1 *$\dot{V}O_2$ Calculation Method When Walking*

Ex. 1 **W is a 51-year-old man with a moderate risk of weight 163 lbs. He has been under high stress and has recently started an exercise program at the company wellness center. He started his treadmill walking load at a comfortable level, with speeds and slopes of 3 mph and 6% grade.**

Q What is the estimated gross oxygen consumption $ml.min^{-1}.kg^{-1}$ of this person, and how much is Net $\dot{V}O_2$ and Net calories burning per minute?

Commentary Initially, convert the units required by the formula. First, convert mph, the unit of speed, to $m.min^{-1}$, and convert lbs, which represents body weight, to kg.

$$3 \text{ mph} \times 26.8 = 80.4 \text{ m} \cdot \text{min}^{-1}$$
$$163 \text{ lbs} \div 2.2 = 74.1\text{kg}$$

$$\dot{V}O_2 = 3.5 + 0.1 \times (\text{Speed}) + 1.8 \times (\text{Speed}) \times (\text{Grade})$$

$$= 3.5 + 0.1 \times (80.4) + 1.8 \times (80.4) \times (0.06)$$
$$= 3.5 + 8.04 + 8.6832$$

Answer 1 **Gross $\dot{V}O_2 = 20.2 \text{ ml} \cdot \text{min}^{-1} \cdot \text{kg}^{-1}$**

Answer 2 **Net $\dot{V}O_2 = 20.2 - 3.5 = 16.7 \text{ ml} \cdot \text{min}^{-1} \cdot \text{kg}^{-1}$**

$$\frac{16.7\text{ml} \cdot \text{min}^{-1} \cdot \text{kg}^{-1} \times 74.1\text{kg}}{1000} = 1.237 \text{ l} \cdot \text{min}^{-1}$$

Answer 3 **$1.237 \text{ l} \cdot \text{min}^{-1} \times 5\text{kcal} \cdot \text{l}^{-1} = 6.2 \text{ kcal} \cdot \text{min}^{-1}$**

Energy consumption during walking increases when speed exceeds the normal rate. If a person is walking very fast, the energy rate increases rapidly. Therefore, the metabolic formula for walking is not applicable to competitive walking, such as race walking, and is used only for normal walking. In particular, this formula is very accurate on a treadmill and walking on level ground.

Example Study 2 Workload Calculation Method When Walking

Ex. 2 P(male/34 years old) is a patient who received a heart transplant. There is little change in heart rate from resting to exercise, and $\dot{V}O_2max$ is 32 mℓ · min^{-1} · kg^{-1}. Therefore, the doctor encouraged him to exercise under supervision at a cardiac rehabilitation center, with 40 to 60% of $\dot{V}O_2R$.

Q If Mr. P feels comfortable walking at 2.5 mph, how much should the grade of the treadmill be adjusted to achieve the recommended intensity?

Commentary1 Initially, convert the units required by the formula. First, convert mph, the unit of speed, to $m.min^{-1}$, and use the VO_2R formula to calculate the minimum and maximum range of exercise.

$$2.5 \text{ mph} \times 26.8 = 67 \text{ m . min}^{-1}$$

$$\text{Target } VO_2 = (\text{Intensity}) \times (VO_2max - 3.5) + 3.5$$

$$\text{Effective limit } VO_2 = (0.40) \times (32 - 3.5) + 3.5 = (0.40) \times (28.5) + 3.5$$
$$= 11.4 + 3.5 = 14.9 \text{ ml.min}^{-1}\text{.kg}^{-1}$$

$$\text{Safe limit } VO_2 = (0.60) \times (32 - 3.5) + 3.5 = (0.60) \times (28.5) + 3.5$$
$$= 17.1 + 3.5 = 20.6 \text{ ml.min}^{-1}\text{.kg}^{-1}$$

Commentary2 In Table 4.3, select the walking formula and assign VO_2 of effective and safe limits, which you already know.

$$\mathbf{VO_2 = 3.5 + 0.1 \times (Speed) + 1.8 \times (Speed) \times (Effective\ limit\ grade\ \chi)}$$

$$14.9 = 3.5 + 0.1 \times (67) + 1.8 \times (67)\ \chi$$
$$14.9 = 3.5 + 6.7 + 120.6\ \chi$$
$$14.9 = 10.2 + 120.6\ \chi$$
$$14.9 - 10.2 = 120.6\ \chi$$
$$4.7 = 120.6\ \chi$$
$$4.7 \div 120.6 = \chi$$

$$\mathbf{VO_2 = 3.5 + 0.1 \times (Speed) + 1.8 \times (Speed) \times (Safe\ limit\ grade\ \chi)}$$

$$20.6 = 3.5 + 0.1(67) + 1.8(67)\ \chi$$
$$20.6 = 10.2 + 120.6\ \chi$$
$$20.6 - 10.2 = 120.6\ \chi$$
$$10.4 = 120.6\ \chi$$
$$10.4 \div 120.6 = \chi$$

Answer 1	$\chi = 0.039$ or 3.9 %	The grade according to the exercise prescription of P is about 4% ~ 9%.
Answer 2	$\chi = 0.086$ or 8.6 %	

Running

Running is done when a subject's adaptive ability improves after walking. Running is easy to control the speed, it produces a significant effect in a short amount of time, and has many benefits without the need to learn difficult techniques. However, it is advisable to wear appropriate running shoes to absorb impact and to run at a speed that allows conversation with another person. A running distance of 16~25 ㎞ per week is recommended because it does not give joints any load. Beginners should walk or run 100 meters for 50 seconds, intermediate runners for 45 seconds, and advanced runners for 40 seconds. The formula for running is different from that of walking because there are times when both legs are off the ground. In other words, 0.2 ㎖ of oxygen is required to move the body weight horizontally, while 0.9 ㎖ of oxygen, which is half compared to walking, is consumed during vertical movements along a grade [Table 4.3]. However, the formula for running can be applied when on a treadmill or outdoor slope, but not going downhill.

Example Study 3 $\dot{V}O_2$ Calculation Method for Running

Ex. 3 **C is a 26-year-old female member of a low-risk group with a weight of 118 lbs. Currently she is working on a treadmill with a speed of 7 mph and a 3% grade.**

Q What is the gross oxygen consumption and net calories converted by her MET?

Commentary Convert mph, the unit of speed, to $m.min^{-1}$, and convert lbs, which represents body weight, to ㎏.

$$7 \text{ mph} \times 26.8 = 187.6 \text{ m} . \text{min}^{-1}$$
$$118 \text{ lbs} \div 2.2 = 53.6 \text{ kg}$$

$$VO_2 = 3.5 + 0.2 \times (\text{Speed}) + 0.9 \times (\text{Speed}) \times (\text{Grade})$$

$$= 3.5 + 0.2 \times (187.6) + 0.9 \times (187.6) \times (0.03)$$
$$= 3.5 + 37.52 + 5.0652$$
$$\text{Gross } VO_2 = 46.1 \text{ ml.min}^{-1}.\text{kg}^{-1}$$

Answer 1

46.1 ÷ 3.5 = 13.2 METs

$$\text{Net } \dot{V}O_2 = 46.1 - 3.5 = 42.6 \text{ ml.min}^{-1}.\text{kg}^{-1}$$

$$\frac{42.6 \text{ ml} \cdot \text{min}^{-1} \cdot \text{kg}^{-1} \times 53.6 \text{ kg}}{1,000} = 2.283 \ \ell \cdot \text{min}^{-1}$$

Answer 2

$$\mathbf{2.283 \ \ell \cdot min^{-1} \times 5 kcal \ \ell^{-1} = 11.4 \ kcal \cdot min^{-1}}$$

Example Study 4 Workload Calculation Method for Running

Ex 4 **Mr. W (female / 57 years old) is a skilled runner. She is of moderate risk due to her age, but is very healthy and runs 50 to 60 miles per week. She runs on a flat surface, and the pace is about six and a half minutes per mile. W wants to know how much pace he has to maintain to climb the long hills of the upcoming race. For reference, the grade of the hill is 8%, and the $\dot{V}O_2max$ of W is 62 mℓ · min^{-1} · kg^{-1}.**

Q Assuming she can run 75~85% of the VO_2R to extend the race time, what is the speed when climbing the hill?

Commentary1 Initially, convert the units required by the formula. First, convert mph, the unit of speed, to m.min^{-1}, and use the VO_2R formula to calculate the minimum and maximum range of exercise.

$$\text{Target } VO_2 = (\text{Intensity}) \times (VO_2max - 3.5) + 3.5$$
$$\text{Effective limit } VO_2 = (0.75) \times (62 - 3.5) + 3.5 = (0.75) \times (58.5) + 3.5$$
$$= 43.9 + 3.5 = 47.4 \text{ ml.min}^{-1}.\text{kg}^{-1}$$
$$\text{Safe limit } VO_2 = (0.85) \times (62 - 3.5) + 3.5 = (0.85) \times (58.5) + 3.5$$
$$= 49.7 + 3.5 = 53.2 \text{ ml.min}^{-1}.\text{kg}^{-1}$$

Commentary2 Select the running formula in Table 4.3 and assign the lowest and highest values of VO_2 already known.

$$\text{Effective limit } VO_2 = 3.5 + 0.2 \times (\text{Speed}) + 0.9 \times (\text{Speed}) \times (\text{Grade})$$
$$47.4 = 3.5 + 0.2 \times (\text{Speed}) + 0.9 \times (\text{Speed}) \times (0.08)$$
$$47.4 = 3.5 + 0.2 \times (\text{Speed}) + 0.072 \times (\text{Speed})$$
$$47.4 = 3.5 + (0.2 + 0.072) \times (\text{Speed})$$
$$47.4 - 3.5 = 0.272 \times (\text{Speed})$$
$$43.9 = 0.272 \times (\text{Speed})$$
$$43.9 \div 0.272 = \text{Speed}$$
$$\text{Speed} = 161.4 \text{ m . min}^{-1}$$

$$\text{Safe limit } VO_2 = 3.5 + 0.2 \times (\text{Speed}) + 0.9 \times (\text{Speed}) \times (\text{Grade})$$
$$53.2 = 3.5 + 0.2 \times (\text{Speed}) + 0.9 \times (\text{Speed}) \times (0.08)$$
$$53.2 = 3.5 + 0.2 \times (\text{Speed}) + 0.072 \times (\text{Speed})$$
$$53.2 = 3.5 + 0.272 \times (\text{Speed})$$
$$53.2 - 3.5 = 0.272 \times (\text{Speed})$$
$$49.7 = 0.272 \times (\text{Speed})$$
$$49.7 \div 0.272 = \text{Speed}$$
$$\text{Speed} = 182.7 \text{ m . min}^{-1}$$

Commentary3 Use [Table 60] to convert m . min^{-1} to mph.

$$161.4\text{m . min}^{-1} \div 26.8 = \quad \text{mph}$$
$$182.7\text{m . min}^{-1} \div 26.8 = 6.8 \text{ mph}$$

Commentary4 To convert pace mph to mph per minute, divide 60 by mph and change the decimal point to 'minutes: seconds'.

Lower Speed : 60 min/hr ÷ 6.0 miles/hr = min/mile

Upper Speed : 60 min/hr ÷ 6.8 miles/hr = 8.82 min/mile

= 8 min = 0.82 × 60 sec/mile

= 8 min 49 sec/mile

Answer **The speed at which Mr. W can climb the hill with 8% grade is calculated between 8:49 ~ 10:00.**

Cycle Ergometer

In a cycle ergometer, the weight of the upper body is not transmitted to the legs due to the saddle, but this can also contribute to cardiopulmonary endurance as well as the strength of the lower legs as a whole body exercise. It is possible to exercise watching TV, listening to music, or reading the newspaper at home, regardless of the cold winter or hot summer. It provides a convenient way to exercise. While sitting on the saddle, let the knees extend to about 120° and adjust the pedals to make the subject feel comfortable. Also, gently hold the handle in a relaxed posture.

Example Study 5 VO_2 Calculation Method of Indoor Biking

Ex. 5 G is a 37-year-old female member of a moderate-risk group with a weight of 173 lbs. Currently, she is working on a Monark bike for weight loss with a rotation speed of 50 rpm and a resistance value of 3 ㎏.

Q How many minutes does she need to ride a bicycle to burn 1 lbs of fat?

Commentary1 Convert lb, representing body weight, to ㎏.

$$173 \text{ lbs} \div 2.2 = 78.6 \text{ kg}$$

$$\begin{aligned}\text{Workload} &= (\text{Resistance value}) \times (\text{Flywheel distance per revolution}) \times (\text{Number of rotations})\\ &= 3 \text{ kg} \times 6 \text{ m} \times 50 \text{ rpm}\\ &= 900 \text{ kgm} \cdot \text{min}^{-1}\end{aligned}$$

Commentary2 Select the bicycle formula in [Table 4.3] and calculate VO_2.

$$\begin{aligned}VO_2 &= 7 + 1.8 \times (\text{Workload}) / (\text{Weight})\\ &= 7 + 1.8 \times (900) / 78.6\\ &= 7 + 1620 / 78.6\\ &= 7 + 20.6\\ &= 27.6 \text{ ml} \cdot \text{min}^{-1} \cdot \text{kg}^{-1}\end{aligned}$$

Commentary3 As a problem of weight loss, VO_2 is marked as Net VO_2, and later converted to $\ell \cdot \text{min}^{-1}$ and $\text{kcal} \cdot \text{min}^{-1}$.

$$\text{Net } VO_2 = 27.6 - 3.5 = 24.1 \text{ ml} \cdot \text{min}^{-1} \cdot \text{kg}^{-1}$$

$$\frac{24.1 \text{ ml} \cdot \text{min}^{-1} \cdot \text{kg}^{-1} \times 78.6 \text{ kg}}{1000} = 1.894 \ \ell \cdot \text{min}^{-1}$$

$$1.894 \ \ell \cdot \text{min}^{-1} \times 5 \text{ kcal} \cdot \ell^{-1} = 9.47 \text{ kcal} \cdot \text{min}^{-1}$$

Answer Since 1lbs of fat corresponds to about 3,500 ㎉, 3,500 ㎉ / 9.47 ㎉min^{-1} = 370 min (About 6 hours)

Riding a no-load cycle requires much more work than sitting comfortably. In fact, cycling consumes about 1MET (3.5 ㎖/kg/min) of oxygen when peddling at 50~60 rpm (revolution/meter).[4-6] Therefore, the bicycle metabolic formula presented in [Table 4.3] calculates about 7 mℓ/kg/min, plus the resting oxygen uptake of 3.5 mℓ/kg/min and the no-load pedaling oxygen uptake of 3.5 mℓ/kg/min. On the other hand, 1.8 mℓ of oxygen per workload (kg · m) is required for the load of cycling, which corresponds to a vertical workload during walking or stepping. However, this figure is converted based on 60 rpm, and if people peddle faster than 60 rpm, the oxygen consumption of the no-load cycle will be even higher. However, the factor for cycling with a load decreases compensatively when the number of revolutions (cadence) increases. Therefore, when increasing the number of revolutions to at least 90 rpm, a single formula needs to be rationalized. The cycling performed in most facilities does not show the power, but only the resistance (kg) and RPM (cadence). The workload can be calculated by work-rate as follows.

Work-rate = (Resistance value) × (Flywheel distance per revolution) × (Number of revolutions)

In the formula, the unit of work-rate is kgm/min. Moreover, the flywheel is calculated as a meter (m) when pedaling once, which is converted to almost 6 m using only the Monark leg ergometer. The other model is about 3 m. Many cycles show power in watts (1 watt is approximately 6 kgm/min).

Muscle Strength Exercise

Muscle strength refers to how force can be exerted through one contraction. It is proportional to the muscle's thickness or cross-sectional area. That is, the larger the muscle volume, the greater the force. The reason for the increase in muscle strength through exercise is that the contractile protein of the muscle fiber increases, the muscle becomes thicker, the mobilization ability of the muscle fiber is improved, and many muscle fibers can contract simultaneously. The details are as follows.

Factors of Muscle Strength

Cause of Hypertrophy

Exercise for muscle strengthening results in muscular hypertrophy. Muscles are composed of many muscle fibers. Among them, thin fibers range from 10~60 μ, and thick fibers are about 150 μ. Thin and thick muscle fibers are both involved before exercise, but during exercising, the proportion of thick fibers generally increase. So far, muscular hypertrophy is thought to be caused by the thickening of muscle fibers. However, in recent years, the growth in the number of muscle fibers has been proven through animal experiments.

Strength and Protein

During muscle strength training, protein acts as an energy source that can supply ATP for muscle contraction. Proteins are used as a fuel for exercise. It was found that protein supplies only 3~6% of total energy expenditure during exercise and 4.8% of total energy expenditure in protein metabolism. These results are relatively small compared to the use of 14.1% at rest. Thus, it can be seen that protein is not a relatively important energy source during endurance exercise compared to fat and carbohydrates. On the other hand, amino acids play a very important role in endurance exercise as a precursor of glucose synthesis to prevent hypoglycemia. Hypoglycemia has been considered as a factor in increasing fatigue, and this fact indicates the importance of glucose homeostasis in neural tissue. Blood glucose is supplied from liver glycogen in the early stages of endurance exercise. However, when the liver glycogen is depleted, glucoseneogenesis is gradually activated. In other words, protein plays a supporting role as an energy source during exercise.

Increase in Capillary Network Distribution

The hypertrophy of skeletal muscle, which occurs during muscle strength exercise, is generally increased with the number of capillary blood vessels. To sustain exercise or to exert more power, the transport of an energy source is required. The blood flow responsible for the transport of this energy source must increase flow to the deepest part of the muscle. Muscle vessels developed through muscle strength training surround each motor fiber, whereas untrained fibers have a small amount of capillaries surrounding the muscle fibers. The increase in muscle fibers is proportional to the increase in the capillary network. Increased capillary vessels per muscle fiber allows for more active oxygen and nutrient supplies and the removal of byproducts from muscles.

Types of Exercises to Improve Muscle Strength

Everyone gets weaker with age. As a result, the development of poor posture results in injuries associated with the muscle joints. A simple and basic method for preventing and treating muscular weakness is through muscle strengthening exercises. There are two

Upper Body Exercise

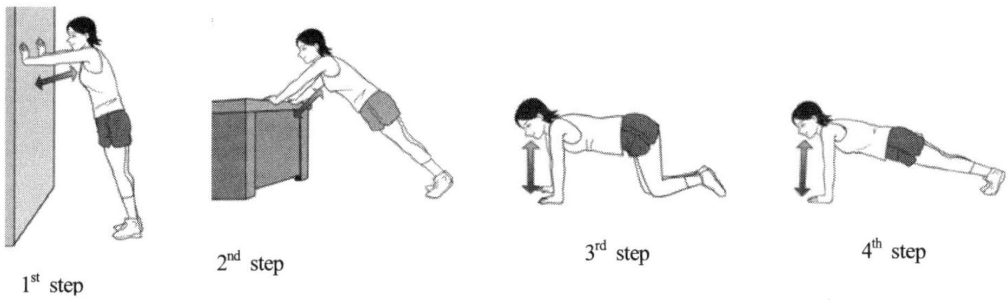

Fig. 4.3 ***Upper body exercises***

① Stand up against the wall and push up, ② Push up on desk, ③ Knee push-up, ④ Push up on the ground. You have to start with the steps that are right for you and try to develop them into difficult steps. The main stimulus and developmental muscles are pectoralis muscle, triceps, and anterior deltoid.

Trunk Exercise – I

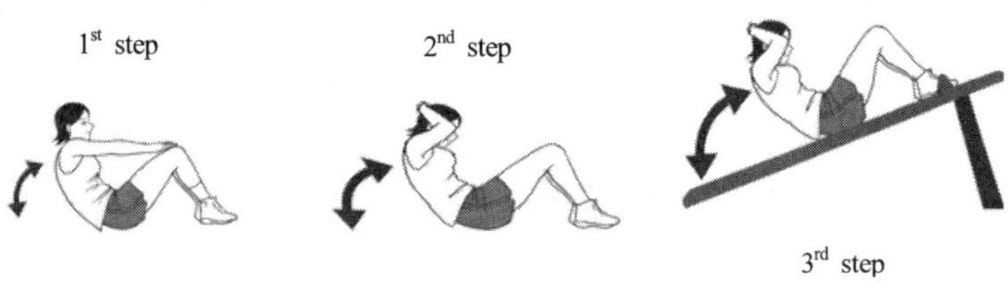

Fig. 4.4 ***Abdominal exercises***

① Lie down and stretch arms toward knees, ② Lying down, put both hands on the head and sit-ups, ③ Sit-ups in sloping places. You have to start with the steps that are right for you and try to develop them into difficult steps. The main stimulus and developmental muscles are the rectus abdominis muscle, external oblique muscle of abdomen, quadriceps muscle and musculus tensor fasciae latae.

Trunk Exercise – II

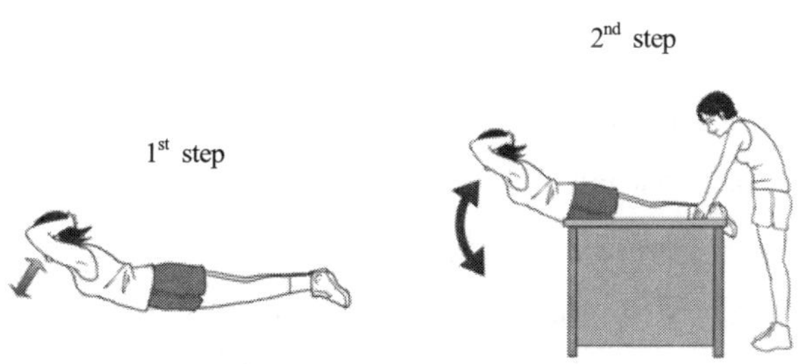

Fig. 4.5 ***Trunk exercises***

① Lie on one's stomach and raise upper body, ② Lie on one's stomach on the desk and raise upper body. You have to start with the steps that are right for you and try to develop them into difficult steps. Major stimulus and developmental muscles are gluteus maximus, semimembranosus muscle, biceps femoris, Iliocostalis lumborum, iliocostris thoracis, spinal erector muscle and lumbar quadrate muscle.

Lower Body Exercise

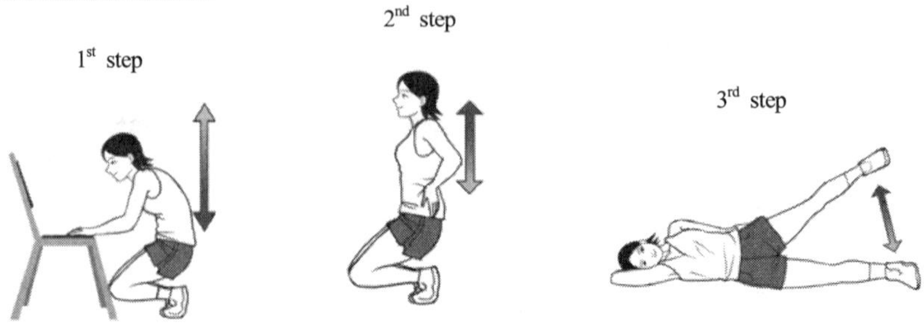

Fig. 4.6 Lower body exercises

① Standing and sitting on the floor grasping a chair and ② Standing and sitting on the floor grasping waists can develop gluteal muscles and leg muscles (quadriceps and hamstrings). ③ Raising legs on sideways gluteal maximum, gluteal medium, and tensor fasciae latae.

types of exercises for improving muscle strength: 'weight bearing training' using body weight and 'weight training' using weights. In general, for a beginner who starts exercise for the first time, it is more effective to maintain and improve muscle strength while avoiding injury by using their own weight, without using special equipment.

Weight Bearing Training

Weight bearing training starts from the easiest of the various types of exercises listed in [Fig. 4.3] to [Fig. 4.11] and proceeds to more difficult types. The number of repetitions for each exercise should be 1 or 2 sets of 8~10 repetitions. Once accustomed, the difficulty can be raised by performing 3~4 sets of 12~15 repetitions.

Weight Training

It is desirable to perform resistance training using a free weight or a machine after weight training using body is completed. Specifically, the speed is repeated at a rate of about once every two seconds while maintaining a constant rhythm. During exercise, take about 1~2 minutes to relieve fatigue. It is effective to perform this training initially for 1~2 days per week, gradually increasing to 3~4 days per week for at least 4~8 weeks. It is recommended to perform regular exercise at least once or twice a week because muscle strength reduces rapidly when training is stopped for a long period of time. Beginners should be careful because muscle pain or spasticity can occur if excessive training is performed from the beginning. In order to avoid such an unfortunate event, it is essential to receive proper training in posture from experts before exercise, and to warm-up and cool-down before and after work-out. It is also essential to adequately stretch the muscle group before exercise. Before exercising with equipment, be sure to perform 1RM test and the necessary training to accomplish the goal. It is recommended to consult with experts about what muscle function components to focus on, which are presented in [Table 4.5].[2]

Table 4.5 ***Relationship between maximum percentage of muscle strength and maximum number of repetitions***

※ The set is 3~4 times, but it increases with the trainers.

Type	Speed	Workload	Ratio (%)	Repetition (times)	Rest Time (min)	Myofunctional Component (muscle fiber)
Endurance	Low to Medium	Low	40	80~100	1~2	Muscle endurance (Type I)
			50	40~50	1~2	
Muscle strength	Low to Medium	Medium	60	25	2	Muscular hypertrophy (Type IIa/IIb)
			65	20~25	2	
			70	15	2	
			75	10~12	2	
	Low to Medium	Heavy	80	8~10	3~5	Maximum muscle strength Muscle power (Type IIb)
			85	6	3~5	
			90	4	3~7	
			95	2~3	3~7	
Power	Low	Maximum	100	1	4~5/7	

Precautions for Strength Training

- Dressing during training should be comfortable and should be made from cotton that has good sweat absorption.
- After relaxation of the muscle joints by stretching, perform the weight machine or free-weight exercise 8 times lightly.
- When finishing the strength training, cool down by stretching and take moderate amounts of water.
- If you stop breathing while giving strength to your muscles, it may cause temporary dizziness, so breathe naturally.
- Breath out when contracting muscles and breath in when relaxing muscles.
- Severe strength training is a great burden on the heart, so people with hypertension or heart problems should avoid.
- Exercising after a meal is a burden on the digestive system and restricts exercise, so it should be done an hour after a meal.

1RM Direct Measurement Method

Direct measurement is time-consuming but relatively accurate. However, if the 1RM test is not possible, it is preferable to set the weight according to the indirect measurement method.

1RM Indirect Measurement Method

Indirect measurement is a method that can estimate 1RM using only one repetition frequency by using a randomly selected weight. When planning weight training exercises for a team, it has the advantage of being able to determine each individual's maximum strength within a short time. Indirect measurement is applied to the general public rather than athletes. It is used as an estimation method when weight training is performed to promote health through muscle strengthening.

For example, assume that a person has been given 30 ㎏ of W0 (random weight) 15 reps. Then, the weight that the person can lift is W1 = 30 ㎏ × 0.025 × 15 reps, or 11.25 ㎏. 1RM = W0 + W1, so 30 ㎏ + 11.25 ㎏ = 41.25 ㎏, which is 1RM. Strength exercises have many benefits for everyone. However, since it is easy to incur injuries, it is advisable to keep in mind the precautions to be followed during exercise.

Isometric Muscle Strength Training

Isometric strength training is used when there is no time to exercise or for rehabilitation when there is a problem with a specific muscle joint. As a matter of note, isometric training can cause Valsalva maneuver, so be sure to breathe out during training and keep it for less than 10 seconds. Repeat this method three to five times.

Procedures and Precautions for Direct Measurement

- Choose a light weight and prepare doing 6~10 reps, then rest for 5 minutes.
- Select any weight that can be lifted more than 4 reps.
- Rest in 1~2 minutes in the middle of the measurement and increase the weight by 5 ㎏ each one.
- Once the weight that can be lifted at most once is determined, it is called 1RM.
- Train the muscle function to develop with reference to the items in [Table 4.5].

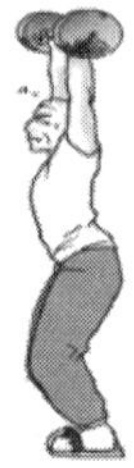

Procedures and Precautions for Indirect Measurement

- Select the random weight (the weight that can be lifted to 10 reps or less).
- After performing the maximum repetitive exercise, the random weight and the number of repetitions are substituted into the estimated equation below.
- 1RM = W0 (random weight) + W1 (weight lifted)
- W1 = W0 × 0.025 × R (the number of repetitions)

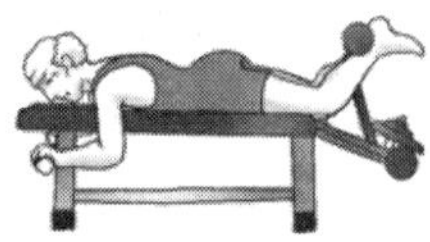

Upper Extremity Exercise – I

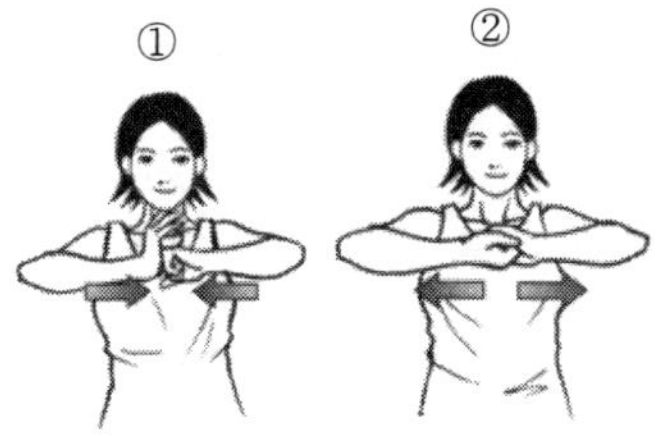

Fig. 4.7 ***Upper extremity exercise 1***

① Two-handed Push : Hold your arms horizontally and bend your arms. One hand holds your fist, and the other hand gives strength to each other. Change the shape of the hand and repeat. The stimulation site is the thorax and the shoulder. ② Two-handed Pull : With both arms flat, bend your arms and pull your left and right fingers together. Repeat with changing hand shape up and down. Stimulation sites are upper back and forearm muscles.

Upper Extremity Exercise – II

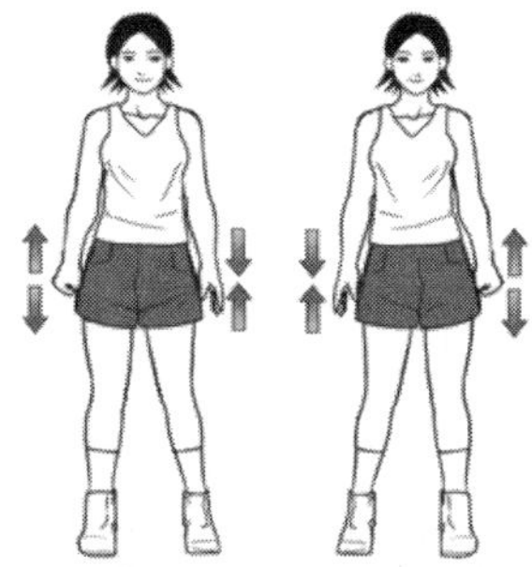

Fig. 4.8 ***Grasping a fist***

With both arms naturally lowered, hold your fist and hold your fist as tight as possible. The stimulation site is the forearm muscles

Upper Extremity Exercise - III

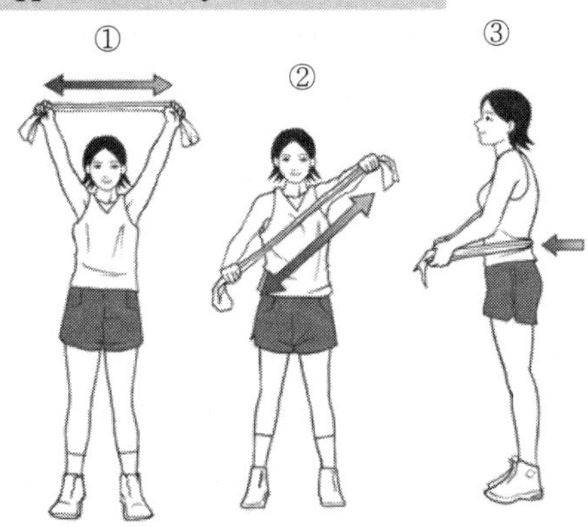

Fig. 4.9 ***Upper extremity exercise 3***

① Spread Arms over Head : Raise your arm over your head, hold the towel or strap with your hands and pull it outward. Change the direction of the palm and repeat. Developmental sites are the neck and forearm. ② Pull the Arms Apart : Squeeze the towel and pull it up and down. Developmental sites are the shoulder and neck. ③ Waist Pull : Naturally, in a posture that gives strength to the waist, hold the towel behind your waist with both hands and slowly pull it forward. Stimulation areas are abdomen, back, chest, and forearm.

Trunk and Lower Extremity Exercise

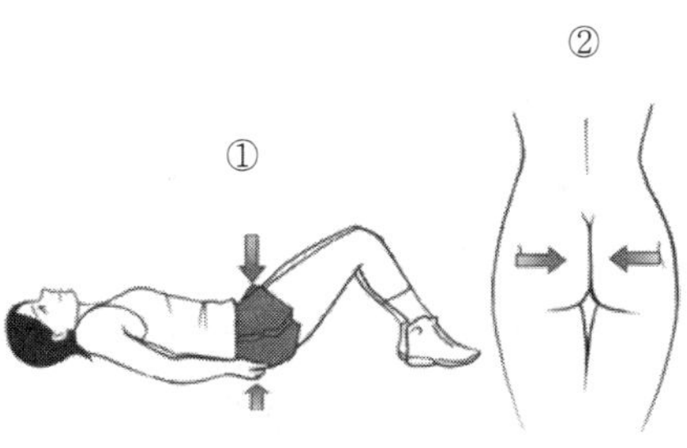

Fig. 4.10 ***Trunk and lower extremity exercise***

① Lie Down and Press Pelvis : Naturally lie down, kneeling, and pushing the belly and buttocks with force. Stimulation sites are the upper arm, the forearm, and the femur. ② Tighten and Loosen Hip : Lie down on the stomach naturally and apply force to my buttocks. The developmental region is the buttocks.

Lower Extremity Exercise

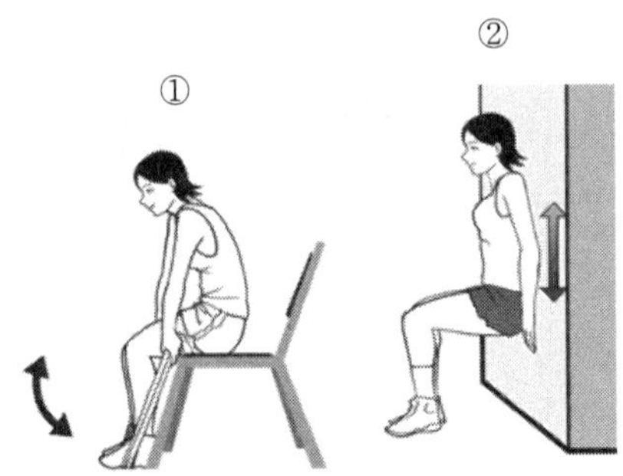

Fig. 4.11 ***Lower extremity exercise***

① Unfold and Fold Legs : With your knees flexed slightly, step on foot with a cord or a towel, then hold it with both hands and naturally unfold your legs. Developmental sites are shoulder, leg, and buttocks.

② Sit Down and Stand Up with the Back on the Wall: Sit down with the back against the wall. Do not bend your knees too much at first, but gradually bend your knees as you become accustomed. Developmental areas are the femur, lower leg, and buttocks.

Weight Training

Weight training involves adding weight to increase muscle strength. Since muscle strength depends on the magnitude of the tension exerted by muscle contraction, the training method varies depending on the target muscle type. In general, the types of muscle contraction can be divided into isotonic, isometric, and isokinetic contractions. The effect of muscle training methods for each muscle contraction type has unique characteristics and their pros and cons. In order to carry out the weight training safely and effectively, it is preferable to exercise according to specific, progressive, and overloading principles of exercise prescription.

Specific Principle

Strength training requires high-intensity static training or high intensity and low repetition programs. In order to perform strength training properly, it is necessary to understand the specific principle. First, the increase in muscle strength through weight training differs depending not only on the muscle group, but also on the type of motion. In other words, when you want to improve the strength of a specific muscle, only the corresponding part develops, and the body adapts only to that specific training. Therefore, if a patient does not have a particularly unbalanced wound or injured area, it is recommended to perform training each body part evenly. Second, the specific principle applies to the speed of muscle contraction and ROM. In other words, isometric movements mainly develop only at the moving joint angles, and isokinetic movements develop only at the applied contraction speed. In order to compensate for this, isometric exercise must be performed at various angles and isokinetic exercise should be performed at various angular speeds.

Progressive Principle

Strength training improves muscle strength by performing a number of sets and repetitions according to the load imposed at the beginning. However, if the number of sets and repetitions initially imposed do not increase and the fixed program continues, it is hard to expect further progress. Therefore, the proper number of sets and repetitions should be re-prescribed. In other words, the number of sets and repetitions prescribed at the beginning of training must be increased deliberately because they become low loads over time. Generally, in the conditioning phase, 1~2 sets of 8~10 repetitions is prescribed depending on the weight, and then 2~3 sets of 12~15 repetitions is prescribed in the improvement phase. For reference, if the initially prescribed weight can be lifted more than 15 reps, the weight should be increased according to the overload principle.

Overload Principle

Muscle strength improves when training with loads greater than those at rest. Exercise intensity to develop muscle strength is about 60~95% of 1RM. Specifically, a load of 60~75% improves muscle strength, and a load of 80~95% improves maximum muscle strength and muscle power. For example, according to the principle of overload, when a patient with low back pain starts exercising at 60% of 1RM on a back extension machine to develop the lumbar extension muscle around the backbone erector, increasing the weight to 70% after 4 weeks of exercise will improve muscle strength. For reference, the overload principle should be considered after the number of sets and repetitions have increased.

Composition of Training

An ideal weight training program should include at least one motion for the body's limbs, trunk, chest, and other major muscles. In order to avoid accumulation of fatigue in the muscles, the exercise sequence should be arranged so that the same muscles are not used consecutively. The general training sequence is shown in [Table 4.6].

Table 4.6 ***General sequence of training***

Order	Training site	Equipments
①	Femur and hip joint	Leg curl/ squats
②	Thorax and upper arm	Bent-arm pullover/ bench press/ incline press
③	Back muscle and hamstring	Squats/ stiff-legged dead lift/ back extension
④	Lower legs and ankles	Toe raise/ squats
⑤	Shoulder and Triceps	Bent-over row/ press behind neck/ triceps
⑥	Abdomen	Bent-knee sit ups
⑦	Forearm	Arm curl
⑧	Wrist	Wrist curl/ wrist rollers

Muscle Endurance Exercise

Muscle endurance refers to the ability to move certain muscles for a prolonged period of time without becoming exhausted. It is necessary to strengthen muscular endurance in order to exercise more effectively or to improve athletic ability. The muscle endurance strengthening method includes using one's own weight, and a method using weights and resistance equipment. The former provides a method for those who do not exercise regularly without the need for special equipment, and the latter is effective for those with a special purpose of training specific muscles.

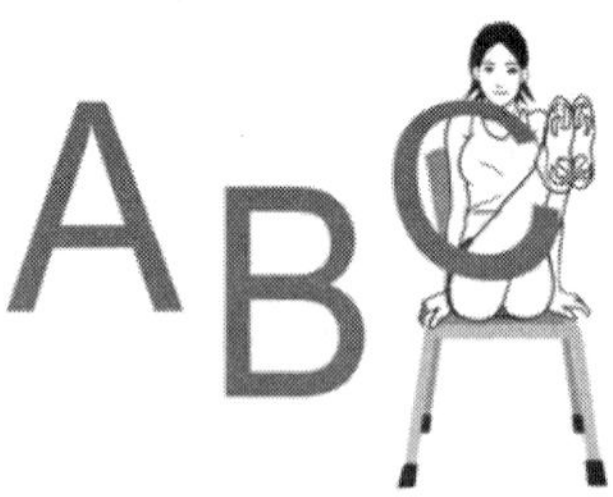

In order to improve muscular endurance, it is effective to reduce resistance and increase the number of repetitions as much as possible. At first, perform each type of exercise at the easiest level of 1~2 sets of 10~15 repetitions. Once the body adapts, bring it up to the next level of 3~4 sets of 20~30 repetitions. For each motion, the movement should be repeated at a rate of about once every 2 seconds, maintaining a constant rhythm. In this way, beginners should exercise one or two times a week for the first time, and then train every other day when they get used to it. Most muscle endurance training is almost identical to weight bearing strength training. That is, the training exercises are the same, but their attributes are different. As a matter of note, muscle endurance training using body weight can be somewhat boring, so it is advisable to apply abdominal exercises to interesting movements as shown in the picture. The details are as follows.

- Muscle endurance refers to the ability to move certain muscles for a long time without exhaustion.
- Muscle endurance training includes weight bearing and resistance training in the same way as strength training.
- Muscle endurance training uses the same motions and instruments used for strength training.
- It is the difference from strength training exercises is that the weight is decreased and the number of repetitions is increased.
- Begin with 1~2 sets of 10~15 RM, then increase 3~4 sets of 20~30 RM.
- It takes a lot of time and is a good idea to include interesting motions to keep subjects interested.

Factors of Muscle Endurance

Increase in Rate of Muscle Blood Flow and Capillaries

Muscle endurance refers to how long a muscle can sustain muscle contraction. In other words, the improvement of this ability is based on the improvement of the energy transport system and the consumption system. In fact, muscle blood flow should be increased to improve oxygen delivery capacity in the muscles. Increased muscle blood flow during exercise is possible by increasing the number of capillaries. An increase in capillary blood flow means that blood vessels that are closed are opened. Through training, the number of capillaries can be increased by about 50%.

Increase in Intramuscular Oxygen Consumption

The intramuscular oxygen consumption is the difference in oxygen content between the arterial blood and the venous blood. This is called 'arteriovenous oxygen difference'. The larger the difference, the greater the oxygen utilization of the muscles and the better the muscular endurance. The intramuscular oxygen uptake increases in proportion to the intensity of exercise, but there is a limit, so the increase in muscle blood flow as described above is a prerequisite.

Increase in Oxygen Diffusion Capacity

The oxygen that the blood carries is spread to the muscle tissue by the difference of the oxygen partial pressure between the arterial blood and the tissue. The diffusion capacity of muscle tissue depends on the degree of capillary development. Increased capillary blood circulation allows the contact surface of arterial blood and muscle tissue to become wider, making oxygen exchange easier.

Psychological Tolerance

The ability of human beings to exert their power has the physiological threshold of the human body and the psychological limit point which depends on the excitement level of the cerebral cortex or central nervous system. In fact, even if the physiological limits are the same, the psychological limits vary greatly depending on the individual's desire or will. Therefore, the power of human beings can be greatly restricted by psychological limits. In particular, muscular endurance exercises, which maintain long-term muscle contractions, cannot achieve good results unless psychological resistance (or willpower) is high. Therefore, to develop muscular endurance, patients need to strengthen their minds.

Considerations for Muscle Endurance Training

The weight training prescription for muscle endurance generally reduces the load intensity and lengthens the exercise time compared to the exercise prescription for muscle strength. For reference, muscular endurance type weight training for general people or patients who are not athletes, is circuit training. Specific considerations are as follows.

Exercise Intensity

In the exercise prescription for muscle endurance, it is important to choose a weight that does not inhibit muscle blood flow during exercise. That is, a light load should be used. According to one study, 25%, 33%, and 50% of maximum strength were used for endurance training, and the most effective load was 25%. In other words, a load of 25% of the maximum strength is a weight that does not inhibit blood flow and is an effective load that can develop muscle endurance.

Exercise Duration

Exercise duration is the most important factor in muscular endurance training. According to one study, the maximum repetition frequency was measured at a rate of 60 repetitions per minute with an exercise intensity corresponding to 1/3 of the maximum strength, with the exercise being repeated at 25%, 33%, and 50% until fatigue. The results showed the improvement of muscle endurance in the exercise method that had the longest exercise time. In addition, the relationship between the intensity of muscular contraction and blood flow during muscle endurance training showed that the increase in blood flow was observed from the start of exercise to about 60 seconds and thereafter, blood flow did not increase significantly. Ultimately, the exercise duration for muscle endurance training should be more than 60 seconds, which is sufficient for vasodilation, and should be sustained until exhaustion at a rate of 60 repetitions per minute.

Exercise Frequency

According to studies on exercise frequency for muscle endurance training, it is appropriate to exercise almost every day of the week. Because muscle endurance training is the training of local muscle groups, even though exercise continues until exhaustion unlike cardiopulmonary endurance training, fatigue recovery speed is fast. According to one study, an intensity of 1/3 of maximum strength, performed until exhaustion at a rate of 60 repetitions per minute, 6 times a week, was more effective than 3 days per week.

Circuit Weight Training

Circuit weight training is a method that combines circuit training concepts with weight training. While circuit training emphasizes the development of various physical factors centered on cardiopulmonary function, circuit weight training aims to enhance cardiorespiratory function along with muscle endurance and other muscular system development. Although the training described so far is primarily single-purpose training, circuit weight training is multipurpose and can be called 'comprehensive training' covering most of the fitness elements. Because circuit weight training is able to address most of the fitness factors, it is thought to be a suitable method for basic physical strength and rehabilitation training that is time-efficient in clinical practice. On the other hand, an example of circuit weight training is shown in [Fig. 4.12], and the factors to be considered for the load are as follows.

Arrangement of Activities

The goal of circuit weight training is muscle endurance training of the entire body. Therefore, it should be arranged so that the load is not concentrated on a specific muscle group, but in a way that promotes balanced development of various parts. If the aim is to strengthen the upper limb muscles through bench presses, it is important to perform squats to enhance lower limb muscles and to develop balance between flexor and extensor muscles.

Circuit Stations and Order

In circuit weight training, the short-term, mid-term, and long-term types include 6, 9, and 12 stations, respectively. Training should be based on the functional ability and physical strength of the patients and the general public. The order of physical factors to be emphasized are muscle endurance, cardiopulmonary endurance, and muscle strength.[7]

Determination of Training Volume

In regards to the training volume of circuit weight training, 25~30% of 1RM is appropriate for exercise intensity, but should be adjusted to 40~50% if the subject can lift more than once per second. At this time, if the number of repetition is 30, the exercise time should be one muscle contraction / relaxation per second. On the other hand, it is necessary to shorten the rest time between each item to prevent the decrease of muscle blood flow. The number of sets can vary depending on the subject's physical fitness level, but in the case of the general public, two or three sets are preferred. Lastly, it should be performed for at least six weeks in order for results to appear.

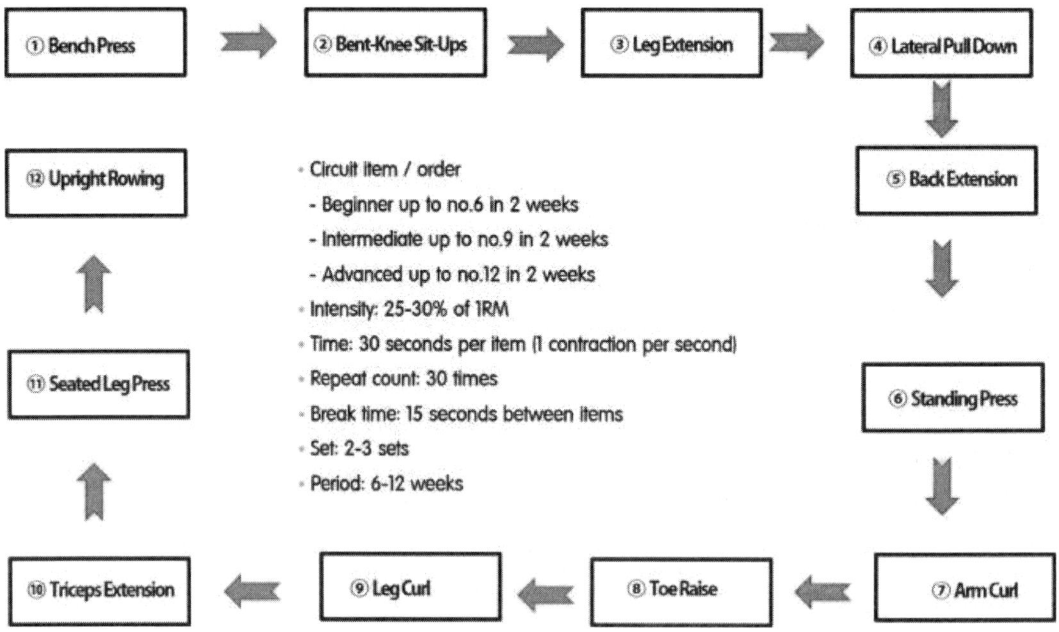

Fig. 4.12 ***Circuit weight training***

❖ Study Questions

1. What is the preferred stretching method in the hospital? (*A*)

   A. Static stretching
   B. Dynamic stretching
   C. PNF
   D. All Stretching

2. Which type is not PNF? (*C*)

   A. Hold-relax technique
   B. Hold-relax-contract technique
   C. Hold-contract technique
   D. Hold-relax-swing technique

3. Which method is wrong with the static stretching method? (*B*)

   A. Gently stretch the muscles and hold the state for 10 seconds.
   B. Breathing maintains inspiration when the muscles are stretched.
   C. If you feel pain, stretch a little less.
   D. In the case of the elderly, the total stretching time should be reduced by 20%.

4. When a beginner starts to exercise, a weight bearing method is recommended first. It is desirable to perform (*1~2*) sets of (*8~10*) repetitions of initial exercise.

5. If a beginner starts using muscle strength exercise, he must measure 1RM. Which statements are wrong with that? (*A, C, D*)

   A. Using a light weight, warm up with 6 to 10 exercises and then rest for 1 minute.
   B. Lift the random weights that can be lifted more than 4 repetitions.
   C. Place the appropriate rest in the middle of the measurement and increase the weight by 10 kg and lift it one time.
   D. Muscular hypertrophy requires 80~95% of 1RM and 8~12 repetitions.

6. If 1RM cannot be measured directly, the indirect measurement should be used. Assuming that A person lifts 50kg and repeats 20 reps, the weight that person can actually lift is (*75*) kg.

7. What are the precautions for strength training? (*A, D*)

   A. If you stop breathing during muscle contraction, you will have a temporary stroke, so you should breathe naturally.
   B. It is recommended that patients with hypertension or heart disease should refrain from using excessive exercise because it stimulates the heart.
   C. Athletic attire should not limit exercising and be made of sweat-absorbing cotton.
   D. Exercising after meals is a burden on your heart, so it is best to do it in 1 to 2 hours.

8. Muscle endurance exercise is performed by one or two sets of easy initial steps 10 to 15 reps, and when skillful, it is increased to (*3~4*) sets (*20~30*) reps.

9. Cardiopulmonary endurance exercise is in other words called aerobic capacity or (*systemic*) endurance exercise.

10. Changes in the human body through cardiopulmonary endurance training include increased $\dot{V}O_2max$, (*maximum cardiac output*), and respiration volume.

11. (*Fartlek training*) is a method of training athletes or trained people using natural environments such as coastal roads and lawns.

12. MET is the term to describe calories consumed by your body weight per hour, also called metabolism equivalence or (*energy expenditure*).

13. When managing patients with MET, the level of expert observation required is less than (*8*) METs.

14. A is a 45-year-old male, weighing 170 lbs, treadmill walking with a speed of 4 mph and a 7% grade. The gross oxygen consumption of this person is (*27.7*) $m\ell \cdot kg^{-1} \cdot min^{-1}$, Net $\dot{V}O_2$ is (*24.2*) $m\ell \cdot kg^{-1} \cdot min^{-1}$, Net calories are (*9.4*) $kcal \cdot min^{-1}$.

15. B is a 30-year-old male, weighing 200 lbs, treadmill walking with a speed of 5 mph and a 3% grade. The gross oxygen consumption of this person is (*24.1*) $m\ell \cdot kg^{-1} \cdot min^{-1}$, Net $\dot{V}O_2$ is (*20.6*) $m\ell \cdot kg^{-1} \cdot min^{-1}$, Net calories are (*9.3*) $kcal \cdot min^{-1}$.

16. C is a 22-year-old male, weighing 150 lbs, treadmill walking with a speed of 4.5 mph and a 5% grade. The gross oxygen consumption of this person is (*26.4*) $m\ell \cdot kg^{-1} \cdot min^{-1}$, Net $\dot{V}O_2$ is (*22.9*) $m\ell \cdot kg^{-1} \cdot min^{-1}$, Net calories are (*7.8*) $kcal \cdot min^{-1}$.

17. A (male / 32) is a patient who underwent heart transplantation. There is little change in heart rate from rest to exercise, and $\dot{V}O_2max$ is 40 $m\ell \cdot kg^{-1} \cdot min^{-1}$. Therefore, the doctor encouraged him to exercise under supervision at the cardiac rehabilitation center, 40~60% of $\dot{V}O_2R$. If A feels comfortable walking at 3 mph, treadmill slope should be adjusted to (*4.3*) ~ (*9.3*)%.

18. B (male / 35) is a patient who underwent heart transplantation. There is little

change in heart rate from rest to exercise, and $\dot{V}O_2max$ is 30 mℓ·kg^{-1}·min^{-1}. Therefore, the doctor encouraged him to exercise under supervision at the cardiac rehabilitation center, 40~60% of $\dot{V}O_2R$. If B feels comfortable walking at 2 mph, treadmill slope should be adjusted to (*5.4*) ~ (*10.9*)%.

19. D is a 28-year-old female who is a member of a low-risk group with a weight of 120 lbs. Currently, she is working on a treadmill with a speed of 7 mph and a 2% slope. Her gross oxygen consumption in terms of her METs is (*12.7*) METs, and her net calorie consumption is 11.2 ㎉·min^{-1}.

20. C (female / 46) is running 70~80 miles per week on a flat surface, and the pace is 10 seconds per mile. The slope of the hill is 6%, and $\dot{V}O_2max$ is mℓ·kg^{-1}·min^{-1}. Assuming she can run 80~90% of the $\dot{V}O_2R$ to extend the time of the race, the speed of climbing the hill should be adjusted from (*4*) minutes (*41*) seconds to (*5*) minutes (*19*) seconds.

21. G is a 35-year-old woman who is a member of the moderate-risk group with a weight of 180 lbs. Currently, she is working on a Monark bicycle for weight loss at 65 rpm and a resistance of 2 ㎏. In order for her to burn 1 lbs of fat, she must ride a bicycle for about (*413*) minutes.

22. B is a 21-year-old woman who is a member of the moderate-risk group with a weight of 125 lbs. Currently, she is working on a Monark bicycle for weight loss at 80 rpm and a resistance of 6 ㎏. In order for her to burn 1 lbs of fat, she must ride a bicycle for about (*130*) minutes.

23. F is a 60-year-old woman who is a member of the moderate-risk group with a weight of 100 lbs. Currently, she is working on a Monark bicycle for weight loss at 33 rpm and a resistance of 5 ㎏. In order for her to burn 1 lbs of fat, she must ride a bicycle for about (*360*) minutes.

24. J is a 24-year-old woman who is a member of the moderate-risk group with a weight of 200 lbs. Currently, she is working on a Monark bicycle for weight loss at 26 rpm and a resistance of 8 ㎏. In order for her to burn 1 lbs of fat, she must ride a bicycle for about (*273*) minutes.

25. I is a 44-year-old woman who is a member of a moderate-risk group with a

weight of 144 lbs. Currently, she is working on a Monark bike for weight loss at 55 rpm and a resistance of 7 kg. In order for her to burn 1 lb of fat, she must ride a bicycle for about (*160*) minutes.

26. To develop muscle endurance with weight training, exercise intensity should be (*40~50*) percents.

27. To develop muscular hypertrophy with weight training, exercise intensity should be (*60~75*) percents.

28. To develop muscle power with weight training, exercise intensity should be (*80~100*) percents.

29. The order of weight training is ① the femur and hip joint ② the thorax and upper arm ③ (*latissimus dorsi and hamstring muscle*) ④ the lower leg and ankle ⑤ the shoulder and triceps ⑥ (*the abdomen*) ⑦ the forearm and ⑧ (*wrist*).

30. Weight training that can comprehensively develop the physical fitness level including cardiopulmonary function is called (*circuit*) training.

Chapter 5

Clinical Sports Medicine

Goals

- To understand the causes of metabolic diseases such as obesity, diabetes, and hyperlipidemia and to learn the advantages of exercise.
- To understand the causes of heart disease, including hypertension, and to learn how to treat them accordingly.
- To understand the causes and types of lung diseases and to learn how to deal with them.
- To understand the causes of musculoskeletal disorders such as joint disease, osteoporosis, and back pain and to learn the principles of exercise prescription.
- To understand the causes of cancer and strokes and to learn about coping strategies.

Obesity

Definition and Causes of Obesity

Obesity is a disease that occurs when the energy intake exceeds the energy expenditure, which is a serious disease that can cause of all kinds of chronic degenerative

Table 5.1 *Normal range of BMI according to age*

Age	BMI (kg/m²)
19~24	19~24
25~34	20~25
35~44	21~26
45~54	22~27
55~64	23~28
65≤	24~29

diseases.[1] The definition of obesity refers to when the body fat mass exceeds 25% of the body weight for men and 30% for women.[18] When the body mass index (BMI) exceeds 30 kg/m^2 regardless of gender, it is called obesity. However, since the normal range of BMI (18.5~24.9 kg/m^2) is affected by age, it is recommended to refer to [Table 5.1].[57]

The fat distribution of obese patients varies according to gender. However,

What is Heredity?

DNA (Deoxyribose Nucleic Acid)

DNA consists of a double helix strand in which two long chains are connected by deoxyribose and phosphate. These chains are composed by four bases: adenine (A), thymine (T), guanine (G), and cytosine (C). Adenine binds to thymine and guanine binds to cytosine.

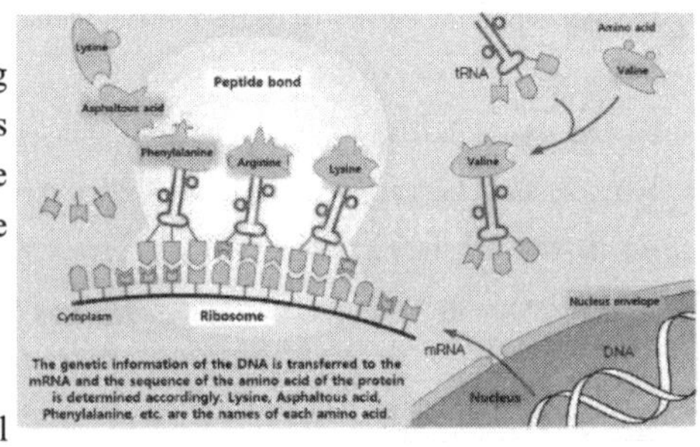

The genetic information of the DNA is transferred to the mRNA and the sequence of the amino acid of the protein is determined accordingly. Lysine, Asphaltous acid, Phenylalanine, etc. are the names of each amino acid.

What is Genetic Information?

A gene is a physical or functional unit through which all biological information of an individual is transmitted from one generation to the next. From a genetic point of view, the origin of the gene is in DNA. The DNA sequences (A, T, G, and C) are transcribed into RNA and then mapped to each other in three pairs to determine the amino acid sequence. This amino acid constitutes a protein so that the gene information is expressed. All the organs and tissues in the body have the same genes in the cells, even though they have different shapes or functions. Genes are often examined from a strand of hair, an oral cell, or a hemocyte, but they all contain the same gene. On the other hand, genetic information is expressed when certain conditions are met. In other words, normal cells contain obesity genes and when they are exposed to a certain environment or condition (such as lack of exercise or overnutrition), obesity genes are expressed, which results in obesity.

What is Gene Polymorphism?

It refers to various types of genes, that is, kinds of structures by variation. Specifically, when a variation occurs in the structure of the DNA (such as insertion, deletion, or repetition of the base sequence), it appears to be genetically diverse in humans. In other words, if a variation occurs in a specific gene region, it means that the same body region can display various traits depending on the individual.

What is Genome?

It is a mixture of genes and chromosomes, which refers to all the DNA in the nucleus. The genome is stored in 46 chromosomes in 23 pairs in the nucleus of the cell and consists of 3.5 billion base combinations. Recently, the National Institutes of Health has completed the Human Genome Project, which analyzes the base sequence of over 100,000 genes in 23 pairs of human chromosomes. The purpose is to treat human hereditary diseases by mapping the DNA base sequence of a human and mapping out which genome sequence of a certain chromosome has certain genetic information. A chromosome is a collection of each gene (each cell has 46 chromosomes in 23 pairs) and refers to the structural form of a gene that is tightly stored in a protein to compress the genetic information of the DNA chain.

progesterone, estrogen, lipoprotein lipase, and related hormones in other body parts also affect fat distribution. In this context, the fat distribution of males and females with different hormone composition ratios varies widely. In the case of women, fat is accumulated in the femur and hips when weight gain occurs, resulting in a 'pear type obesity', whereas, in males, fat accumulates in the abdomen, resulting in an 'apple type obesity'. To date, many researchers have found that android obesity is likely to cause metabolic disease, which is associated with a greater risk of exposure to diabetes, hypertension, stroke, and CAD.

The causes of obesity known to date are inherent factors that can be influenced by parents and acquired factors due to overnutrition and hypokinetic disease. In addition, it is thought to be caused by abnormalities of the hypothalamus, endocrine system, and thyroid function.

In addition to the causes mentioned above, obesity is affected by cultural, ethnic, socioeconomic, and seasonal factors, and may also be influenced by individual psychological factors. In fact, there are various causes of obesity that cannot be conclusively ranked in terms of their effect. However, some studies have emphasized that genetics play a particularly significant role. A survey of 540 obese patients investigating biological BMI revealed that the cause of obesity was more closely related to genetic factors than environmental factors.[6]

- Genetic factors: Family history by parents
- Acquired: Overnutrition and hypoactivity
- Medical endocrine factors: Hypothalamus and endocrine control problems
- Metabolic factors: Decrease in basal metabolic rate such as thyroid function
- Cultural factors: Excessive eating habits and culture / high-calorie food preferences of Western cultures
- Ethnic factors: Black people have a higher prevalence of obesity
- Socioeconomic factors: The middle-class prefer higher calorie foods
- Seasonal factors: Lack of activity and overnutrition during winter
- Psychological factors: Depression or personality Type B (easy-going personality)

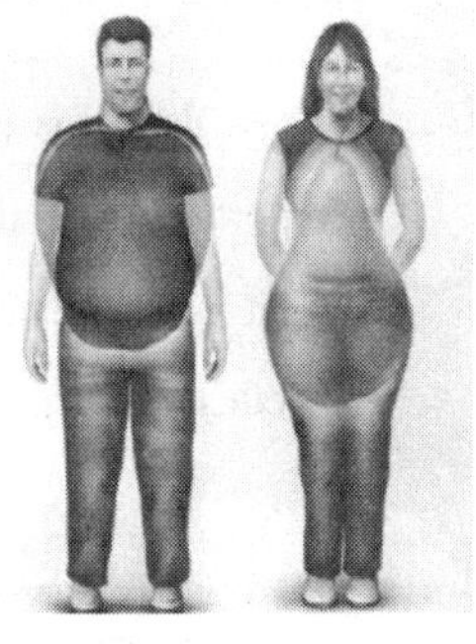

Obesity and Psychological Disorders

Many women, as they gain weight, think of feminine beauty as "thin" and are eager to lose weight. However, in reality, beauty and fashion models are far thinner than normal. As a result of this extreme concept of beauty, women may view themselves negatively, which can develop into psychological problems. For obese patients, psychological problem can be severe, however, they are often overlooked or ignored due to cultural prejudice and stereotypes. Two psychiatric conditions that can cause obesity are bulimia[15] and depression. Specifically, severe depression is usually associated with weight loss, but mild depression is affected by seasonal factors. In other words, patients with mild depression are prone to weight gain due to binge eating during the autumn and winter.

Obesity-related Genes and Exercise Prescription

In terms of the genetic characteristics of obesity, more than 200 factors have been proposed, which mainly consist of genes and chromosomal abnormalities affecting energy consumption, dietary intake, and fat metabolism. The major genes for such variation are leptin, leptin receptors, beta-3 adrenergic receptors, Neuropeptide Y, Uncoupling protein (UCP), Pro-opiomelanocortin (POMC), Tubby like protein (TULPs), and Peroxisome proliferator activated receptor (PPAR). Two beta-3 adrenergic receptors are expressed in the adipose tissue and show three polymorphisms: Trp/Trp, Trp/Arg, and Arg/Arg. It was reported that when the Arg allele was present, the WHR and body fat mass were higher than normal subjects. Since Arg/Arg and Trg/Arg are more likely to indicate obesity than Trp/Trp, when obese parents with an Arg allele give birth to a child, it is necessary to examine the baby's beta-3 adrenergic receptor gene. It is also desirable to have healthy eating habits, lifestyle, and regular exercise from youth so that the gene is not expressed.[15]

Relationship between Antidepressants and Weight

- Serotonin Inhibitors: amitriptyline, chlorpromazine, lithium ➜ serotonin ➜ appetite ↑ ➜ weight ↑
- Serotonin activators: fluoxetine, fenfluramine, dexfenfluramine ➜ Serotonin ↑ ➜ appetite ↓ ➜ weight ↓

To date, the pathological cause of obesity and depression is not clear, but it has been reported to be related to neurotransmitters, including serotonin.[16] Medication is used to treat depression, activate or inhibit serotonin, and lower appetite to induce weight loss. Medications such as amitriptyline[17], chlorpromazine[18], and lithium[19] cause weight gain

---

15) Bulimia: Pathological starvation status. It often occurs in women and is a mental disorder that occurs early in puberty or adults. Patients continue to eat a lot of food until abdominal pain, sleep, spontaneous vomiting occurs. It is characterized by fear of not stopping voluntarily, self-blame and depression after eating a lot. Unlike anorexia nervosa, there is no extreme weight loss.

16) Serotonin: Vasoconstrictors. It is released from platelets in humans and exists at high concentrations in many tissues including the mucosa, pineal gland, and central nervous system. It has physiological properties such as inhibition of gastric secretion and smooth muscle stimulation, and acts as a central neurotransmitter.

17) Amitiptyline: Antidepressants. White, odorless nodular powder that is soluble in water, alcohol, chloroform, and methanol.

18) Chlorpromazine: Used as a powerful mental stabilizer and antiemetic.

by decreasing serotonin-mediated neurotransmitter activity and increasing appetite. Fluoxetine[20], on the other hand, can increase appetite suppression and weight loss by increasing serotonin-mediated neurotransmitter activity. In addition, antidepressants inhibit serotonin reuptake and stimulate tryptophan[21] and serotonin, while fenfluramine[22] and dexfenfluramine increase serotonin levels to lower carbohydrate phagomania and cause weight loss. Some studies have suggested that obese people with depression frequently intake carbohydrates because it activates inhibited serotonin resulting in an increase in satiety and a decrease in discomfort.

Obesity and Elderly

It would not be an exaggeration to say that one or more degenerative diseases occur in the elderly. Fortunately, the chronic diseases of the elderly can be prevented or improved through exercise, which is beneficial for daily life. However, in order to gain the greatest benefits of exercise, it is best to start exercising at a younger age. The proverb, 'What is learned in the cradle is carried to the tomb' indicates the importance of habits learned in childhood.

Obesity is the most common cause of weight loss among the degenerative diseases described above and is the main cause of disorder in the human body. As a result, obesity is recognized as a terrible disease that causes complications such as diabetes, hypertension, heart disease, and gallbladder disease, leading to a shortened lifespan.[54]

Many studies have measured obesity in the elderly, but most of the indicators need to be modified for the elderly [Table 5.1]. The reason for this is that as age causes height loss, the reliability of the BMI using height and weight is lowered, and the skinfold method is inaccurate because aging causes the skin to slacken. [Table 5.2].

Table 5.2 ***Elderly BMI (㎏/㎡)***

Category	Male	Female
Normal	24~27	23~26
Overweight	28~31	27~32
Obesity	≥32	≥33

19) Lithium: It is effective for the treatment of bipolar disorder and has preventive effect on recurrence.
20) Fluoxetine: Antidepressants.
21) Tryptophan: Amino acids essential for proper development of infants and nitrogen metabolism in adults.
22) Fenfluramine: Temporary oral appetite suppressant for obesity.

Fortunately, the recently developed BIA method, CT, and Dexa tests are highly reliable, easy to measure, and are used in many hospitals because they quantitatively measure lean body mass, including muscle mass and fat mass. For reference, lean body mass, which is obtained from the BIA method, is body weight minus body fat, which refers to muscle mass, bone mass, and total body fluid.

Obesity in the elderly population continues to increase despite numerous efforts to date. The main causes include sedentary lifestyle, unhealthy diet, and lack of exercise. By reversing these causes, an effective prevention plan can be derived. In other words, you can reduce your chances of obesity and developing a degenerative disease by leading an active lifestyle, oriental diet, and hyperkinetic behavior rather than an passive lifestyle, westernized diet, and hypokinetic behavior. The two methods for this are as follows.

First, adopting a proper diet is important. Many people may think that decreasing calories or starving can reduce weight and fat mass. However, an extreme weight-loss diet does not only decrease lean body mass, which is very important for our bodies, but it also has a detrimental effect by inducing dehydration. Furthermore, attempting to lose body weight by suddenly reducing the intake of food can actually lead to an increase in body weight due to dehydration. Therefore, elderly women should consume 1,200 ㎉/day and elderly men, 1,500 ㎉/day. The composition ratio should be 50% carbohydrate, 30% fat, and 20% protein. For example, in the case of elderly men, the recommended daily carbohydrate intake should consist of 750 ㎉ of carbohydrates (equivalent to 2 ½ bowls of rice), 450 ㎉ of fat, and 300 ㎉ of protein.

Second, it is necessary to take up an active lifestyle through regular exercise. For this purpose, a light to moderate intensity exercise is effective in treating obesity. Nutrients that are used as energy in our bodies are typically carbohydrates and fats. Among them, carbohydrates are mainly used in oxygen limited conditions, such as running 100~400 meters, while fat is mobilized in low and light exercises. It is good to engage in walking or brisk walking, which can be done at a leisurely pace for a longer durations. In addition, light to moderate intensity exercise for the elderly is highly recommended because it reduces the risk of injury by half compared to high-intensity exercise. In the case of the elderly (BMI $\geq$ 32~33 kg/m^2),exercising before meals is more effective because it reduces appetite. Walking and brisk walking are the most recommended types of exercise. During the winter, it is recommended to ride a stationary bicycle in a professional facility or home. Exercising at an intensity between 40~60% of $\dot{V}O_2max$ with a duration of 20~30 minutes per exercise session 2 times a day at least five days a week, is effective in reducing fat.

Table 5.3 ***Daily exercise program for elderly obese patients***

Category	Item	Time	Repetition	Unit calorie	Per week	Calorie	Purpose/Advantage
Warm up	13 types Calisthenics	10 min	10 sec 2 set	40㎉	× 5 d	200 ㎉	. Postural balance / flexibility . Improved coordination
Aerobic Exercise	Brisk walk	40 min	1 times	200㎉	× 5 d	1,000 ㎉	. Cardiopulmonary development . Decrease of fat
	Walk	10 min	After meals, 3 times	70㎉	× 7 d	490 ㎉	. Lifestyle correction . Fat burning
Cool down	18 types stretching	10 min	For 15 sec	50㎉	× 5 d	250 ㎉	. Fatigue recovery . Prevention of potential diseases
						Total 1,940㎉	

For the elderly, a reduction of 1 ㎏ per month is desirable, and this amount is equivalent to 7,700 ㎉. So if the plan is to exercise 5 days a week, calorie intake must be limited to 380 ㎉ per day (380 ㎉ x 5 days x 4 weeks ≒ 7,700). Exercise programs for older people with obesity are shown in Table 5.3, which indicates how 1 ㎏ of fat mass can be reduced in about one month (7,700 ÷ 1940 ㎉).

Management of Obesity

Exercise for the treatment of obesity is aimed at decreasing body fat mass and increasing lean body mass. For weight loss and body fat mass loss in obese patients, a combination of diet and exercise therapy is more effective than exercising alone. However, if the patient does not exercise after reaching their desired weight, and their food intake is the same, weight gain can eventually result. Therefore, if the patient does not exercise, dietary intake should be reduced.[12]

Suitable types of exercise for obese patients are those that can be carried out continuously for more than 15 minutes, such as walking, brisk walking, stationary bicycle riding, and swimming. Movements that may cause joint strains or injuries should be avoided. Exercise intensity should be between 40~60% of $\dot{V}O_2$peak, with a frequency of 5 days or more per week, and an exercise duration of 30~60 minutes for effective fat reduction.[83] Ultimately, in the case of young adults, a reduction in fat mass of 500 g per week is desirable, which amounts to a required calorie intake of 3,500 ㎉. Therefore, when exercising 7 days a week, it is appropriate to consume 500 ㎉/day. It is most important to exercise with a high total calorie expenditure. This means that it is better to engage in a relatively light exercise that can last longer than a vigorous exercise that causes fatigue in a shorter amount of time.

Table 5.4 *Calorie consumption for 30-minutes of physical activity and exercise*[29]

Type	Calorie Consumption (㎉)	Type	Calorie consumption (㎉)	Type	Calorie Consumption (㎉)
Climbing	250	Fencing	300	Sitting / Writing	50
Badminton	200	Football	300	Standing / Easy Activity	80
Baseball	160	Golf (using cart)	120	Skiing (steep)	350
Basketball	300	Golf (carrying clubs)	200	Cross-country	300
Cycling at 8.8kph	150	Handball	330	Soccer	300
Cycling at 10.2kph	200	Hiking	180	Softball	150
Cycling at 17.2kph	310	Horse riding	200	Swimming (Freestyle)	180
Bowling / Dancing	150	Racquetball	300	Walk at 3.2kph	120
Canoeing at 6.4kph	220	Running at 8.8kph	375	Walk at 6.4kph	220
Tennis (singles)	270	Running at 10.2kph	500	Walk at 8.0kph	270

Table 5.5 *Exercise test, drug, and specific considerations for obese patients*

<table>
<tr><th colspan="2">Test item</th><th>Measurement</th><th>Recommended Stopping Point</th><th>Remarks</th></tr>
<tr><td rowspan="4">Aerobic Power Ability</td><td rowspan="4">■ Treadmill (1～2METs/ 3min stage)
■ Cycle (25～50watt/ 3min stage)</td><td>■ 12 lead ECG</td><td>■ Severe arrhythmia appearance
■ ST segment depression / elevation > 2 mm
■ Ischemic threshold
■ T wave inversion with ST change</td><td rowspan="4">Obese patients have a high risk for CAD / hypertension.</td></tr>
<tr><td>■ HR</td><td>■ Maximal heart rate > (220 - age)</td></tr>
<tr><td>■ BP</td><td>■ SBP/DBP > 250/115 ㎜Hg</td></tr>
<tr><td>■ RPE</td><td>■ Sudden increase of psychological fatigue</td></tr>
<tr><td>Flexibility Exercise</td><td>■ Goniometer</td><td>■ ROM</td><td></td><td>ROM tends to be reduced compared to normal people.</td></tr>
<tr><td>Neuromuscular Exercise</td><td>■ Gait analysis
■ Balance analysis</td><td></td><td></td><td>Walking is slower than normal, gait pattern is irregular, and balance is reduced.</td></tr>
<tr><td>Pharmacotherapy</td><td colspan="4">■ It is important to remember that reducing fat mass while preserving lean body mass is the primary goal of obesity management.
■ Drugs recommended by the FDA are sympathetic stimulants (amphetamines, isoindoles, caffeine).
■ Serotonin inhibitors cause appetite suppression, but are not recommended by the FDA (clinical trials are inadequate).
■ Thyroid hormones can cause cardiovascular disease and osteoporosis, so it is dangerous to use in weight management.</td></tr>
<tr><td>Considerations</td><td colspan="4">■ It is desirable to classify patients according to the age group.
■ Obese patients are at high risk for exposure to orthopedic injuries.
■ Obese patients are at high risk for exposure to cardiovascular disease.
■ Obese patients are very vulnerable to the warm environment.
■ In the case of obese patients with psychological disorders such as depression, the exact physiological change of the drug being administered should be known.</td></tr>
</table>

Table 5.6 ***Management program for obese patients***

	Type	Goal	Intensity/Frequency/Time	Period
Aerobic Exercise	■ Major muscle exercises · Walking · Brisk walking · Rowing · Cycling · Aquatic exercise	■ Decrease in body fat ■ Increase in functional ability ■ Reduction of CAD	■ Peak oxygen uptake 40～60% ■ using RPE and HR ■ 5 days or more per week ■ 30～60min (intermittently 20～30min × 2 times/day) ■ Emphasis on extending exercise time rather than intensity	■ 9~12 mon
Flexibility Exercise	■ Stretching · Extension/ Flexion type	■ Increased ROM	■ Daily or 5 days per week	
Functional Exercise	■ Activity orientation correction	■ Activities of daily living ■ Change in job style ■ Satisfaction with the body	■ 10 minutes walk after each meal ■ commute by walking	■ Lifetime
Pharmacotherapy	■ It can be considered when BMI is more than 2 degrees obesity (≥35kg/m²). ■ Sympathomimetic drugs recommended by the FDA may be prescribed by a physician.			
Considerations	■ Select low shock type for joints. ■ Low intensity exercise is desirable for cardiac relationships. ■ The risk of hyperthermia should be considered. ■ Be able to modify exercise equipment to fit the body size (such as a large saddle on a bicycle or rowing equipment). ■ Strength exercises are an essential requirement to maintain or increase lean body mass, which provides resilience to the body. ■ For strength enhancement, high intensity / low repetition times should be considered after the patient has fully adapted to the program.			

For example, as shown in [Table 5.4], walking at 8.0 kph for 30 minutes leads to an expenditure of 270 ㎉ with fatigue. On the other hand, walking at 6.4 kph for 60 minutes leads to burning 440 ㎉ with less fatigue. So, low-intensity, but a longer duration of exercise, is very effective in terms of body fat loss. It is also helpful to refer to the caloric expenditure of each type of exercise listed in [Table 5.4] when obese patients perform general outdoor activity programs. Exercise prescribers should refer to [Table 5.5, 5.6] and provide a detailed plan for examinations and management methods for obese patients.[3,5,10,17,22,88]

Diabetes Mellitus

Definition and Causes of Diabetes Mellitus

Diabetes mellitus (DM) is a metabolic disease characterized by a deficiency of the hormone, insulin, or insulin resistance, leading to hyperglycemia. Younger people, including children, are affected by a lack of insulin hormone production due to the physical destruction of the Langerhans islets in the pancreas, which is referred to as Type 1 DM or insulin dependent diabetes mellitus (IDDM). It accounts for 10 to 15% of all diabetics. Characteristically, 90% of IDDM patients have antibodies that inhibit insulin secretory cells in the pancreas, suggesting that people with diabetes can easily become infected with viruses such as Coxsackie[23]or Mumps[24].

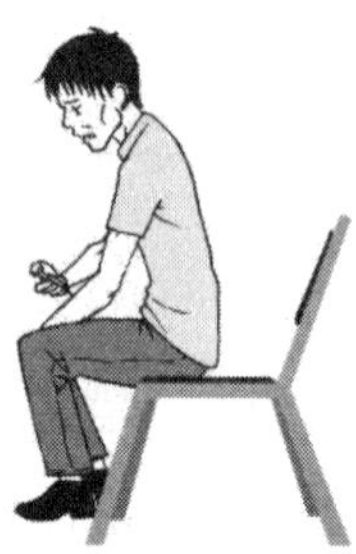

Adult diabetes is caused by the inability to accept insulin in tissue cells, which leads to increased resistance. This phenomenon is caused by diminished insulin receptors, decreased sensitivity, or the failure of the second messenger to cause intracellular glycogen synthesis. It is called Type 2 DM or non-insulin dependent diabetes mellitus (NIDDM), accounting for 85~90% of diabetic patients. Characteristically, NIDDM occurs mainly after 45 years of age and progresses slowly. It is reported that 6% of the population aged 45 or older and 10% of the population aged 65 or older have NIDDM, which is caused by a number of factors such as insulin resistance due to genetic factors, obesity, and lack of exercise. It does not require insulin at the onset of the disease and ketosis[25] does not occur, except in extreme situations. However, insulin therapy is essential for NIDDM patients who do not recover through exercise, diet, weight loss, and oral hypoglycemic agents.

The two types of diabetes mentioned above have changed somewhat over time. First, IDDM can occur in all age groups, including children. In other words, IDDM usually appears suddenly before age 30, but 10 to 20% may not be thought to be caused by inheritance, since it may occur after age 35. Second, the term 'non-insulin dependent' has been used because it literally does not use insulin. In fact, it is somewhat confusing to

23) Coxsackie virus: One of the diverse groups of intestinal virus. It causes polio but does not cause paralysis.

24) Mumps virus: Mainly found in children. It causes infectious paramyxovirus diseases that cause persistent immunity. It is infected by the inspiration, and the most intensive virus infection occurs in the salivary gland. It is severe especially in the parotid gland than in the submaxillary gland or sublingual gland.

25) Ketosis: In patients with type 1 diabetes, glucose is not used, but fat is used as an energy source in the liver, which causes scum to cause metabolic complications.

use the term because most people with NIDDM often need to use insulin during the treatment process.

Ultimately, both types of diabetic patients have common symptoms such as polyuria, polydipsia, polyphagia, weight loss, and increased fatigue. Symptoms of tachycardia, dyspnea, nausea, vomiting, confusion, syncope can result when the disease is not recognized and treated. Severe cases lead to complications in the nervous system, cardiovascular system, retinas and kidneys, and eventually death. The cause of diabetes is not known to date but it is reported to be connected to abdominal obesity, aging, pregnancy, stress, increase in sympathetic nervous system activity, hypokinetic disease, increased adipose tissue, reduced lean mass and habitual activity.

- Abdominal obesity
- Aging
- Pregnancy
- Vigorous stress
- Sympathetic activity
- Hypokinetic activity
- Increase in adipose tissue
- Reduction of lean mass
- Reduced habitual activity

Although the procedures and criteria for diagnosing diabetes differ slightly depending on authors, the data can be summarized as shown in [Table 5.7].[57] Impaired glucose tolerance is in the middle range between 'not normal' and 'diabetes.' It can be defined as a temporary phenomenon caused by excessive alcohol abuse, stress, lack of sleep, and a large amount of caffeine ingestion. However, despite the discovery of impaired glucose tolerance, if the patient continues with unhealthy habits, diabetes is more likely to develop.

***Table 5.7* Diagnostic criteria for diabetes**

<table>
<tr><th></th><th>Fasting</th><th>Postprandial 2 hours</th><th>Various test methods and blood glucose levels for diagnosing diabetes mellitus</th></tr>
<tr><td>Normal</td><td>60~110 mg/dℓ</td><td>≤ 140 mg/dℓ</td><td rowspan="3">. Blood glucose level is 126 mg/dl or more when more than 2 time fasting
. With the symptoms of diabetes, 200 mg/dl or more in the random glucose test
. After 2 hours of ingestion of 75g of glucose, blood glucose is 200 mg/dl or more
. 2 hours after the meal, the level of blood sugar is 200 mg/dl or more</td></tr>
<tr><td>Impaired glucose tolerance</td><td>111~125 mg/dℓ</td><td>140~199 mg/dℓ</td></tr>
<tr><td>Diabetes</td><td>≥126 mg/dℓ</td><td>≥ 200 mg/dℓ</td></tr>
</table>

Diabetes-Related Genes and Exercise Prescription

The genes involved in the induction of diabetes are FABP2 and IRS-1. First, FABP2 is one of the substances that regulates the absorption, transport and metabolism of fatty acids in cells and is a protein that binds to long chain fatty acids in the cells. This gene is based on the fact that the mutation from alanine to threonine in codon54 is associated with insulin resistance. It acts as a transcytoplasmic fatty acid carrier, a transmitochondrial fatty acid carrier, or to mitigate the degradation of intracellular enzymes. In particular, FABP2 is known to be present in the epithelial cells of the small intestine and cause insulin resistance by affecting fatty acid metabolism. Second, IRS-1 is present on chromosome 2 and is known to delay growth or to cause insulin resistance when lost. Among the polymorphisms of the IRS-1 gene, the polymorphism of codon972 gene from GGG to AGG has been reported to be most relevant to diabetes. FABP2 and IRS-1 can be expressed by extreme stress, excessive carbohydrate / alcohol consumption and lack of exercise. Therefore, healthy lifestyles and regular exercise should be performed to prevent the expression of two genes.[52]

Characteristics of Adult Type Diabetes Mellitus

Adult type diabetes, Type 2 diabetes, is characterized by insulin resistance and excess glucose secretion in the liver. In other words, beta cells in the pancreas of patients secrete more insulin to compensate for insulin resistance, but the amount of insulin produced does not overcome insulin resistance. Even in tissues like muscles, there are less insulin receptors and the insulin resistance increases. Ultimately, the liver, which must produce an energy source, causes hyperglycemia, which secretes and utilizes glucose excessively, thereby rapidly raising blood sugar levels. Patients with insulin resistance and hyperinsulinemia have metabolic problems with fat and cholesterol[26]. Thus, there is an increase in very-low-density lipoprotein cholesterol (VLDL-C) and triglyceride (TG), a decrease in high-density lipoprotein cholesterol (HDL-C), and an increase in low-density lipoprotein cholesterol (LDL-C), resulting in atheroma and blocked arteries. Ultimately, these patients may experience gout due to hyperuricemia. In addition, patients with NIDDM have visceral obesity, leading to hypertension. The presence of obesity and hypertension increases the risk of vascular disease by more than ten times.

The causes of insulin resistance and hyperinsulinemia, which are characteristic of NIDDM, are environmental factors such as lack of exercise and obesity. On the other hand, metabolic abnormalities that cause insulin resistance are considered to be genetic factors very similar to those that cause obesity.

26) Cholesterol: A pearl-color fat-like monohydric alcohol. It is found in animal fats, bile, blood, brain tissue, milk, yolk sac, myelin sheath, liver, kidney, adrenal gland. It constitutes the majority of gallstones, or is present in atherosclerosis, various tumors and cancerous tissues. Most cholesterol in the body is synthesized in the liver and some are absorbed in food. This is very important for the synthesis of steroid hormones.

Diabetic Complication

Diabetes reduces arterial elasticity and raises blood pressure, leading to heart disease, kidney disease, stroke and other diseases listed below. The details are as follows.

Diabetes and Heart Disease

Diabetes weakens the heart muscle and causes CAD. It can also lead to ischemia and a heart attack without causing chest pain. People with hypertension, smoking, and blood lipid abnormalities or those who have stem family members who have had CAD before the age of 50 are at high risk for a heart attack.

Diabetes and Kidney Disease

About 25% of diabetic complications result in renal failure. The incidence of developing kidney disease in patients with Type 1 DM over 20 years of age is 30~40%, and about 15~20% with Type 2 DM patients throughout their lives. An early symptom of kidney disease is the detection of protein in urine. This is because hypertension and LDL-C levels are raised to increase the amount of proteinuria. ACE inhibitors are used to treat these two diseases, which have the effect of lowering blood pressure as well as protecting the kidneys. For reference, patients with diabetes should undergo kidney function tests and blood tests every year to prevent complications from kidney disease.

Diabetes and Eye Disease

Diabetic patients are vulnerable to microvascular injury. Because micro vessels are most commonly distributed in the eyes of the human body, the risk of exposure to diabetic complications such as retinopathy and glaucoma as well as cataracts is high. In other words, it is no exaggeration to say that cataracts are the main cause of blindness in diabetic patients. Because of this, diabetics are advised to conduct an eye test every year.

Diabetes and Nervous Disease

Diabetes also affects peripheral and autonomic nerves. Peripheral neuropathy is common in the hands and feet. It is usually accompanied by tingling, burning, and pain, characterized by a low sensitivity to temperature and equilibrium, which becomes more severe at night. Taking amitriptyline or capsaicin cream to the affected area 2~4 times helps relieve pain.

Autonomic neuropathy is usually a condition in which the nerves distributed in the heart are infected and cause a transient incapacitated state during exercise so that heart rate does not increase or the patients do not feel pain even with myocardial infarction. In the case of neuropathy in the stomach, it is common to have nausea and chest pain accompanied by delayed digestion time or decreased digestive capacity. However, when all the organs are infected, internal diseases, diarrhea, or constipation may be induced. For treatment, high-fiber diets and diarrhea and constipation medicine are prescribed.

Diabetes and Foot Disease

Diabetic patients are susceptible to foot damage due to complex problems of the nerves and arteries. In particular, the infection and necrosis rate is 20 times higher, and the toes and legs may need to be cut. Therefore, if the skin shows redness, swelling or lesions, immediate antiulcer treatment is required. When diabetics buy new shoes, they should choose a comfortable and appropriate size. After washing their feet, they need to dry them well and apply oil cosmetics. [Table 5.8] summarizes the management guidelines for the complications listed above.[3,5,7,10,,22,33,88]

Table 5.8 ***Guidelines for the management of diabetic complications***

Items	Guidelines	Items	Guidelines
① Body weight	· Less than 120% of ideal body weight	⑦ ECG	· Constant waveform / ST segment / PVC Caution
② Blood glucose level	· Before meals : 80~120 ㎎/dℓ · After meals 1.5~2 hr : 180 ㎎/dℓ or less · Fasting : 100~140 ㎎/dℓ	⑧ Blood pressure	· 135/85 ㎜Hg or less · Measurement every year · Frequent measurement if abnormal
③ HgA1C (Reflects blood glucose level for 3 mon)	· Below 2% of normal upper limit · IDDM every 3 mon/ NIDDM measurement on demand · Older people with hypoglycemia should control blood glucose before meals less than 200 ㎎/dℓ and HgA1C within 3%	⑨ Lipid level	· LDL 130 ㎎/dℓ or less · HDL 35 ㎎/dℓ or more · TG 200 ㎎/dℓ or less
④ Assessment of visual acuity	· Annual mydriasis test	⑩ Urine component / albumin	· Every year
⑤ Smoking cessation/ Counseling	· Family Counseling / Patient Education	⑪ Creatinine /clearance rate	· Every year
⑥ Urinalysis	· Every year	⑫ Exercise	· 3 d/wk 20~45 min

Management of Diabetes Mellitus

Diet Therapy

People with diabetes should consume between 2,000 ㎉ and 2,500 ㎉ daily to maintain their ideal body weight. In particular, even if NIDDM patients are obese, calories should not be limited to less than 1,200 ㎉. Excessive calorie restriction results in hypoglycemia, decreased muscle mass, and a deficiency of vitamins and minerals.

Diet therapy for glycemic control emphasizes the intake of complex carbohydrates, such as vegetables, corn, starch and fruit, and limits the intake of simple carbohydrates, such as candy or cookies, that rapidly increase blood sugar. High levels of fat and protein intake are also detrimental. Proteins should consist of 20% of total calories, 50% for carbohydrates, and less than 30% for fat (less than 10% for saturated fats). Because diabetic patients have abnormally high cholesterol levels, it is desirable to restrict high-fat dietary intake and limit cholesterol to less than 300 ㎎ per day.

Exercise Therapy

Exercise is an important factor in the treatment of diabetes and is more important for NIDDM patients. For diabetics, exercise offers benefits such as increased physical fitness, prevention and reduction of obesity, improved lipid levels, improved metabolic control of blood sugar, reduced risk factors for CAD, and reduced stress.

Because there is a strong relationship between diabetes and CAD, a graded exercise test must be performed prior to exercise. Various exercise methods are recommended for the management of diabetes, but careless exercise can lead to health deterioration such as aggravating glucose metabolism, hypoglycemia, retinopathy, musculoskeletal and soft tissue injury, complex foot injury, and myocardial infarction. Therefore, exercise prescription and proper exercise based on the person's fitness level is important. For novices in particular, blood sugar test should be done before, during, and after exercise for about a month to prevent hypoglycemia and ensure safe exercise. If the regulation of blood glucose is stable, the measurement interval may be reduced weekly. [Table 5.9] shows a guideline on how exercise is to be applied according to the results of pre-exercise blood glucose measurements.

In [Table 5.9], when the blood glucose level is higher than 300 ㎎/㎗, exercise is contraindicated because it exacerbates the metabolic state since the appropriate blood glucose level before exercise is 150~249 ㎎/㎗. In the case of IDDM, blood glucose should be measured before, during, and after exercising since exercise affects insulin.

Before exercising, insulin injections should be decreased by 1~2 units or 10~15 g of carbohydrates 30 minutes before exercise should be consumed. When injecting insulin, it should avoid body parts that are used primarily for exercise.[57] On the other hand, when exercising for the first time, exercising with a person who is knowledgeable about treatment, symptoms, and signs of hypoglycemia is a good idea in order to prevent possible hypoglycemia during exercise.

To date, the effects of exercise on IDDM patients have been reported to reduce risk factors for cardiovascular disease, and improve weight control and the quality of life rather than improving the control of blood glucose. However, the role of exercise is very significant in the treatment of NIDDM patients. Particularly, low-intensity exercise, such as walking, is very effective in increasing insulin sensitivity.

Table 5.9 ***Guidelines for applying exercise according to results of pre-exercise blood glucose measurement***

Blood glucose level	Guidelines for applying exercise
300 ~ ≥ 400 mg/dℓ	Do not exercise. Consult with a specialist for more detailed blood glucose control.
250 ~ 299 mg/dℓ	Exercise with caution. Re-measure after 10 minutes of exercise and stop the exercise when the value goes up. Consult with a specialist for more detailed control.
150 ~ 249 mg/dℓ	Exercise possibly. The extent to which the patient can exercise safely, although it is not consistent with the purpose of the treatment.
100 ~ 149 mg/dℓ	Exercise with caution, although it is not consistent with the purpose of the treatment. Watch for signs and symptoms of hyperlipidemia. Re-measure if necessary or provide 10 to 15 g of juice.
≤ **100**mg/dℓ	Do not exercise. (Consultation about drug and food intake habits before exercise) Taking complex carbohydrates is recommended. After 15 minutes, re-measure. If it is over 100 mg / dℓ, exercise carefully.

Exercise Program

Exercises Type

Aerobic exercise, such as walking, is an easy and preferred method of exercise, but stationary or outdoor cycling and swimming are also recommended exercises. In order to improve insulin sensitivity, it is also desirable to increase muscle mass with an appropriate intensity weight training program. Weight training is effective for major muscle-oriented movements, such as bench presses and leg presses.

Exercise Intensity

The degree of exercise intensity can be measured using heart rate, blood pressure, subjective symptoms, ECG, and oxygen consumption during the graded exercise test. The recommended exercise intensity for diabetic patients is 50~80% of the maximal heart rate, 50~80% of the maximal oxygen uptake, and a RPE range of 10~16. In particular, exercise prescriptions using RPE is a very desirable method for autonomic patients with unstable heart rates. On the other hand, when performing muscle strength exercise, a light weight that can be repeated 10~15 reps with 1~2 sets for each muscle group should be used. It is recommended not to exceed a RPE of 16 for aerobic exercises as well. The elderly who have led a sedentary lifestyle for a long time have many difficulties and limitations when it comes to exercise, so the initial exercise intensity should be set at 30~40% of $\dot{V}O_2max$. Provided that the average fitness level of 65 year-olds is 7 METs, the elderly should walk with 2~3 METs. The increase in exercise intensity is lower than in the general population, increasing only up to 50~70% of $\dot{V}O_2max$.

Exercise Frequency

Exercise should be done 4~7 days per week to maximize calorie consumption and adjust blood sugar levels. The elderly should also exercise at least three times a week, although daily exercise is recommended in order to control blood glucose and improve health.

Exercise Time

An exercise time that is comfortable for the subject should be selected. Initially, it should start at around 10 minutes and gradually increase to 20~60 minutes from 2~4 times per week. Because the physiological adaptation time or recovery time for exercise is very slow, the elderly should avoid a sharp increase in the amount of exercise and have enough time for warm-up and cool-down. Energy consumption per exercise is recommended to be about 10% of calorie intake per day. When the daily calorie intake is 1,800~2,200 ㎉ per day, an average of 200 ㎉ is appropriate for the elderly. For an elderly person to consume 200 ㎉, it takes 30 minutes to 1 hour, depending on the intensity of exercise. Exercise time should be increased gradually according to the individual's fitness level, starting at 30 minutes. Ultimately, exercise prescribers should familiarize themselves with various types of exercise, testing and management methods listed in [Tables 5.10, 5.11], and present specific plans to patients.[3,5,7,10,,22,33,88]

Table 5.10 ***Exercise test, drug, and specific considerations for diabetic patients***

Test item		Measurement	Recommended Stopping Point	Remarks
Aerobic Power Ability	■ Treadmill (1~2METs/ 3min stage) ■ Cycle (25~50watt/ 3min stage) Ramp protocol	■ 12 lead ECG	■ Severe arrhythmia appearance ■ ST segment depression / elevation > 2 mm ■ Ischemic threshold ■ T wave inversion with ST change	※Diabetes patients are at high risk for CAD, stroke, hyperlipidemia.
		■ HR	■ Maximal heart rate 85%	
		■ BP	■ SBP/DBP : 250/115mmHg excess	
		■ RPE	■ The emergence of peripheral tissue pain	
Myofunction	■ Isotonic / Isokinetic	■ 1RM or peak torque		※Excessive blood pressure increase is a serious problem in the presence of vascular complications.
Flexibility	■ Goniometer ■ Sit-and-reach	■ ROM ■ Degree of muscle relaxation		
Neuromuscle	■ Gait analysis ■ Balance analysis ■ Nerve conduction			※Applied when looking for signs of peripheral neuropathy or considering correction tools.
Pharmacotherapy	■ The management goal of diabetic patients is to normalize their blood glucose levels, but they can be managed through dieting and exercise therapy rather than rely on drugs alone. ■ Insulin / oral hypoglycemic / other hypoglycemic agents: Excessive use may cause hypoglycemia. ■ Antihypertensives, lipid-lowering agents and analgesics can be used as well as hypoglycemic agents. ■ Oral hypoglycemic agents stimulate the pancreas to secrete many insulin, reduce glycogen degradation in the liver, and increase insulin sensitivity.			
Considerations	■ If the blood glucose level is > 250 mg/dℓ, or if the blood ketone level is high, the test may be delayed. ■ Carbohydrates should be ingested if the patient has a blood glucose level of 80~100 mg/dℓ. ■ Because autonomic nervous system neuropathy is common, there may be latent ischemia, orthostatic hypotension, or no change in heart rate for exercise. ■ Peripheral nervous system neuropathy is often present, leading to numbness, limb tingling, and reduced equilibrium. ■ Microvascular complications may be affected by excessive blood pressure. ■ Peripheral vascular disease can result in intermittent claudication, infection, or ulceration in a not well-healed leg. ■ Insulin dosing and meal planning should be considered at the time of testing. ■ Hypoglycemia may also occur several hours after the end of the exercise (if hypoglycemia is observed at the exercise prescription center after exercise, the patient should be checked for hypoglycemic symptoms by telephone at 5 hours after he or she returns home). ■ Angina or latent ischemia may occur.			

Table 5.11 ***Management program for diabetic patients***

	Type	Goal	Intensity/Frequency/Time	Period
Aerobic Exercise	■ Major muscle exercises · Walking · Brisk walking · Rowing · Cycling · Aquatic exercise	■ Increased aerobic capacity ■ Reduced fatigue induction time ■ Increased exercise capacity ■ Improvement of blood pressure response to exercise ■ Reduction of cardiovascular risk factors	■ HR peak 50～80% ■ $\dot{V}O_2$peak 50～80% ■ using RPE ■ 4～7 d/wk ■ 20～60 min/bout	■ 4～6 month
Myofunction Exercise	■ Free weight (bar / dumbbell) ■ Weight equipment ■ Isokinetic equipment	■ Increase of lean body mass ■ Increase of lean body mass ■ Maintain bone density levels	■ Low resistance, many repetitions ■ High-resistance exercise is also good for patients with well-controlled blood glucose.	■ 4～6 month
Flexibility Neuromuscular Exercise	■ Stretching / Yoga ■ Yoga (neuromuscular exercise)	■ Increased ROM ■ Improvement of walking level ■ Improved balance / co-ordination	■ 2~3 days per week	■ 4～6 month
Functional Exercise	■ Activity orientation correction ■ Weight management	■ Increase in activities of daily living ■ Increase of job ability ■ Increase of job ability	■ 10 minutes walk after each meal ■ Commute by walking	

Pharmacotherapy

Insulin type		Effect Point	Peak time (No Exercise)	Duration	Remarks
Regular*		30 min~1 hr	2~3 hr	3~6 hr	*Regular=CZI: crystalline zinc insulin † NPH: neutral protamine Hagedorn
Intermediate	NPH †	2~4 hr	4~10 hr	10~16 hr	
Intermediate	Lente	3~4 hr	6~16 hr	18~30 hr	
Ultralente		6~10 hr	14~26 hr	32~36≥ hr	

Considerations

■ Snacks are needed.
■ Insulin dose should be adjusted 30~60 minutes before exercise.
■ Observation of blood glucose levels before and after exercise.
■ Exercising late at night can lead to nocturnal hypoglycemia.
■ Angina or latent ischemia may occur.

Hyperlipidemia

Definition and Causes of Hyperlipidemia

Hyperlipidemia refers to a state in which the amount of lipoprotein in the serum is increased above normal levels. Lipoprotein includes TC, TG, phospholipid, and protein. It is classified according to the density of lipoprotein cholesterol: HDL-C, LDL-C, and

VLDL-C. TC level is the overall amount of cholesterol found in the blood, in which HDL-C accounts for about 17%, LDL-C 70%, and VLDL-C 13%.[80]

Cholesterol is not a bad substance. Rather, it is an important ingredient for energy storage, transport, and cell membrane formation. However, an abnormally high accumulation of lipid components in blood vessels can result in various vascular diseases. Hyperlipidemia refers to the accumulation of high levels of cholesterol and triglycerides in blood vessels. Hypercholesterolemia is a high accumulation of cholesterol, while hypertriglyceridemia is a high accumulation of triglycerides.[65] A high accumulation of either or both of them is called hyperlipidemia. It is divided into three stages: mild, moderate, and severe [Table 5.12].

Table 5.12 ***Classification of hyperlipidemia***

	TC	LDL-C	HDL-C	TG
High risk	≥ 240 mg/dl	≥ 190 mg/dl	≤ 40 mg/dl	≥ 500 mg/dl
Moderate risk	-	160 ~ 189 mg/dl	-	200 ~ 499 mg/dl
Mild risk (Borderline high)	200 ~ 239 mg/dl	130 ~ 159 mg/dl	-	150 ~ 199 mg/dl
High normal	< 200 mg/dl	100 ~ 129 mg/dl	-	-
Low risk (optimal)	-	< 100 mg/dl	≥ 60 mg/dl	≤ 150 mg/dl

* Hypertriglyceridemia increases the risk of pancreatitis and abdominal pain.

† Recommendation of ACSM (2014)[88]

Types and Roles of Lipoprotein

Since cholesterol in plasma is not soluble, it is transported in combination with proteins, which is the role of lipoprotein. Lipoprotein is composed of cholesterol ester and TG, which are hydrophobic lipids in the center, while phospholipid, cholesterol, and apoprotein are hydrophilic lipids on the surface. The main lipoproteins that bind easily to cholesterol are HDL-C, LDL-C, and VLDL-C. LDL-C mainly contains apoprotein B, and HDL-C contains apoprotein A. These cholesterols are released from the liver and go through their metabolic processes. HDL-C transports cholesterol in the blood vessel wall to the liver where it can be broken down, whereas LDL-C has the opposite effect. On the other hand, TG are potentially used as an energy source for muscle activity.[38]

Specifically, HDL-C in the blood is small in size (90Å in diameter), has a high specific gravity, and is a hard lipoprotein. It consists of 50% apoprotein A, 25% phospholipids, 20% cholesterol, and 5% triglycerides.[82] Human peripheral tissue cells have receptors for HDL-C, and the activity is regulated by the intracellular cholesterol content. It plays an important role in eliminating cholesterol in the cell. In particular, HDL-C is classified into HDL_1, HDL_2, and HDL_3 according to the specific gravity. Increased HDL_2 transports plaque in the peripheral tissue to the liver for decomposition, or inhibits LDL-C from adhering to cells, thereby preventing arteriosclerosis.[30] In this context, it has been reported that the risk of the cardiovascular system decreases by 50% when HDL-C increases by 10 mg/dℓ, and 2~3% when HDL-C increases by 1 mg/dℓ.[31] It is known that HDL_2 among HDL-C, which is beneficial to the human body, is increased by high fitness levels or regular training.[33]

Blood LDL-C is a substance produced by VLDL-C which releases most of the triglycerides by lipoprotein lipase (LPL). That is, it consists of 50% fat and 70% cholesterol.[85] LDL-C is about 210~250Å in size and its main component is apolipoprotein B. Its function is to transport cholesterol, ester-type cholesterol, and triglycerides from the liver to various peripheral tissue cells and accumulate it. There is an LDL-receptor on the cell surface that absorbs LDL-C, but if it is overfilled, the absorption function is either lost or macrophages take in cholesterol, eventually leading to atherosclerosis. In other words, VLDL-C and LDL-C increase the risk of CAD by transporting lipids to the vascular wall.[7] The prevalence of CAD and most of the deaths from the disease are high among elderly people over 65 years of age. It is thought that the risk of disease is high because of high levels of LDL-C and low levels of HDL-C in the blood vessels. In particular, the 1% : 2% rule applies to middle-aged patients, including the elderly. The rule means that a 1% reduction in blood cholesterol reduces the risk of cardiovascular damage by 2%. Such health-damaging LDL-C can be reduced through long-term exercise.

Hyperlipidemia related Gene and Exercise Prescription

When the lipase is congenitally deficient, the body can not function, and the lipid of the blood increases, resulting in hyperlipemia. In other words, hyperlipidemia is also genetically related. The gene associated with hyperlipidemia is a polymorphism of the lipoprotein lipase (LPL) gene, a protein involved in energy input into the body. There are more than 90 mutations and genetic polymorphisms in the LPL gene, among which exon 9-Hind I, intron 6-Pvu II, and intron 8-LPL Hind III can be analyzed in Korea. Any researchers reported that the group with H2 alleles in the Hind III region of LPL had high serum triglyceride and low HDL. They also reported that the group with H2 alleles had higher triglyceride among the CAD groups, but no differences in triglyceride in the normal group.[90,91] Ultimately, hyperlipidemia, which can manifest as a genetic mutation, can be detected by analyzing the LPL gene and thereby prevent serious atherosclerosis or stroke early.

Hyperlipidemia-related Diseases

Plaques containing LDL-C are important pathologically because they are not only a major cause of hyperlipemia, but are also recognized as major risk factors for arteriosclerosis, fatty liver, and other CAD.[21] Some studies have shown a negative correlation between the incidence of CAD and HDL-C levels in the blood, but a positive correlation with triglycerides and LDL-C. For example, if a person has died of CAD despite low LDL-C levels, the cause may be excessive hypertriglyceridemia. On the other hand, hyperlipidemia can lead to strokes, CAD, arterial sclerosis in the peripheral tissues such as intermittent claudication, and the disruption of fat metabolism caused by fatty liver.

Management of Hyperlipidemia

Diet and regular exercise are essential to prevent or treat hyperlipidemia. Diets should aim to reduce the intake of saturated fatty acids, encourage the consumption of carbohydrates, and promote fat burning through regular, continuous aerobic exercise. Exercise therapy, however, is only applicable if the level of lipid in the blood presented in [Table 5.12] is below the mild risk level. If the level is a moderate or higher risk group, the exercise program should be avoided until it falls below the mild risk level through medication.[65]

Walking, brisk walking, climbing, jogging, stationary bicycle riding, and swimming are suitable for hyperlipidemic patients. It is good to refrain from exercises with heavy physical contact. Exercise intensity is determined at 40~70% of the maximum work rate. If it is difficult to measure heart rate, exercise should be performed in the RPE range of 11~16. Exercise time and frequency should be between 15~40 minutes, depending on the intensity of exercise, and performed 5~7 days per week.

Management of Hyperlipidemia-related Diseases

Atherosclerosis

Atherosclerosis is a condition in which the arteries are weakened by hyperlipidemia,[65] aging, hypertension, smoking, lack of exercise, obesity, diabetes, and hyperuricemia, or the blood supply is reduced due to the accumulation of lipids in the arteries. Having many of these risk factors can lead to life-threatening complications.[23] Cerebral infarction or cerebral stroke may occur in the cerebral artery, and myocardial ischemia or myocardial infarction may occur in the coronary arteries, resulting in disabilities or a shortened life span. In order to prevent atherosclerosis and to restore patients already suffering from the disease, a vegetable-based diet should be adopted, and recumbent cycling and brisk walking should be recommended to increase blood flow with a constant increase in blood pressure. At this time, the exercise intensity and the exercise time should be 40~70% of the $\dot{V}O_2max$ for a duration of 40 minutes, 5~7 days per week, respectively.

Fatty Liver

Another disease related to hyperlipidemia is fatty liver. The liver, which plays a key role in our bodies, stores most of the nutrients that come into the body or supplies them to other tissues as needed. It also detoxifies toxins from drugs, food, or the body, and helps to build up bile to help fat oxidation. However, when the liver is inflamed or the liver cells are destroyed due to excessive taking an alcohol, fat is not decomposed, which accumulates and causes fatty liver.

Table 5.13 ***Exercise test, drug, and specific considerations for hyperlipidemia patients***

Test Item		Measurement	Recommended Stopping Point	Remarks
Aerobic Power Ability	▪ Treadmill (1~2METs/ 3min stage) ▪ Cycle (25~50watt/ 3min stage) Ramp protocol	▪ 12 lead ECG	▪ Peak oxygen uptake/ power ▪ Severe arrhythmia appearance ▪ ST segment depression / elevation > 2 mm ▪ Ischemic threshold ▪ T wave inversion with ST change	Patients with hyperlipidemia are at high risk for CAD and stroke.
		▪ HR	▪ Maximal heart rate 85%	
		▪ BP	▪ SBP/DBP >250/115 mmHg ▪ Hypotensive reaction	
		▪ RPE	▪ Sudden rise of psychological fatigue	
Endurance	▪ 6-min walk	▪ Distance	▪ Time, distance, and symptoms at rest are criteria.	Useful as training time.
Pharmacotherapy	▪ HMG (hepatic hydroxymethylglutaryl) CoA reductase inhibitor and fibric acid may cause muscle damage. ▪ The damage to the muscle protein can be observed through urinalysis.			
Considerations	▪ It has high risk for cardiac system and arterial system failure. ▪ Xantomas may cause biomechanical problems. ▪ Extremely high triglyceride and cholesterol levels may precipitate on the vessel wall and cause ischemic disease.			

Table 5.14 ***Management program for hyperlipidemia patients***

	Type	Goal	Intensity/Frequency/Time	Period
Aerobic Exercise	■ Major muscle exercises · Walking · Brisk walking · Rowing · Cycling · Aquatic exercise	■ Increase exercise capacity ■ Increase of endurance ■ Reduction of cholesterol ■ Reduction of triglycerides ■ Increased Calorie Consumption ■ Reduced body fat	■ Peak power 40～70% ■ RPE 11～16 ■ 1~2 times per day × 5~7 days per week ■ 40 min ■ Emphasis on extending exercise time rather than intensity	■ 4 month (Fitness ↑) ■ 9～12 month (Lipid profiles ↓)
Flexibility Exercise	■ Stretching · Extension/Flexion type	■ Increase of ROM	■ Daily or 5 days per week	
Functional Exercise	■ Activity orientation correction	■ Activities of daily living ■ Change in job style	■ 10 minutes walk after each meal ■ Commute by walking	
Pharmacotherapy	■ Lipid reduction or lipid synthesis inhibitors are often used in combination with each other and are likely to cause side effects. ■ Side effects include toxicity of muscles and rhabdomyolysis of muscle proteins. ■ Niacin(nicotinic acid) : Inhibit the synthesis of VLDL-C. Niacin lowers vasodilation and blood pressure. ■ Cholestyramine/Colestipol (Bile acid sequestrants) : reduce LDL-C by absorbing bile acids in the small intestine and reducing bile acid reabsorption. ■ Gemfibrozil/Clofibrate(fibric acid series) : Increases the activity of lipoproteinases and reduces VLDL-C and LDL-C. However, clofibrate may cause arrhythmias and angina in patients with myocardial infarction. ■ Lovastin(hepatic HMG coA reductase inhibitor) : It suppresses cholesterol synthesis resulting in an increase in LDL receptor. It decreases LDL-C, but can cause 'rhabdomyolysis' when used with fibric acid series drugs. ■ Probucol : increases lipid removal rate, but may also result in prolongation of QT interval. ■ Beta-blocker : It reduces endogenous sympathetic hyperactivity, but results in an increase in TG and a decrease in HDL-C. ■ Thiazide diurethcs : It increase TC, VLDL-C, LDL-C and TG. ■ Oral hypoglycemics : It reduces TG and increases HDL-C in patients with unregulated diabetes. ■ Levothyroxine : It increase LDL receptor in the liver and reduce LDL-C in hypothyroid patients. Side effects may include increased heart rate and blood pressure, arrhythmia. Angina is caused in CAD patients. ■ Sex steroids : If used as an oral contraceptive, it tends to increase cholesterol. ■ Estrogen : There is a tendency to increase HDL-C and VLDL-C and TG in postmenopausal women. ■ Progesterone : It reduce TG and HDL-C.			
Considerations	■ Obesity with hyperlipidemia may limit exercise training. ■ See considerations for obese patients.			

In the case of fatty liver patients, it is necessary to induce weight loss through a proper lifestyle, a vegetable-based diet, and to oxidize fat through aerobic exercise. Exercise should begin after the GPT level drops to 100 IU/L. Equipment that can maintain the level of exercise intensity, such as the recumbent cycle, is suitable. Exercise intensity and time should be between 40~60% of the maximum heart rate and performed every day for about 30 minutes.

Ultimately, many related diseases such as hyperlipidemia do not improve in a short time, so it is important to be patient and develop a habit of constantly exercising for 9~12 months. Exercise prescribers should be familiar with the tests, medications, and considerations of exercises given in [Table 5.13], and to explain the management methods presented in [Table 5.14] to patients with hyperlipidemia and related diseases.[3,5,7,10,,21,22,33,88]

Heart Disease

Hypertension

Symptoms and Characteristics

Hypertension is defined as the period when SBP is greater than 140 ㎜Hg and DBP is greater than 90 ㎜Hg. The prevalence of hypertension increases with age. South Korea has a prevalence of about 12% (5.4 million people), while the US has about 45 million people with hypertension, as much as the entire population of Korea. In the past, mild SBP was not taken seriously. However, many specialists in the field today claim that even mild hypertension (140/90 ㎜Hg) should be treated. The reason for this is that when SBP is 140~150 ㎜Hg, the risk of stroke is increased by 42% and the risk of heart disease is increased by 56%.

The one-time measurement is not important unless the blood pressure is significantly elevated in the initial measurement. Hypertension is diagnosed when blood pressure is consistently high three times over several months. If the SBP is between 140 and 150 ㎜Hg and the DBP is between 90 and 99 ㎜Hg, it should be remeasured within two months. However, if the SBP is 160 ㎜Hg and the DBP is greater than 100 ㎜Hg, the evaluation should be done within one week to one month, and if it is consistently high, it must be reevaluated and treated.[32,57]

In some studies on the pathogenesis of hypertension, salt intake, heredity, and obesity are among the most important factors. According to some studies, hypertension does not exist in societies with low salt intake. This suggests that high salt intake can lead to hypertension, but other studies suggest that some people do not develop hypertension despite a high-salt diet. So, there is no conclusive connection between salt intake and hypertension. Heredity and obesity also play a major role in the development of hypertension. In particular, a family history of hypertension further increases the risk of hypertension. Smoking, drinking, contraceptives, and nonsteroidal anti-inflammatory drugs are also reported as major causes of hypertension.

Examination and Classification of Hypertension

There is much controversy regarding the baseline and normal range of hypertension, but the criteria set out in a report of the Joint National Committee (JNC) published by the National Institute of Health is used. The standard of hypertension is gradually decreasing. In 1993, JNC 5th report and 1995 ACSM 5th version defined SBP 130~139 ㎜Hg and DBP 85~89 ㎜Hg as 'high normal'. However, in the 2003 JNC 7th report, SBP 120~139 ㎜Hg or DBP 80~89 ㎜Hg was classified as a pre-stage of hypertension [Table 5.15].[44]

Table 5.15 ***Blood pressure levels in adults over 18 years (㎜Hg)***

Category	SBP	DBP
Normal	< 120	< 80
Pre-hypertension	120~139	80~89
Stage 1 hypertension	140~159	90~99
Stage 2 hypertension	≥160	≥100

*Target blood pressure when there is chronic kidney disease or diabetes : <130/80

After determining hypertension, a blood test, kidney function test (by measuring mineral components), and urine test are performed. Electrocardiography should be performed on all hypertensive patients, and echocardiography should be performed on patients with complications.[16] If an abnormality is found in the previous examination, or if complications are suspected and blood pressure is not controlled, an endocrine test, X-ray, and kidney sonography are performed.

Heart Disease Gene and Exercise Prescription

The heart 's health status, the cardiovascular gene, is the ACE gene. This gene is expressed in blood vessels, organs and hormones. It converts angiotensin1 into angiotensin2, which has various physiological functions such as strong vasoconstriction, aldestherone secretion, and cell proliferation. ACE is present on the 17th chromosome (17q23band) and has 26 exons. The size is about 21kb, and there is I allele and a deleted D allele with about 289bp segment inserted at the end of Intron 16. Polymorphisms include II, ID, and DD. Type II belonging to the dominant group has a high maximum oxygen uptake associated with cardiovascular function, while DD type has been reported to have a low level and is also called a fitness gene. That is, in the case of DD type, ACE increases and vasoconstrictive action becomes active, which is likely to lead to hypertension, myocardial infarction, cardiomyopathy, left ventricular hypertrophy, CAD and heart attack. Ultimately, early detection of the DD type, a recessive factor for ACE, to prevent serious conditions can be an area of exercise prescription.

Complications of Hypertension

Hypertension is a major risk factor for many other diseases. If the DBP increases by 6 ㎜Hg, the risk of complications is doubled. Therefore, the goal of hypertension treatment is to prevent complications related to hypertension. In addition, if severe hypertension is maintained at normal blood pressure through appropriate treatment, complications can be considerably reduced. In addition, if mild hypertension is maintained at normal blood pressure, the mortality rate can be greatly reduced. The following cases show the degree of reduction of complications when hypertension is lowered to normal.

- Stroke: 35~40% reduction
- Myocardial infarction: 20~25% reduction
- Heart failure: 50% reduction

Alzheimer's Dementia-associated Genes and Exercise Prescription

The gene associated with dementia is ApoE. ApoE becomes soluble after tightly coupling with amyloid protein, which is difficult to decompose in the cell, so it makes plaques in the nervous system and promotes neurodegeneration. The ApoE2, ApoE3, and ApoE4 gene types are polymorphic and the presence of the ApoE4 gene is considered to have a high risk of developing Alzheimer's disease. Genetic testing can compare the polymorphisms of protein genes that have the greatest impact on the onset of Alzheimer's disease and predict whether or not the person is susceptible to developing dementia. This can allow early management measures to be taken in order to prevent dementia from being expressed.

Hypertensive Cardiovascular Disease

Circulatory system disease caused by hypertension is called hypertensive cardiovascular disease. Heart disease can be diagnosed by ECG or echocardiography. If the thickness of the myocardial wall is increased in the ECG or sonogram, it is judged as left ventricular hypertrophy. Those who make such judgments should know that the risk of heart disease is high and a specialist should be consulted. Indeed, effective antihypertensive medications can protect or improve such cases.

Hypertensive Cerebrovascular Disease

The brain circulatory system disease caused by hypertension is called hypertensive cerebrovascular disease. Systolic hypertension is the leading cause of dementia caused by stroke. It has recently been revealed that patients with Alzheimer's dementia are most likely to have hypertension.

Hypertensive Renal Disease

Renal disease caused by hypertension is called hypertensive renal disease and is commonly seen in black people. Hypertension and diabetes lead to kidney disease, and kidney disease exacerbates hypertension. Therefore, early diagnosis and treatment of hypertensive kidney disease and diabetes are important.

Peripheral Vascular Disease and CAD

Hypertension also hardens the arteries in the human body, which is called atherosclerosis.27) Generally, genetics, diabetes, hypercholesterolemia, and smoking also cause atherosclerosis. Because arteriosclerosis is caused by a number of factors, treatment of hypertension does not necessarily lead to the prevention of arteriosclerosis.[87] However, treating hypertension can reduce CAD, aortic aneurysm28), and other diseases.

Classification of Hypertension

Hypertension can be divided into two categories, essential and secondary. 95% is essential (inherited type) hypertension, but its cause is unknown. The remaining 5% are

27) Atherosclerosis: The deposits of yellow plaque (atheroma) contain cholesterol, lipid and fat-storing cells. Deposits occur in the endothelium and midgut of the aorta and middle artery.[87]

28) Aneurysm: It is a pocket in which the walls of arteries, veins and heart are enlarged and relaxed. Because blood is filled in the arteries, pulsatile noise and beating occurs, and the surrounding tissues are pressed to cause pain and paralysis.

secondary (acquired cause) hypertension due to endocrine abnormalities or kidney disease.

Management of Hypertension

The goal of hypertension treatment is to reduce or prevent cardiovascular disease, CAD, peripheral vascular disease, cerebrovascular disease, and renal failure. These goals are achieved when SBP is lowered below 140 mmHg and DBP to below 90 mmHg without adverse effects or reducing the quality of life. However, caution should be exercised when lowering SBP to 160 mmHg or lower in elderly patients since side effects may occur. Unfortunately, hypertension is also a contributing factor to metabolic or endocrine disorders that are not related to hypertension. These factors lead to the elevation of insulin and abnormal lipid levels in the blood, resulting in the activity of renin-angiotensin that constricts the arteries. Above all, ideal hypertension management does not use many kinds of medicine, but lowers blood pressure without side effects.[34]

Although the selection of drugs for hypertension is controversial, 40~50% of the hypertensive period can be controlled with one drug, and 80~90% can be controlled by mixing two or more drugs. Specifically, the physiological effects of the drug are as follows. Control of blood pressure results from cardiac output and peripheral resistance. Blood pressure can be decreased by reducing one or both of the two variables. First, beta-blockers and diuretics are the primary drugs used in patients with hypertension. Beta-blockers reduce cardiac output while diuretics decrease blood volume and peripheral resistance. Beta-blockers tend to be less preferred because they increase blood lipids and cholesterol, insulin resistance, and insulin levels. However, among the beta-blockers, labetalol and acebutolol are lipid-neutral and are considered as exceptional drugs.

The angiotensin converting enzyme inhibitor (ACE inhibitor), which reduces angiotensin-II[29] and aldosterone[30], has been increasingly used because it does not adversely affect blood lipids. To date, ACE inhibitors have been regarded as the most effective drug in the treatment of hypertension. In addition, ACE inhibitors are recommended for athletes with hypertension because they do not cause a reduction in the $\dot{V}O_2max$ that are affected by beta blockers. All ACE inhibitors have the same effects, including similar side effects, and are also recommended for its low cost.

A 25 mg of hydrochlorothiazide, a small amount of diuretic, decreases blood pressure by reducing plasma volume and lowering vascular resistance without causing significant

---

29) Angiotension-Ⅱ: A substance acting like an adrenaline.

30) Aldosterone: A hormone that maintains moisture and sodium by the kidneys.

changes in blood lipids. The drug is more effective for black people, obese patients, and the elderly. For women, hydrochlorothiazide can also have additional benefits that reduce the risk of osteoporosis. The side effect of this drug is hypokalemia, which is uncommon in small doses and can be prevented by adequate intake of fruits and vegetables.

With the exception of some ethnic groups, about 50% of hypertensive patients can control blood pressure with small amounts of diuretics. In fact, the choice of drugs for hypertensive patients depends on many factors. For example, young white people respond well to beta-blockers, ACE inhibitors, and calcium channel blockers. Older white people may experience positive effects from diuretics, beta-blockers, and calcium channel blockers. Blacks are known to respond well to diuretics and calcium channel blockers, so there is no need to emphasize ACE inhibitors.

Table 5.16 ***Factors for selecting antihypertensive agents***

Factors	Antihypertensive treatment
■ People without hypertension related diseases, young people, white people	⇨ Thiazide or beta-blocker
■ Elderly patients with hypertension, single systolic hypertension, black people	⇨ Thiazide (long-acting nifedipin)
■ Diabetes	⇨ Angiotensin converting enzyme inhibitor
■ Heart failure	⇨ Angiotensin converting enzyme inhibitor, diuretic
■ CAD	⇨ Beta-blockers without sympathetic action

People with CAD can benefit from beta-blockers, and patients with diabetes or heart failure can benefit from ACE inhibitors in addition to blood pressure reduction [Table 5.16].

Follow-up Care of Hypertension Patients

Patients often need to visit their physician at an early stage to control blood pressure. If the blood pressure is below 180/100 ㎜Hg, the patient should visit the clinic every 1~2 months to get information about antihypertensive agents. If the blood pressure level is higher, the patient will often need to see a doctor. If blood pressure is well controlled, the number of visits can be reduced to once a year.[57]

Seven Lifestyle Rules to Prevent Hypertension
(Korean Society of Hypertension, 2001)

- Eat a bland and balanced diet.
- Maintain an ideal body weight so that you do not gain weight.
- Proper exercise for 30 minutes or more every day.
- Abstain from smoking and drinking alcohol.
- Reduce fat and consume a lot of vegetables.
- Avoid stress and keep calm.
- Regularly measure blood pressure and consult with a physician.

Patients with hypertension need to learn how to measure blood pressure and frequently measure blood pressure. If the blood pressure is consistently high, the patient should seek another measurement by a physician. Follow-up tests are indicated according to individual needs. Particularly, patients taking beta-blockers should be tested for blood lipid levels every year and should undergo ECG every 2~4 years, depending on the risk factors for heart disease. Patients with hypertension should not expect immediate effects after treatment, but should aim to live a normal life and increase their life expectancy by preventing the occurrence of complications in the long term. In order to do this, the following seven rules must be observed.

Non-medicinal Treatment of Hypertension Patients

Mild hypertension can be treated without drugs. The 'antihypertensive program', which is performed by the general clinic's exercise prescription department, emphasizes weight loss, regular exercise, ingestion of high contents of potassium and magnesium, and abstaining from alcohol, smoking, and salty foods. Potassium plays a role in lowering blood pressure by expanding the arteries and because bananas have a high potassium content, eating one a day also helps lower blood pressure.

It is reported that doctors did not recommend exercise to hypertensive patients in the past. According to the US National Health Interview Survey, only 48% of hypertensive patients were encouraged to exercise by an attending physician and 46% were recommended to lose weight. Moderate exercise can lower blood pressure and may treat patients with mild hypertension below 145/90 mmHg at rest. Some studies have reported that blood pressure decreased by 2 mmHg when body weight was reduced by about 1 kg. This reduction is more pronounced in patients with secondary hypertension due to renal failure.[57] Along with regular exercise, blood pressure can be lowered even if patients quit smoking, suppress salt intake, and reduce alcohol drinking.

Hypertension and Exercise

Regular exercise reduces the incidence and severity of cardiovascular risk factors, including hypertension, and may mitigate the risk of premature death by cutting down the intake of antihypertensive medications. The treatment of patients with mild hypertension depends on the outcome of exercise therapy. Recently, a number of studies have reported that a high level of fitness is associated with a decrease in SBP at rest, while weight loss, smoking cessation, and alcohol withdrawal further lower blood pressure.

Light physical activities such as walking and gardening are not effective in lowering blood pressure, except for the elderly with a sedentary lifestyle. Only moderate exercise helps reduce blood pressure. For example, moderate exercise, which is 50% of $\dot{V}O_2max$ or maximal capacity, is a good way to prevent blood pressure from rising in the morning. In fact, lowering blood pressure is very important because the prevalence and mortality of cardiovascular events increase in the morning when the parasympathetic nervous system is transferred to the sympathetic nervous system.

The frequency, type, time, and intensity of exercise are not significantly different from those of healthy people. However, exercise between 40~70% of maximum heart rate or between a RPE of 11 (moderate) to 13 (somewhat hard) is more effective than at high intensity. The reduction of exercise-induced blood pressure occurs within 4~5 weeks and is maintained for the duration of the exercise program. Patients with resting SBP of 180~209 ㎜Hg and DBP of 110~119 ㎜Hg should not exercise until drug therapy is started.[34] If the patient is taking vasodilators, it may be desirable to have a longer cool-down time, since blood may be drawn into the veins after suddenly stopping exercise.

Exercise Prescription for Hypertension Patients

Aerobic Exercise

Exercise is considered to be a non-pharmacological antihypertensive method because hypertension patients can prevent blood pressure and complications as time goes by when they perform aerobic exercise. If blood pressure rises sharply, aerobic exercise should be considered after medical treatment. Exercise can further decrease blood pressure and reduce drug administration, thereby lowering the risk of premature mortality. In particular, when blood pressure is lowered in combination with weight loss, salt intake restriction, and antihypertensive therapy, it is desirable to prescribe an appropriate exercise program through a GXT.

Blood pressure responses during exercise provide prior information about the risk of hypertension. For example, if the blood pressure increases to at least 180/90 ㎜Hg at 50% of maximal exercise capacity or 225/90 ㎜Hg at maximal exercise, it could indicate mild hypertension. It is also dangerous if hypertension develops before or at the beginning of exercising and falls to normal blood pressure at rest, or if it increases to maximal blood pressure at the time of exercise or immediately after exercise. On the other hand, in patients who are taking beta-blockers to lower blood pressure, heart rate and maximal exercise capacity may be reduced. Therefore, if the patient is taking beta-blockers, measuring exercise intensity by RPE is better than by heart rate.

The types of exercise for hypertensive patients include aerobic exercises such as walking, brisk walking, swimming, and stationary bicycling. It is good to refrain from exercising that requires intense temporary exertion such as short-distance running or tug-of-war. In particular, an exercise that increases blood pressure by 200 ㎜Hg or more should be avoided.

Ultimately, the intensity of aerobic exercise for hypertensive patients should be 40~80% of maximum heart rate or 40~60% of $\dot{V}O_2$ reserve. It is also desirable to exercise at a reasonable blood pressure range by applying the "target blood pressure formula" (see Example 1 and Appendix A). Exercise for hypertensive patients should be in the range of 700~2,000 ㎉ per week, with a daily exercise time of 30~60 minutes at a frequency of 4~7 days per week. However, if blood pressure increases to over 250/120 ㎜Hg or the RPE exceeds 'somewhat hard' during exercise, it is necessary to lower the intensity or stop the exercise.

[Example 1] In the exercise test, the SBP was 152 ㎜Hg and the maximum SBP was 215 ㎜Hg at rest. When we try to exercise 40~70% of these hypertensive patients, the target blood pressure during exercise is calculated as follows.

Target SBP = %Intensity × (maximum SBP – resting SBP) + resting SBP
= 0.40 (or 0.70) × (215 - 152) + 152
= 0.40 (or 0.70) × (63) + 152
= 25.2 (or 44.1) + 152
≒ 177~196 ㎜Hg

Life Therapy	SBP (㎜Hg)
■ Reduce weight by 10㎏: maintain standard weight	5~20 ⇩
■ Diet: Fruit, vegetables, low fat	8~10 ⇩
■ Salt limit: 6g per day or less	8~10 ⇩
■ Regular exercise: 30 minutes a day aerobic exercise	8~10 ⇩
■ Moderation in drink : Less than 2 cups per day	8~10 ⇩

Blood pressure levels suitable for exercise are 140/90~159/99 ㎜Hg. Patients with a resting SBP of 180~209 ㎜Hg and a DBP of 110~119 ㎜Hg should refrain from exercising until blood pressure falls to suitable levels after medication. However, if there are no complications, walking at 2~3 METs is considered to present no risk and good results. It is well known that other lifestyle strategies, including exercise, can reduce SBP.

Resistance Exercise

Weight loading exercise, such as weight training, is not recommended as a form of primary exercise to treat hypertension, but a high number of repetitions of strength training using light weights is worth considering. There are some precautions when the level of physical fitness increases to the point where weight training is possible. The most important thing is not to hold the breath when lifting the weight. Holding the breath and lifting weights can lead to Valsalva maneuvers, which can double blood pressure and endanger life.

It is advisable to avoid weight loading exercise in patients with hypertension (> 160/100 ㎜Hg) whose blood pressure is not controlled. It should be noted that isometric exercise such as tug of war, or anaerobic exercise such as 100 m running may further increase DBP. In addition, if the patient has any of the factors listed below, the patient should refrain from weight loading exercise.

- Congestive heart failure[31)]
- Unregulated arrhythmia[32)]
- Severe valve disease
- Metabolism capacity of less than 5 MET[33)]

A suitable weight training method for patients with hypertension is circuit training. It is done by performing one exercise after another with regular intervals. Circuit training can develop muscle endurance, strength, and cardiopulmonary endurance.

Circuit training should be done to control blood pressure and reduce burden on the heart,[48] so when lifting weights, the patient should use proper breathing techniques and

---

31) Congestive heart failure: Clinical syndrome due to heart failure, characterized by poor breathing, edema, and abnormal retention of sodium and water.

32) Arrhythmia: Includes changes in normal rhythm of the heartbeat, sinus arrhythmia, exophthalmus, cardiac block, atrial fibrillation, atrial flutter, alternation, paroxysmal tachycardia.

33) MET: Metabolic EquivalenT (1 MET = 3.5 ㎖/kg/min)

adjust the weight accordingly so that the movements do not stop in the middle of the action.[36] At this time, it is better to select the weight based on individual ability rather than random weights. That is, 1RM should be calculated. In this case, using the modified 1RM calculation formula (m1RM, modified one repetition maximum) shown in [Table 5.19] is the safer method for patients with hypertension than the 1RM formula given above. Based on the results, exercise intensity should be 60~80% of 1RM, and the weight that the patient can lift 15 repetitions at the beginning is selected. If the patient is comfortable with 15 repetitions, increase the weight to the point where the patient can complete 12 repetitions. If the patient can only perform 8 repetitions, remeasure the maximum muscle strength with m1RM.

The above methods for determining exercise intensity can be used for all resistance training, such as free weights (e.g., dumbbells and barbells), weight equipment, hand weights, and elastic bands. However, it is recommended that the RPE be maintained between 11 (fairly light) to 13 (somewhat hard) during weight loading exercise. Ultimately, exercise prescribers should be familiar with the tests, medications, and considerations of the exercises presented in [Table 5.17] and based on this, explain the management method presented in [Table 5.18] to hypertensive patients in detail.[3,5,22,25,88]

Table 5.17 ***Exercise test, drug, and specific considerations for hypertensive patients***

Test Item		Measurement	Recommended Stopping Point	Remarks
Aerobic Power Ability	■ Treadmill (1~2METs/ 3min stage) ■ Cycle (25~50watt/ 3min stage) (17watt/min) Ramp protocol	■ 12 lead ECG	■ Severe arrhythmia appearance ■ ST segment depression / elevation > 2 mm ■ Ischemic threshold ■ T wave inversion with ST change	Drugs should be avoided during exercise.
		■ HR	■ Maximal HR 85%	
		■ BP	■ SBP/DBP >250/115 mmHg ■ Headache or other risk symptoms	
		■ RPE	■ Sudden increase of psychological fatigue	
		■ Gas analysis	■ $\dot{V}O_2max$	
Strength	■ Free weight ■ Machine	■ 1RM ■ MVC		SBP/DBP >250/115 mmHg
Pharmacotherapy	■ Beta-blocker : It can cause a low chronotropic reaction of about 30 times per minute. ■ See pharmacotherapy for myocardial infarction patients.			

Table 5.18 ***Management program for hypertensive patients***

	Type	Goal	Intensity/Frequency/Time	Period
Aerobic Exercise	■ Major muscle exercises · Walking · Brisk walking · Rowing · Cycling · Aquatic exercise	■ Increase in maximal oxygen uptake ■ Increased levels of ventilation threshold ■ Maximum workload / increase in endurance ■ Increase in calorie consumption ■ Blood pressure response control	■ Maximal HR 40∼80% ■ $\dot{V}O_2R$ 40∼60% ■ RPE 11∼13 ■ 4∼7 day per week ■ 30∼60 min/bout ■ Consumption of 700∼2,000 ㎉ per week	■ 4∼6 month
Strength Exercise	■ Circuit training	■ Increase in muscle strength	■ 8∼12 times × 1 set ■ 60∼80% 1RM	
Pharmacotherapy	■ Beta-blocker : Heart rate can be reduced about 30 bpm. ■ alpha1 blocker/ alpha2 blocker/ calcium channel blocker/ vasodilator : Causing hypotension after exercise.			
Considerations	■ See the program for patients with myocardial infarction. ■ If resting SBP> 200 ㎜Hg or DBP> 115 ㎜Hg, avoid exercise. ■ Participate in exercise when the blood pressure response is well controlled by the drug. ■ It reduces resting blood pressure when exercising at 40~60% of the oxygen intake reserve. ■ Exercise at high intensities should also be avoided as it may reduce blood pressure, but may lead to other cardiovascular events. ■ Consumption of 700 ㎉ per week should be the initial target and consumption of 2,000 ㎉ should be the long term target.			

Table 5.19 ***Example of modified 1RM measurement***

① Formula : 100 - (Number of repetitions× 2) = %1RM
② If the patient lifts 40 pounds 10 times,
③ Using the formula, {100 - (10 × 2)}= %1RM
④ 100 - 20 = 80%
⑤ That means 40 pounds is 80% of 1RM.
⑥ So {40 pounds ÷ 0.80} = 50 pounds will be 1 RM.

※ Initially, 30~50% of the 1RM is compatible with the weight of 15~25 pounds.

Antihypertensive Mechanism for Exercise

Blood Pressure Response to Acute Exercise

During intense aerobic exercise, SBP increases and DBP decreases or remains the same, which is a typical blood pressure response. During maximum exercise, SBP increases to 180~210 ㎜Hg and DBP to 60~85 ㎜Hg. Excessive blood pressure response to exercise, along with resting blood pressure, is likely to lead to future hypertension.[59] In addition, blood pressure during exercise can predict the progression of CAD. In healthy adult men, blood pressure during exercise is highly correlated with myocardial infarction morbidity and mortality and can be classified between severe and mild hypertension. Men with a high blood pressure response during exercise (≥ 230/100 ㎜ Hg) and high-risk factors are less sensitive to peripheral resistance and inhibit exercise-induced vasodilatation as a mechanism of hypertension in the future.

Exercise and Blood Pressure Control Mechanism

In many cross-sectional studies, although regular physical activity and exercise are known to play an important role in the prevention and treatment of hypertension, the specific mechanisms for the relationship are unclear.

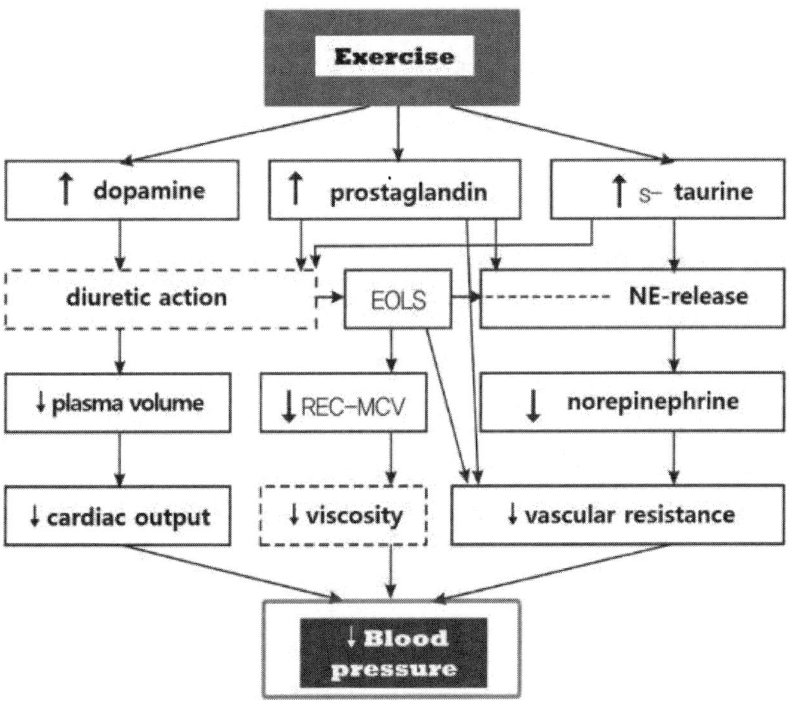

Fig. 5.1 ***Mechanism of Blood Pressure Reduction by Exercise (Arakawa, 1994):*** *S(serum), RBC(red blood cell), NE(norepinephrine), EOLS(endogenous ouabain-like substance)*

Decreased bioavailability and secretion of nitrogen oxide, one of the features of hypertensive patients, reduces vascular relaxation capacity. However, regular exercise increases the shear stress of the blood vessels, activates the cell signaling system, and promotes the secretion and bioavailability of nitric oxide. This induces vascular relaxation, which leads to a decrease in peripheral resistance and can have a positive impact.

Elevated blood pressure may be caused by one or both of increased cardiac output and increased total peripheral resistance.[72] In terms of hemodynamic mechanisms, exercise directly or indirectly affects blood pressure by causing nutritional and metabolic changes. There are several possibilities for hemodynamic mechanisms in which regular exercise can lower blood pressure. First, after regular long-term exercise, the cardiac output and peripheral resistance at rest or given exercise intensity are lowered. Second, the activity of serum catecholamine and plasma renin decreases after regular long-term exercise. Third, prostaglandin E, which enlarges the blood vessels, and dopamine, which causes diuretic action, increase, while plasma and cardiac output decrease. As a kind of amino acid, taurine, which is a vasodepressor, increases and norepinephrine decreases, leading to a reduction in peripheral vascular resistance. Taken together, exercise can reduce blood pressure because norepinephrine is reduced, tensions in the autonomic nervous system are relaxed, blood vessels are expanded, baroreflex is readjusted, and peripheral resistance is lowered [Fig. 5.1].

Coronary Artery Disease

Symptoms and Features

Coronary arteries supplying oxygen and nutrients to the cardiac muscles become narrower like other blood vessels when lipid components are deposited on the inner walls of the coronary arteries. A series of such diseases is called CAD. That is, when oxygen and nutrient supply to the heart muscle is reduced, angina and myocardial infarction are induced.

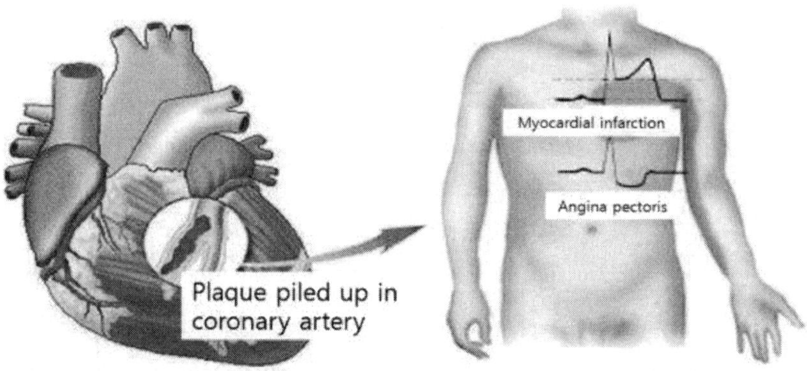

Fig. 5.2 ***Induction of Angina and Myocardial Infarction***

The main symptom of angina is uncomfortable and painful pain on the left chest, shoulders, arms, neck and jaw, lasting 20~30 minutes. On the other hand, myocardial infarction has symptoms similar to angina, but it is severe, lasts more than 60 minutes, and does not easily disappear [Fig. 5.2].[27]

Specifically, when angina occurs during severe exercise, the coronary artery is occluded by more than 50~70%, and when angina is observed at rest, 90% is occlude d[34]. On the other hand, the blood flow of the coronary arteries increases 5 times more during exercise than at rest. However, blood flow in patients with CAD does not flow into damaged coronary beds, resulting in an imbalance between myocardial oxygen consumption[35] and supply. The cause of this imbalance is further exacerbated by the contraction of the coronary arteries and the deposition of platelets. Characteristically, platelet viscosity decreases in moderate intensity exercise, whereas in high-intensity exercise, platelet viscosity increases. Although there is no angina on the ECG, silent ischemia[36] and an elevated emotional state may constrict the blood vessels and cause angina even at rest.

As a reaction phenomenon due to exercise, localized muscle contraction activity causes blood vessel expansion and skeletal muscle mechanoreceptor activation, whereas in inactive blood vessels, they contract. When the vasoconstrictor acts on the inactive vascular bed, it activates the baroreceptor, and other receptors located in the myocardial layer cause neurogenic vasodilation, leading to the reduction of vasoconstriction.[2,8] Ultimately, due to the combined action of vasoconstrictor and vasodilator, blood flow in active muscles increase significantly, blood pressure increases, and systemic vascular resistance decreases.[55] In patients with CAD, an increase in myocardial oxygen consumption causes a contraction of the damaged coronary artery, resulting in a health hazard.

Management Methods

Medication and Surgery Treatment

There are many medications used for CAD, and the purpose of treatment is to decrease myocardial oxygen consumption and increase coronary blood flow to the

---

34) Angina and exercise: It is necessary to accurately identify the intensity of the symptoms through GXT and to exercise at 10 to 20% lower intensity.

35) Myocardial oxygen consumption: It is assessed by hear rate × SBP. It is also called double product or rate pressure product (RPP). Unit is bmp·㎜Hg.

36) Ischemia: Functional stenosis of blood vessels or partial blood shortage caused by occlusion.

ischemic myocardial layer. β-blockers[37] reduce myocardial oxygen consumption by reducing heart rate, myocardial contractility, and blood pressure. The decrease in myocardial oxygen consumption allows patients taking beta-blockers to perform a high-intensity submaximal exercise capacity without showing myocardial ischemia. Breaking beta-blockers can cause unstable angina.

Table 5.20 ***Exercise test, drug, and specific considerations for CABG/ PTCA patients***

Test Item		Measurement	Recommended Stopping Point	Remarks
Aerobic Power Ability	▪ Treadmill (1~2METs/ 3min stage) ▪ Cycle (25~50watt/ 3min stage) (17watt/min) Ramp protocol	▪ 12 lead ECG	▪ Severe arrhythmia appearance ▪ ST segment depression / elevation > 2 ㎜ ▪ Ischemic threshold ▪ T wave inversion with ST change	▪ Loss of the ST segment is accompanied by restenosis / local block. ▪ It is important to set a safe training intensity. ▪ Chronotropic disorders have a poor prognosis. ▪ Treadmill speed starts at a minimum of 1.0 mph.
		▪ BP	▪ SBP/DBP >250/115 ㎜Hg	▪ Hypotension during exercise (≥20㎜Hg reduction) is not a good prognosis.
		▪ RPE	▪ Sudden increase of psychological fatigue	▪ Concurrent observation of heart rate with intensity.
		▪ Gas analysis	▪ Peak oxygen uptake	▪ If CABG patients show peak power over 9 METs, it is a good prognosis.
Strength	▪ Isokinetic ▪ Isotonic	▪ MVC 90% (Loads up to 2 or 3 reps of lifting)	▪ Repeat 3 consecutive reps	▪ Useful for resistance exercise planning. ▪ The development of muscle function prevents the adverse effects of needle rest. ▪ Strength exercise is prohibited until the sternum is cured.
Pharmacotherapy	▪ See pharmacotherapy in patients with myocardial infarction.			
Considerations	▪ See pharmacotherapy in patients with myocardial infarction. ▪ It takes 4~8 weeks for the chest and lower wound to heal. On the other hand, upper limb arm crank ergometer examination, which can compress the sternum, should be avoided until the wound is cured. ▪ After a maximal or symptom-limited graded exercise test, a prolonged and aggressive cool-down may reduce the risk of cardiovascular complications that can be common after exercise. ▪ The longer the recovery period after CABG, the lower the maximum oxygen uptake. ▪ Graded exercise test after CABG may increase self-satisfaction and self-efficacy. ▪ Within 24~48 hours after PTCA, normal activity can be resumed.			

37) β-blocker: Drugs that cause adrenergic blockade on β_1 or β_2 adrenergic receptors or both.

Table 5.21 ***Management program for CABG / PTCA patients***

	Type	Goal	Intensity/Frequency/Time	Period
Aerobic Exercise	▪ Major muscle exercise ▪ Arm ergometer ▪ Leg ergometer	▪ Increased aerobic capacity ▪ Reduced heart rate and blood pressure during submaximal exercise ▪ Reduced myocardial oxygen demand ▪ Reduced risk factors for CAD	▪ HRR or $\dot{V}O_2max$ 40~80% ▪ RPE 11~16 ▪ Intensity is below the ischemic threshold ▪ 4~7 days a week ▪ 20~60 min/bout	▪ 4~6 month
Strength Exercise	▪ Circuit training	▪ Increase in leisure / work / daily life ability ▪ Increased strength / endurance	▪ MVC 40~50% ▪ 2~3 days per week ▪ 2 to 4 sets / 12 to 15 repetitions ▪ Utilization of 8~10 machines ▪ Start with 1~2 lbs (0.5~0.9 ㎏). To increase weight, it is safe for 3 months after surgery. ▪ The load is increasing incrementally.	▪ 4~6 month
Flexibility Exercise	▪ Upper / lower body ROM activity	▪ Reduced risk of injury ▪ ROM improvement	▪ 2~3 days per week ▪ Static stretching for 10 to 30 seconds	▪ 4~6 month
Pharmacotherapy	▪ See pharmacotherapy in patients with myocardial infarction. ▪ Beta-blocker : It does not affect the exercise / training effects of CABG / PTCA patients. ▪ Calcium channel blocker : It does not affect the exercise / training effects of CABG / PTCA patients.			
Considerations	▪ See pharmacotherapy in patients with myocardial infarction. ▪ Patients with CABG typically can improve at a rapid rate if they start rehabilitation from admission. ▪ Patients with CABG are generally able to concentrate on upper extremity ROM exercises. ▪ Careful observation of signs and symptoms (angina pectoris) of angioblastomas (CABG) or restenosis (PTCA). Periodic intermittent or continuous ECG observations are helpful. ▪ The maximum-limit time point for early exercise prescription (at admission) is set to a range of RPE 11~13 and a 30 times/min rise over resting heart rate.			

Calcium channel blockers[38] have the effect of reducing myocardial contractility. It dilates peripheral blood vessels and reduces myocardial oxygen consumption. In particular, dilatation of the coronary arteries increases the blood flow to the coronary arteries and reduces the contractile force of the coronary vessels. Because of these effects, reducing myocardial oxygen consumption at a specific exercise intensity can significantly delay the onset of ischemia. Verapamil and diltiazem reduce heart rate by slowing the conduction of the sinoatrial node and atrioventricular node. Because nifedipin

38) Calcium channel blocker: A drug that inhibits the entry of intracellular calcium or inhibits the migration of calcium from intracellular stores. It causes atrioventricular conduction or sinoatrial conduction disturbance leading to atrium muscle and myocardial relaxation. It is used as the treatment of angina pectoris, arrhythmia, hypertension.

may cause tachycardia, it may also be used in combination with a beta-blocker that reduces heart rate. Caution is required because taking calcium channel blockers and nitrates together may cause orthostatic hypotension.

On the other hand, nitrates produce nitrogen oxides that expand the arterioles to increase blood flow to the coronary arteries and reduce preload, thereby reducing oxygen consumption and platelet aggregation. However, it is advisable to use nitrates every other day because of the increased tolerance and reduced effectiveness of long-term use of nitrates. If symptoms are not improved despite medication, percutaneous transluminal coronary angioplasty (PTCA) or coronary artery bypass graft surgery (CABG)39) is performed.[24] On the other hand, exercise prescribers should be familiar with the methods of examining and managing patients who have underwent CABG or PTCA and treat them accordingly [Table 5.20, 5.21].[3,5,22,25,88]

Rehabilitation Exercise

Treatment of CAD includes diet, exercise, and life management to lower cholesterol, in addition to drugs and surgery. Clinically, a vegetarian diet, low-fat foods, and regular exercise are recommended. This means that patients should reduce calorie intake by 500 ㎉ and expend 200~300 ㎉ by exercising, which means 700~800 ㎉ can be consumed a day on average. The calorie limit should not be adjusted to less than 1,000 ㎉/day. In fact, exercise is also very effective in preventing angina and myocardial infarction because it helps to control weight and relieve stress. Moreover, these interventions have been applied as a treatment after heart disease.[22] In some studies, patients with cardiovascular disease, including angina pectoris or myocardial infarction, underwent surgery at the clinic and had regular exercise and healthy eating habits. As a result, the recovery time after surgery was several times faster than those who did change their diet and exercise habits. Sequela and recurrence rates were also very low.

Even if the level of activity in everyday life is enhanced, the effect can be increased. In a study published for the first time in the American medical journal 'Lancet', the authors investigated the prevalence of CAD in 'single-row bus drivers' who sat and drove and 'double-decker bus clerks' who were more physically active on the job by having to move around. The clerks reported about 30% less heart disease and 50% fewer

---

39) Coronary artery bypass graft surgery (GABG): Patients with triple CAD, ventricular dysfunction, and left CAD are treated when the condition is not controlled by medication or has severe functional impairment.

myocardial infarctions than the drivers. Surprisingly, after a few years of researching their mortality rates, it was reported that the mortality rate of the clerks was half of that of drivers.[63] Another study reported in the Journal of Circulation found that among 55,000 men in New York, 'those with little activity' had a higher mortality rate than 'those with moderate activity'. According to the journal, those who had moderate activities were people who had walked or climbed stairs every day.[22] In this regard, a study of the worker's electrocardiographic response showed that the 'ischemic ECG response' of people who commute on foot for just 20 minutes or more was reduced to one-third. Recent studies analyzing the correlation between exercise and lethality due to various diseases, have reported that about 30 minutes of exercise every day could reduce lethality by 20~30% and decrease CAD by 30~40%.[74]

Rehabilitation Exercise Phases of Heart Disease

Rehabilitation exercises for heart patients are divided into stages I, II, III, and IV.

Phase I is an inpatient rehabilitative phase, which varies with the degree of myocardial infarction. The goal during this phase is to gradually introduce exercise, even if the patient's level of exercise is limited, unless 'unstable angina' appears. 48 hours after surgery, the patient can get out of bed and start exercising. The exercise involves walking a short distance in the ward 2~3 times between 2~3 METs. It is enough to walk up and down stairs by the time of discharge, which is the end of the phase. In Phase I, there are three important roles of exercise prescribers. First, exercise therapists should train their patients to check their heart rate during exercise and instruct them to increase their heart rate by 20 bpm during exercise. Second, submaximal exercise testing should be performed to allow the patient to exercise independently at home. Third, patients should also be instructed on how to use RPE when they are taking medications which may affect heart rate during exercise, such as beta-blockers.

Phase II is a formalized outpatient rehabilitative phase that takes 4~6 weeks. The goal is to educate people about coronary heart disease and correcting the risk factors for this disease such as smoking cessation and diet. In particular, it is necessary to provide a guidebook to ensure a safe exercise program. The exercise to be presented in the guidebook is to walk a short distance and gradually increase the distance up to 2 km without rest, which is the end point of Phase II. The exercise intensity to be applied at this time starts from a slow pace (about 2 METs) to a fast pace (about 4~5 METs). Heart rate should be increased during exercise by 20 bpm above resting conditions, and should not exceed a RPE of 11 or 12. On the other hand, if the patient's symptoms or fatigue conditions are not good for the prescribed exercise, they should return to the initial stage. For reference, a myocardial infarction patient must visit a clinic and receive a 'symptom-limited GXT' two weeks after surgery [see Appendix B].

Phase Ⅲ is an exercise-based outpatient rehabilitative phase requiring 8~12 weeks. The goal is to alert patients to their safety limits, to recognize the effects of exercise on CAD, and to safely maintain exercise without symptoms. During this phase, the intensity of exercise should be 60~75% of maximum heart rate or a RPE of 12~13. Adjust the warm-up to 20 bpm over the resting heart rate to avoid myocardial ischemia or arrhythmia.

Phase IV is the discharge phase. The goal of this phase is to ensure that patients who are clinically safe and have a functional ability of at least 5 METs will be able to perform exercise themselves. However, if a patient with the above-mentioned ability is determined to be clinically safe, but afraid to exercise independently, it is preferable to meet with an exercise prescription specialist or a person with cardiopulmonary resuscitation (CPR)[40] certificate once or twice a month.

Rehabilitation and Exercise-induced Hypotension

The benefits of exercise in patients who have completed Phase II of cardiac rehabilitation, currently participating, or who are not symptomatic, will experience physiologic changes in the peripheral muscles resulting in increased functional capacity and reduced ischemic response at rest and during exercise. Despite these advantages, however, exercise may cause the cardiac output to drop sharply, resulting in exercise-induced hypotension. For these reasons, researchers have found that the 'abnormal vasodilation' of the inactive vasculature was the main cause of myocardial ischemia. Exercise-induced hypotension may also occur in patients with aortic stenosis, hypertrophic cardiomyopathy[41], or those tested positive for the GXT.[3]

In patients with CAD or valve disease, the prognosis of exercise-induced hypotension or cardiomyopathy is very bad condition. It is not comfortable for people with a healthy heart. However, exercise-induced ventricular arrhythmias are not an independent risk factor for future mortality and coronary heart disease. Rather, the sedentary lifestyle are

---

40) Cardiopulmonary resuscitation (CPR): It is a method of revitalizing the functions of the heart and lungs in the event of cardiac arrest or apparent death caused by electrical shock, drowning, respiratory arrest, or other causes. Generally, it consists of artificial respiration and heart massage.

41) Cardiomyopathy: Myocardial disorders. It means primary myocardial disease and is also used when the cause of the disease is unknown.

the most likely cause of death.[45]

The risk of sudden death associated with exercise is closely related to the severity of disease and exercise intensity, but can be minimized through regular and moderate exercise. Exercise-related accidents are reported in one case per 112,000 people with heart disease, one myocardial infarction per 300,000 people, and one death per 790,000 people. Exercise cardiac rehabilitation programs minimize the need for coronary infarction or CABG. Ultimately, even in patients with CAD, exercising is very safe if the conditions described in [Table 5.22] are met.

Table 5.22 ***When the CAD patient is safe to exercise***

① There is no ischemia at Intensity of 6 METs or less.
② No exercise-induced ventricular tachycardia, hypotension, or cardiac arrhythmia.
③ If you have an ejection fraction of 50% or more.
④ No complication due to myocardial infarction, CABG, angioplasty, or resection.

If the patient does not meet the criteria set out in [Table 5.22], he or she must participate in the program prescribed by the exercise prescriber, as the risk of mortality and unwanted incidences during exercise can be increased. If the patient has unstable ischemia or uncontrolled arrhythmia, do not exercise without a doctor's supervision.

Instructions for Weight Bearing Exercise

Resistance training is safe and effective for patients with a history of heart disease. In fact, most patients experience an improvement in ischemia, angina, and arrhythmias, mainly because of reduced myocardial oxygen consumption ($M\dot{V}O_2$). Hemodynamically, $M\dot{V}O_2$ decreases as the maximum heart rate decreases during maximum isometric exercise. Unlike aerobic exercise, weight loading exercise increases myocardial perfusion by raising DBP and therefore reduces $M\dot{V}O_2$, resulting in less ischemia.

The weight bearing exercise for patients with heart disease slightly increases the submaximal aerobic capacity, but has the advantage of reducing blood pressure in absolute exercise loads because the pressure response to static effort is reduced.[39] In addition to these advantages, weight loading exercise can increase self-efficacy in patients, improve insulin sensitivity due to increased glucose tolerance, and improve lipid composition.[58] However, those with heart disease should participate in weight loading exercise only if they do not fall under the contraindications listed in [Reference 1].

[Reference 1] Patients who are not suitable for resistance exercise

① Patients with uncontrolled hypertension (> 160/100 ㎜Hg)
② Patients with congestive heart failure
③ Patients with uncontrolled arrhythmia
④ Patients with severe valve disease
⑤ Patients with aerobic capacity below 5 METs

On the other hand, circuit training using a light weight that can be lifted a number of times is recommended in weight loading exercise. It improves muscular endurance, muscular strength, and also aerobic capacity. In particular, when performing weight loading exercise, patients should minimize isometric or static movements to control blood pressure and prevent afterload of the heart, and choose a weight that can be lifted without stopping during exercise. The type of weight equipment can be varied depending on the patient's preference and ability. Most importantly, the intensity of exercise should be calculated scientifically. When setting the intensity of the exercise, it is preferable to select a weight based on the individual's ability rather than selecting a random weight. In other words, using the modified 1RM suggested above is a safer method for heart patients [Table 5.23].

Table 5.23 ***Example of modified 1RM measurement***

① Formula : 100 - (Number of repetitions× 2) = %1RM
② If a heart patient lifts 40 pounds 10 reps,
③ Using the formula, {100 - (10 × 2)} = %1RM
④ 100 - 20 = 80%
⑤ That means 40 pounds is 80% of 1RM.
⑥ {40 pounds.÷0.80} = 50 pounds will be 1 RM.

※ Initially, 30~50% of the 1RM is compatible with the weight of 15~25 pounds.

If 1RM is calculated in the formula, choose a weight that can be lifted 10~15 reps at the beginning and repeat it 1~2 reps. After a certain degree of adaptation, the weight should be adjusted so that it can be lifted ten times. However, in order to carry out aerobic exercise by weight loading exercise, RPE should not exceed 12~14.

Ultimately, exercise prescribers should be familiar with the tests, medications, and considerations of the exercises presented in [Tables 5.24 and 5.26]. Based on this, the management methods presented in [Tables 5.25 and 5.27] should be explained in detail to patients with myocardial infarction, angina pectoris, and ischemic heart disease.[3,5,22,25,68,88]

Table 5.24 ***Exercise test, drug, and specific considerations for myocardial infarction patients***

Test Item		Measurement	Recommended Stopping Point	Remarks
Aerobic Power Ability	■ Treadmill (1~2METs/ 3min stage) ■ Cycle (25~50watt/ 3min stage) (17watt/min)Ramp protocol	■ 12 lead ECG	■ Severe arrhythmia appearance ■ ST segment depression / elevation > 2 mm ■ Ischemic threshold ■ T wave inversion with ST change	■ Acute MI patients use low-level Treadmill protocol. ■ Adjust minimum speed of treadmill ≤1.0 mph.
		■ BP ■ Rate-pressure product	■ SBP/DBP >250/115 mmHg	■ It is important to set a safe training intensity. ■ Chronotropic disorders have poor prognosis. ■ Hypotension during exercise (≥20 mmHg) is a bad prognosis.
		■ RPE (6 point scale)	■ Sudden increase of psychological fatigue	
		■ Angina scale	■ +3 (very insecure)	
		■ Radiation nuclear Medicine		■ Sensitivity and specificity are higher than exercise-loaded ECG in estimating ischemic heart disease.
		■ Gas analysis	■ Peak oxygen uptake	■ Utilizing ventilation threshold.
Strength	■ Isokinetic ■ Isotonic	■ MVC 90% (Loads up to 2 or 3 reps of lifting)	■ Repeat 3 consecutive reps	■ Using the modified 1RM. ■ Improvement of myocardial function prevents the adverse effect caused by bed rest.
Pharmacotherapy	■ Beta-blocker : Submaximal / maximum heart rate / blood pressure reduction and reduced exercise capacity when mixed with non-selective drugs. ■ Vasodilator and ACE inhibitor : Generally, it does not affect heart rate during exercise, but it is sensitive to hypotension after exercise. ■ Calcium channel blocker : May cause changes in heart rate response during exercise (Verapamil). ■ Central nervous system-active drug : Effective in heart rate and blood pressure during exercise. Pay attention to low blood pressure, dizziness, syncope. ■ Alpha blocker : Reduces SBP / DBP, but has a small effect on heart rate and oxygen intake during exercise. ■ Digitalis : Promote deformation of the above ST-T wave (note the interpretation). Sometimes it is used to control atrial arrhythmia. ■ Nitroglycerin : Ischemic reaction may be lost or relieved.			
Considerations	■ Orthopedically limited patients can be treated with bicycle, cancer ergometer, and pharmacological stress tests. ■ Patients with CAD are more likely to have symptoms including angina, ischemic ST segment depression, blood pressure abnormalities, and ventricular arrhythmias. ■ Patients with severe peripheral vascular disease can not follow normal load testing (≥85% of predicted maximum heart rate). ■ The maximal exercise test should not be performed before completing a hematologic test. ■ Some cardiovascular drugs also have an effect on body temperature control. ■ It is desirable to have a test after 12 hours fasting or light meal.			

Table 5.25 ***Management program for myocardial infarction patients***

Type		Goal	Intensity/Frequency/Time	Period
Aerobic Exercise	▪ Big muscular exercise ▪ Arm ergometer ▪ Leg ergometer	▪ Increased aerobic capacity ▪ Decrease in heart rate and blood pressure during submaximal exercise ▪ Reduced myocardial oxygen demand ▪ Reduced risk factors for CAD	▪ 40~80% of HRR or $\dot{V}O_2max$ ▪ RPE 11~16 ▪ 3 days or more per week ▪ 20 to 60 minutes/session ▪ 5~10 minutes warm-up and cool-down	▪ 4~6 month
Strength Exercise	▪ Circuit training	▪ Increased strength / muscle endurance ▪ Increase in leisure / work / daily life activity ability	▪ 1RM 30~40% for upper extremity exercise ▪ 1RM 50~60% for lower extremity exercise ▪ 2~3 days per week ▪ 2 to 4 sets, repeating 12-15 reps ▪ The load increases incrementally	▪ 4~6 month
Flexibility Exercise	▪ Upper / Lower body ROM Activity	▪ Reduced risk of injury	▪ 2~3 days per week ▪ Static stretching (10~30 sec)	▪ 4~6 month
Pharmacotherapy	▪ Beta-blocker : It does not affect the exercise / training effects of patients with heart disease. ▪ Calcium channel blocker : It does not affect the exercise / training effects of patients with heart disease.			
Considerations	▪ Observe for abnormalities such as chest pain, irregular blood pressure, dizziness and arrhythmia. ▪ High intensity exercise may cause cardiovascular complications in patients after myocardial infarction. ▪ Observations should be more cautious to middle- to high-risk patients (eg, patients with exercise-induced myocardial ischaemia with obvious ST-segment depression and angina or patients with < 30% left ventricular dysfunction). ▪ After myocardial infarction, the patient is likely to have peripheral artery disease or diabetes. ▪ If possible, you should choose equipment that can adjust the treadmill by 1 MET. ▪ An increase in muscle strength is an important factor for patients with myocardial infarction. As these factors develop, heart rate, blood pressure, and myocardial oxygen demand may be reduced at a given specific strength.			

Table 5.26 ***Exercise test, drug, and specific considerations for angina and ischemic heart disease patients***

Test Item		Measurement	Recommended Stopping Point	Remarks
Aerobic Power Capability	■ Cycle ① 10~25watt/ 3min stage ② 17watt/min Ramp protocol ■ Treadmill (1~2METs/ 3min stage)	■ 12 lead ECG	■ Severe arrhythmia appearance ■ ST segment depression / elevation > 2 ㎜ ■ Ischemic threshold ■ T wave inversion with ST change	
		■ Angina scale	■ Over +3 on the scale of +1 to +4	■ The incidence of angina at low loads is a predictor of ischemic heart disease.
		■ BP	■ Despite the increase in uniformity, SBP shows a plateau phenomenon or decrease tendency. ■ Above SBP/DBP 250/115 ㎜Hg	■ Decrease in SBP during exercise is associated with ischemic heart disease.
Pharmacotherapy	■ Most cardiac medications reduce the sensitivity of the test because it changes the hemodynamic response during exercise.			
Considerations	■ Consult beforehand whether there is any symptom of angina before examination. ■ Unstable angina is a contraindication factor in exercise testing. ■ Inadequate ventricular function may result in dyspnea.			

Table 5.27 ***Management program for angina and ischemic heart disease patients***

	Type	Goal	Intensity/Frequency/Time	Period
Aerobic Exercise	■ Systemic exercise ■ Leg ergometer	■ Improvement of functional ability ■ Reduce CAD risk factors ■ Reduction of blood pressure during submaximal exercise ■ Reduced myocardial oxygen demand	■ Below ischemic threshold (Heart rate less than 10~15 bpm) ■ 3~7 days a week ■ 20 to 60 minutes/session ■ 5~10min warm-up/ cool-down	■ 4~6 month
Strength Exercise	■ Light dumbbell exercise	■ Improvement of functional ability	■ 40~50% of MVV (Valsalva maneuver prohibited) ■ 2~3 days per week ■ 15 to 20 minutes/session	■ 4~6 month
Flexibility	■ Upper / Lower body ROM activity	■ Reduced risk of injury	■ 2~3 days per week	■ 4~6 month
Pharmacotherapy	■ Most cardiac medications cause changes in hemodynamic responses during exercise.			
Considerations	■ See considerations in patients with myocardial infarction. ■ Patients are encouraged to exercise below their ischemic threshold. ■ If symptoms change, visit your doctor as soon as possible. ■ If you are diagnosed with CAD, you should be carrying nitroglycerin. ■ Low intensity walking is highly recommended. ■ Patients with a low ejection fraction, reduced motor ability, or frequent arrhythmias should be closely monitored. ■ Cardiac rehabilitation programs at home may be appropriate only for patients with low risk. ■ Long-term warm-up / cool-down (more than 10 minutes) may provide anti-angiogenic effects.			

Mechanisms of Exercise on CAD

The amount of physical activity and mortality due to all causes have a positive linear correlation. Even if the patient maintains a minimum recommended guideline of expending 1,000 ㎉ a week, it can reduce all-cause mortality by 20~30%. Exercise capacity is a very important prognostic factor for patients with CAD and predicts the mortality of patients with symptoms. Exercise therapy is very useful for those patients who do not require reperfusion of the coronary arteries or those who have severe angina. Exercise training increases exercise tolerance by decreasing heart rate and SBP, resulting in improvement of symptoms. Physical activity is thought to lower the risk of cardiovascular disease by affecting known risk factors for various CAD. The mechanism is shown in [Fig. 5.3]

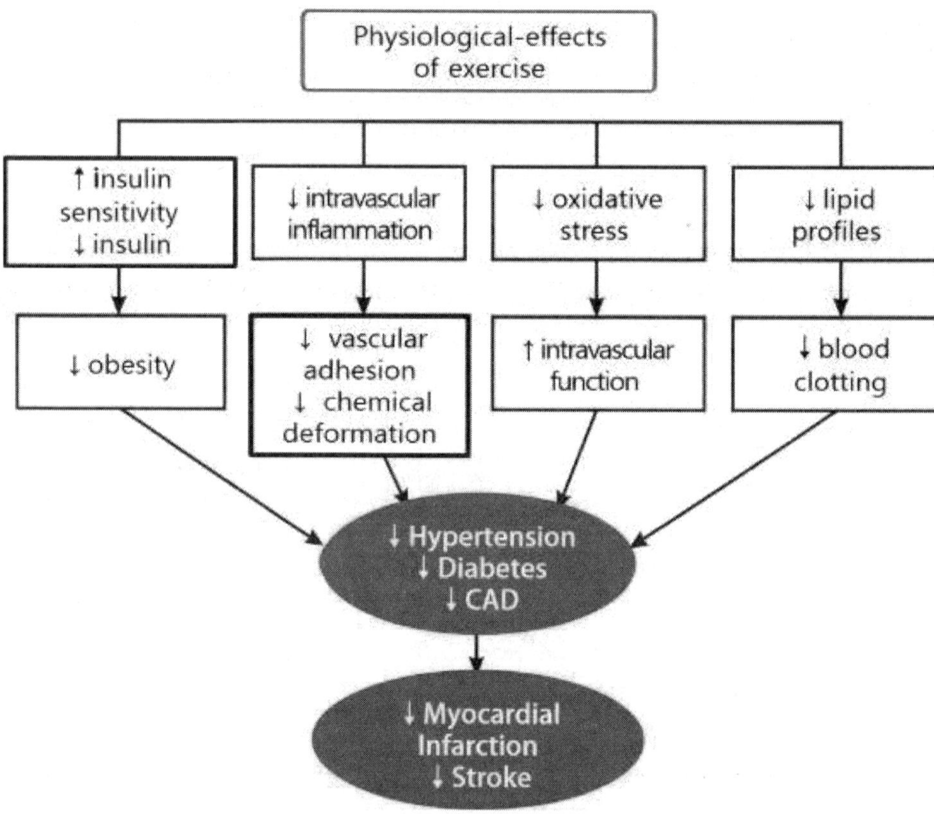

Fig. 5.3 ***Mechanisms of Exercise and Reduction of the Risk of CAD, Hypertension, Diabetes***

Congestive Heart Failure

Symptoms and Features

Heart failure caused by a cardiac pump failure usually has no symptoms, but when starting a physical activity, breathlessness or palpitation can occur. More progress can lead to coughing or phlegm due to lung congestion. This is called congestive heart failure. Congestive heart failure refers to the pathophysiological condition in which congestion occurs in the systemic circulation and the pulmonary circulation due to the inability to pump adequate blood volume to meet the metabolic demand as cardiac capacity gradually decreases.[84] A characteristic symptom is a rapid increase in body weight.[19,25]

Congestive heart failure is divided into systolic dysfunction and diastolic dysfunction according to left ventricular function. Systolic dysfunction is associated with myocardial infarction history, valve regurgitation, Q wave appearance on the ECG, third heart sound, and cardiomegaly. Diastolic dysfunction is associated with a history of hypertension, infiltrative cardiomyopathy or hypertrophic cardiomyopathy, left ventricular hypertrophy on the ECG, fourth heart sound, and small cardiac volume. Once a diagnosis of myocardial hypertrophy is established, exercise programs consisting of more than 60% of $\dot{V}O_2max$ should be contraindicated because they increase the risk of sudden death, and patients with heart failure should undergo echocardiography or radionuclide angiography.

Despite symptoms and signs of heart failure, it is considered that there is diastolic dysfunction if a normal ejection fraction is exhibited. Echocardiographic evidence for diastolic dysfunction are increased diastolic time (measured by closing the aortic valve and opening of the mitral valve), decreased left ventricular filling rate, increased left ventricular wall thickness, and normal or slightly smaller left ventricular volume. The reason for the decreased function of the left ventricle in any cause is due to the increased concentration of catecholamine by the activated sympathetic nervous system. Catecholamine initially improves left ventricular function but contracts the arterioles, resulting in increased systemic vascular resistance, decreased cardiac output, reduced renal perfusion, and increased sodium and water retention. Over time, a deteriorated left ventricular filling pressure causes pulmonary congestion, right ventricular dysfunction, and edema of the peripheral organs.[51] 50% of congestive heart failure patients are reported to die within 5 years of onset. The prognosis depends on the type of disorder or functional ability, but the prognosis is poor if congestive heart failure is caused by systolic dysfunction and CAD.[57]

Mechanism of Heart Failure and Exercise

The main symptoms of chronic heart failure are dyspnea and fatigue during exercise. The lack of cardiac output during exercise can cause blood circulation problems in the skeletal muscle, resulting in fatigue.[60,61] In order to meet the required amount of cardiac output, the left ventricular filling pressure is increased and consequently, lung congestion occurs. Finally, the fluid leaks into the alveoli and dyspnea occurs [Fig. 5.4].

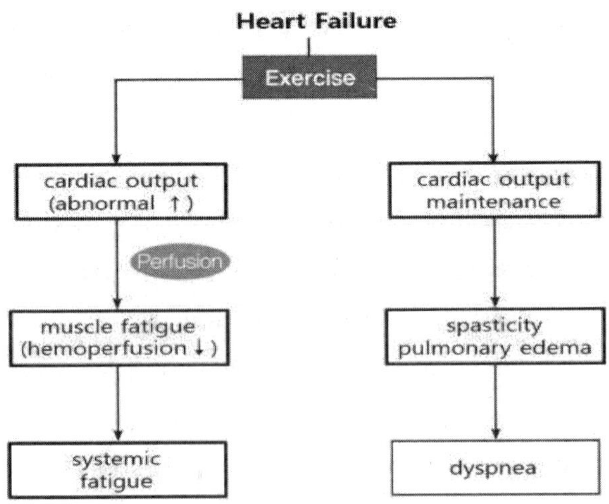

Fig. 5.4 *Hemodynamic Mechanism of Symptom Manifestation in Patients with Heart Failure*

However, this mechanism alone is not enough to explain the symptoms. It has been reported that cardiac function and athletic performance are often discordant, and fatigue and skeletal muscle blood flow abnormalities are not consistent. A recent concept is that changes in the skeletal muscle itself are related to the symptoms of patients with heart failure. In patients with chronic heart failure, skeletal muscle abnormalities are frequently observed, resulting in decreased exercise capacity.[60] In other words, when observing myopathy in patients with heart failure, skeletal muscle volume, muscle strength, and muscle endurance decreases, resulting in increased fatigue. In the end, it invades the respiratory muscles and causes breathing symptoms. The cause of myopathy is an imbalance of catabolism and anabolism (i.e., excessive catabolism), caused by chronic hemodynamic stress. It is accompanied by changes in microstructure (i.e., conversion to type 2 muscle fibers) and mitochondrial abnormalities.

Significance of Exercise Test in Patients with Heart Failure

Symptoms such as dyspnea and fatigue are sometimes difficult to distinguish clearly and are very subjective. Therefore, exercise testing is necessary to objectively assess the functional status of heart failure patients. Metabolic exercise testing or cardiopulmonary exercise testing, which measures the metabolic gas exchange, may be useful to further elucidate the pathophysiology of impaired exercise capacity. Indicators that are frequently used are as follows.

Peak $\dot{V}O_2$

Peak $\dot{V}O_2$ refers to the highest value of $\dot{V}O_2$ attained on GXT. This is a somewhat different concept from the maximal oxygen uptake that can be averaged. Since exercise capacity depends on the degree of cardiac output increase and the degree of oxygen utilization in the skeletal muscle, it is expressed as a numerical value and represents the maximum amount of oxygen that can be used during exercise. Peak $\dot{V}O_2$ can predict the survival rate and is useful for screening patients for heart transplants.[50] Peak $\dot{V}O_2$ varies with age, sex, height, and weight, so the percentage of normalized estimates (% predicted peak $\dot{V}O_2$) is a better indicator.

Carbon Dioxide Emission Slope per Ventilation Equivalent

The carbon dioxide emission slope per ventilation equivalent ($\dot{V}E/\dot{V}CO_2$ slope) is an index of ventilation response to exercise. The slope increases with the deterioration of heart failure symptoms [Fig. 5.5].

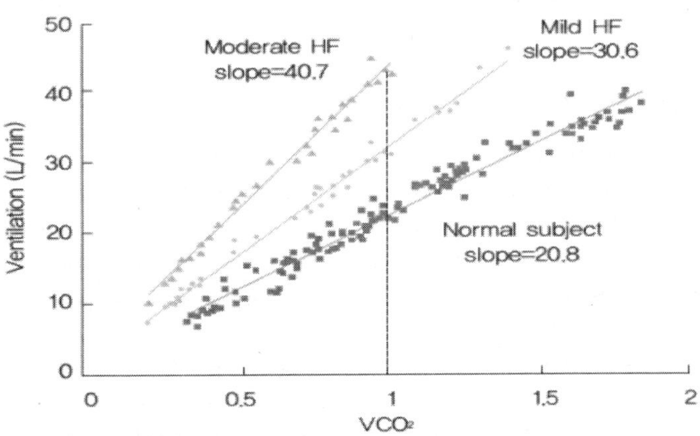

Fig. 5.5 ***Increase in $\dot{V}E/\dot{V}CO_2$ Slope due to Heart Failure***

Anaerobic Threshold

The anaerobic threshold is the point at which the skeletal muscle begins to take non-oxygen metabolism as an energy source. Because of the metabolic acidosis associated with the accumulation of lactic acid, ventilation increases and the production of carbon dioxide increases compared to oxygen consumption. Most daily activities are performed at a lower intensity than the threshold, which is useful for understanding the patient's functional status.

Management Methods

The treatment of patients with congestive heart failure varies greatly depending on the type and severity of the disorder. However, general treatment includes treating the causes of weakening LV function and weight loss, anemia treatment, adopting a low sodium diet, and using diuretics as shown in [Table 5.28].

Table 5.28 ***Treatment guidelines for patients with congestive heart failure***

- Treatment of causes that weaken left ventricular function
- Weight loss for overweight patients
- Anemia treatment
- Thinning eating habits
- Use diuretic

Medication

Medication for patients with congestive heart failure should be divided into two groups: diastolic dysfunction [Table 5.29] and systolic dysfunction [Table 5.30].[57]

Table 5.29 ***Medication for patients with diastolic dysfunction***

- ***Diuretic*** : Control blood volume, improve ventricular relaxation, and regulate heart rate. Digitalis agents and vasodilators are rarely helpful and can be harmful. Patients with diastolic dysfunction should be cautious about the use of diuretics as they are highly affected by total weight. Increased heart rate reduces proper ventricular filling time and weakens tolerance. Heart rate control is very important in patients with atrial fibrillation because these patients can not maintain adequate cardiac output.
- ***Calcium channel blocker β-blocker*** : Controls hypertension and lowers myocardial oxygen demand by lowering my heart rate.
- ***Angiotensin-converting enzyme inhibitor*** : Reduce blood pressure, reduce the activation of renin angiotensin aldosterone system, improve diastolic function, or reduce or prevent myocardial fibrosis. However, vasodilation by an ACE Inhibitor may weaken tolerance. In CAD, nitrate can be treated with beta-blocker or calcium channel blocker to preserve pulmonary edema syndrome and systolic function, but angioplasty or bypass surgery is considered because of its weak effect.

Table 5.30 ***Medication for patients with systolic dysfunction***

- ***Digitalis*** : It is a type of cardiotonics that improves heart muscle function and cardiac function by improving the contractility of the heart. Especially atrial fibrillation and moderate to severe heart failure.
- ***Diuretic*** : Decreased congestion with reduced plasma volume to improve breathing difficulty, edema and improve exercise capacity. Excessive use increases dehydration and vascular resistance, activating renin angiotensin aldosterone system, and causing electrolyte imbalance and arrhythmia.
- ***Isosorbide dinitrate*** : Decreases ventricular filling by intravenous dilator. Use of the denaturation only on the day of systolic dysfunction can reduce or avoid immunity. Used in conjunction with beta-blockers, it is beneficial for patients with myocardial ischemia. The effect on exercise capacity when using only dinitrate is mild. Nitrate improves motor performance and left ventricular contractility when used with the arteriolar expanding agent Hydralazine or an ACE inhibitor. The use of ACE inhibitors in combination with other vasodilators is desirable because of the lack of clinical evidence.
- ***Angiotensin-converting enzyme inhibitor*** : It is the most important drug in the treatment of patients with systolic dysfunction and offers various advantages. First, the renin-angiotensin-aldosterone system is inhibited to reduce ventricular filling pressure and increase cardiac output without increasing heart rate. Second, the degree of improvement in exercise tolerance and athletic performance is greater than when digoxin is used. Third, catecholamine is effective in preventing myocardial infarction and fatal arrhythmia by blocking harmful effects on myocardium. Fourth, it can extend the life of patients with severe congestive heart failure and can be used in place of digoxin in the treatment of mild to moderate patients.
- ***Amoldipine*** : Unlike other potassium channel blockers, amorphodipine (5~10 ㎎ / day) reduces mortality by 46% in patients with nonischemic systolic dysfunction by relieving congestive heart failure. Most heart failure patients with cardiac, hypertensive or atrial fibrillation show good results.
- ***Carvedilol*** : As a selective beta-receptor antagonist, it blocks the alpha-1 receptor and improves the survival rate and reduces the hospitalization rate .While we can not estimate efficacy as compared to other beta-blockers, other beta-blockers may make heart failure worse. While we can not estimate efficacy as compared to other beta-blockers, other beta-blockers may make heart failure worse. Start with small amounts and gradually increase the dose/ week from 25-50 ㎎ twice daily until the target dose is reached.

Rehabilitation Exercise

There is no significant correlation between exercise capacity and ventricular contractility in patients with congestive heart failure, but there is a significant difference in the degree of exercise-induced dyspnea between regularly exercising and non-exercising patients. In particular, the enhancement of skeletal muscle seems to increase exercise capacity in heart failure patients by increasing mitochondrial and capillary density. It is ideal to set the aerobic exercise intensity to the heart rate level below the ventilation threshold. This is because intense exercise above the ventilation threshold may increase the incidence of exercise-induced hypotension and lead to cardiac arrhythmias.[56] Patients with a stable course of treatment can benefit from exercising at 40~70% of HRR or peak $\dot{V}O_2$ or at a controlled intensity of the patient's ability. Exercise time is 20~60 minutes daily, and frequency is 4~7 days per week.

Patients who are not in a compensated state from heart failure may exacerbate exercise-induced pulmonary edema, and those with such unstable conditions should avoid exercise. Also, exercise should be avoided if the patient is not in good condition or if new signs and symptoms appear. Patients taking nitrates may have venous congestion due to sudden ceasing exercise, so it is advisable to perform at least 10 minutes of cool-down. On the other hand, when the exercise load test cannot be performed, the target heart rate can be estimated using age, but this method is less accurate. In particular, it is very unstable when used in patients taking beta-blockers, so exercise should be prescribed with an RPE of 11~14 or 3~5 on the dyspnea scale [Fig. 5.6]. On the other hand, anaerobic exercise, including weight loading exercise, should be contraindicated in patients with congestive heart failure. When patients with heart failure caused by left ventricular dysfunction continue to perform the regular aerobic exercise, the maximal heart rate may be increased to improve oxygen uptake, exercise duration, and exercise tolerance.

Dyspnea scale	
10	Maximal
9	Very, very severe
7	Very severe
5	Severe
4	Somewhat severe
3	Moderate
2	Slight
1	Very slight
0.5	Very, very slight

Fig. 5.6 ***Dyspnea scale***

Ultimately, exercise prescribers should be familiar with the tests, medications, and considerations of the exercises presented in [Table 5.31]. Based on this, the management methods presented in [Table 5.32] should be explained in detail to patients with congestive heart disease.[3,5,22,25,88]

Table 5.31 ***Exercise test, drug, and specific considerations for congestive heart failure patients***

Test Item		Measurement	Recommended Stopping Point	Remarks
Aerobic Power Ability	▪ Cycle (10~15watt/min) Ramp protocol (25~50watt/ 3min stage) ▪ Treadmill (Naughton protocol)	▪ 12 lead ECG	▪ Severe arrhythmia appearance ▪ ST segment depression / elevation > 2 ㎜ ▪ Ischemic threshold ▪ T wave inversion with ST change	▪ Norton protocol, a low-level protocol, is appropriate because the maximum exercise performance is less than 5 METs.
		▪ HR	▪ More than 85% of maximum heart rate	
		▪ BP	▪ Hypotensive reaction	
		▪ Dyspnea scale ▪ RPE	▪ Decreased respiratory function and difficulty ▪ Soaring psychological anxiety	
Endurance	▪ 6-min walk test	▪ Distance	▪ Time	▪ Very useful for whole exercise planning.
Functional Ability	▪ Daily life check	▪ Ability to perform activities related to daily activities		
Pharmacotherapy	▪ Digoxin : Reduces ST effects and improves exercise performance. ▪ Diuretics : It can cause ectopy and lower blood pressure. ▪ Vasodilators : Increase heart rate, lower blood pressure, improve exercise performance. ▪ ACE inhibitors : Lower blood pressure and improve exercise performance. ▪ Antiarrhythmias : It can increase heart rate, but it does not affect exercise performance.			
Considerations	▪ Unbalance of ventilation / perfusion leads to increased mucus, hyperreflexia and dyspnea. ▪ Risk of increased dyspnea.			

Table 5.32 ***Management program for congestive heart failure patients***

	Type	Goal	Intensity/Frequency/Time	Period
Aerobic Exercise	▪ Major muscle exercise ▪ Leg ergometer	▪ Increased peak oxygen uptake ▪ Increased ventilation threshold ▪ Increase in peak work ▪ Increase in maximum muscle endurance	▪ 40~70% of HRR or $\dot{V}O_2$peak ▪ RPE 11~14 ▪ 4~7 days a week ▪ 20~60 min/session ▪ 10~20 min/ 2~3 sessions	▪ 3 month
Strength Exercise	▪ Circuit training	▪ Reduction of muscle atrophy	▪ High repetition / low load exercise	▪ 3 month
Flexibility Exercise	▪ Upper / Lower body ROM activity	▪ Reduced risk of injury	▪ 2~3 days per week	▪ 4~6 month
Functional Exercise	▪ Increase in the type of daily activities	▪ Return to work environment ▪ Improving the quality of life ▪ Maintain independence		▪ 3 month
Pharmacotherapy	▪ Beta-blockers : Reduces heart rate by about 30 times per minute, providing a positive long-term effect. ▪ ACE inhibitors/ Diuretics: When used in conjunction with vasodilators, it may increase exercise performance, but may also cause hypotensive reactions after exercise.			
Considerations	▪ See considerations in patients with myocardial infarction. ▪ Intensity tolerance may be somewhat less for patients with congestive heart failure. ▪ Some patients may feel fatigue after exercise for a long time. ▪ Weight gain and increased breathing difficulty may cause decompensated heart failure.			

Valve Disease

The valve [Fig. 5.7] that prevents blood from flowing back into the heart loses its structure and function due to various causes. If left untreated, it leads to death. Rehabilitation therapy through exercise is also applicable to patients with valve disease, which can be divided into the mitral stenosis, mitral valve regurgitation, mitral valve prolapse, aortic valve stenosis, aortic valve regurgitation, and multiple valve disease.

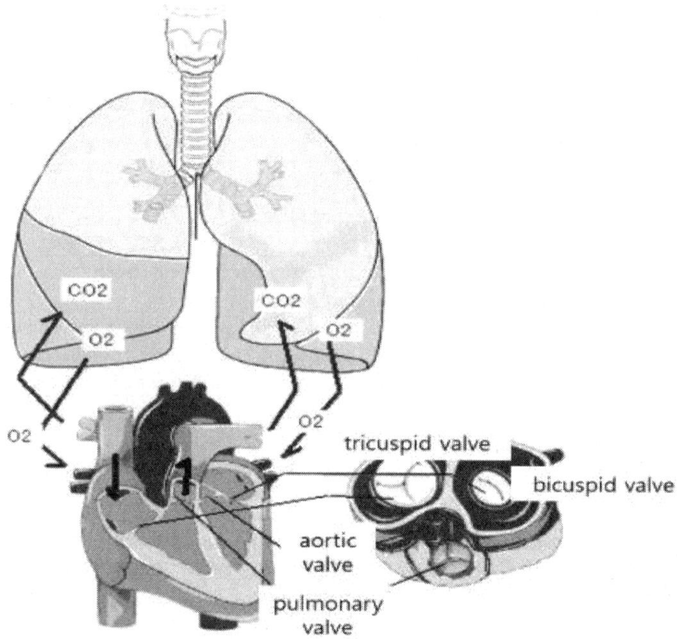

Fig. 5.7 *Types of Valves and Circulation*

Mitral Stenosis

Symptoms and Features

The most common cause of mitral valve stenosis is known to be rheumatic fever. Stenosis is considered to be 'mild stenosis' if the stenosis is over 2 cm^2 according to the transverse area of the mitral valve, and 'severe stenosis' if the stenosis is less than 1cm^2. To maintain normal cardiac output during rest, the left atrial pressure should be around 25 mmHg. However, in the case of severe occlusion, the atrial pressure is significantly increased because the blood flow through the valve increases with minimal activity. Dyspnea during exercise is correlated with the magnitude of atrial pressure during exercise and when the atrial pressure exceeds 25 mmHg, pulmonary vein pressure is increased to cause dyspnea. Exercise intensity causing dyspnea is a good indicator of the severity of stenosis. Dyspnea indicates early symptoms of mitral stenosis. Doppler echocardiography examines the point of failure of the valve and allows the diagnosis of pulmonary artery pressure.[11]

Severe dyspnea or acute pulmonary edema are often associated with atrial fibrillation. In particular, reduced atrial contraction reduces blood flow through the mitral valve by 30%, causing tachycardia and significantly reducing ventricular diastole time. In other words, a great obstacle to ventricular filling occurs. Most patients with mitral valve stenosis, have very mild symptoms. These symptoms may persist for years, and the incubation period can last for about 25 years. Once symptoms begin, they progress rapidly and become a serious disorder within 5 years.

Management Methods

Clinical management of mitral stenosis should consist of eliminating or controlling all causes of tachycardia, such as anemia and atrial fibrillation. Treatment guidelines are shown in [Table 5.33].

Table 5.33 ***Treatment guidelines for patients with mitral stenosis***

- Beta-blockers reduce heart rate and myocardial oxygen consumption and improve athletic capacity.
- Diuretics reduce venous congestion and dyspnea.
- Digitalis only helps patients with atrial fibrillation.
- Digitalis and beta blockers should be used in proper amounts for the goal of 60~65 bpm of resting heart rate.
- Acute patients require surgery.

Mitral Valve Regurgitation

Symptoms and Features

Mitral valve regurgitation42) is caused by the deformation of the annulus, leaflets, chordae tendineae, and papillary muscles that make up the mitral valve. Diseases that dilate the left ventricle cause mitral regurgitation by dilating the mitral annulus. Severe calcification of the annulus is common in hypertension, aortic stenosis, and diabetes, and can lead to mitral valve regurgitation. Mitral valve regurgitation is commonly found in patients with CAD, as rheumatic fever or endocarditis may cause chordae tendineae disorder, papillary muscle is perfused by distal vessels, and is easily damaged by

42) Regurgitation: The heart has aortic, mitral, pulmonic, and tricuspid, which act as a barrier to blood from back to upper. However, if the valve is opened by incomplete occlusion, the blood will flow backwards.

ischemia. The severity of mitral regurgitation depends on the size of the regurgitant orifice, the pressure difference between the ventricle and the atrium, and the resistance of the aortic blood flow.[49]

Generally, about half of the regurgitation is reversed to the left atrium before the aortic valve opens. To compensate for this, the left ventricle attempts to empty the left ventricle completely by increasing the contraction force or accelerating the velocity, but the blood volume of the diastolic phase also increases. In addition, mitral valve regurgitation increases as the ventricles expand. Myocardial contractility and ejection fraction increase beyond normal in a compensated state. For this reason, echocardiography often indicates a mild state. In fact, showing an ejection fraction of 40~50% is not a moderate disability, but actually a serious one. In order to accurately assess myocardial function in patients with mitral regurgitation, measuring the end-systolic volume is considered a good method. Typically, patients with mitral regurgitation do not exhibit early symptoms of mitral stenosis. In other words, it does not show symptoms until it becomes serious, and it remains asymptomatic, often leading to situations in which the left ventricular dysfunction cannot be restored.

Management Methods

Medication is used when surgery is not necessary. Medication may include reducing afterload with ACE-inhibitors or hydralazine and reducing ventricular dilatation with digitalis (cardiotonic) and diuretics. Digitalis is known to be very effective for patients with atrial fibrillation. Because there is no relationship between the manifestation of symptoms and ventricular dysfunction, surgery should be considered if dyspnea occurs during physical activity.[81]

Mitral Valve Prolapse

Symptoms and Features

Mitral valve prolapse is congenital or occurs in patients with CAD in which palpitations are also present. Only 15% of mitral valve prolapse patients have mitral regurgitation. The risk of endocarditis is low, but the risk of cerebral micro embolus, which can be caused by platelet aggregation, is high. Doppler echocardiography can detect mild mitral regurgitation that may be missed in two-dimensional B-mode echocardiography and M-mode echocardiography.

Management Methods

Asymptomatic patients do not require treatment, but should undergo a Doppler echocardiography every four years. The prevention of endocarditis is controversial, but it is a worthwhile method. Patients with palpitation should have a 24-hour ECG or a GXT to determine the function of the myocardium. Phenytoin43) is prescribed to patients with a delayed QT interval, while others are prescribed beta-blockers.

Aortic Valve (Mitral Valve, Tricuspid Valve) Stenosis

Symptoms and Features

Aortic valve stenosis, which is limited to young people, is mostly a congenital problem. Degenerative stenosis is a major cause of aortic valve disease in adults. Diabetes and hyperlipidemia are also a cause.[58] Aortic stenosis associated with mitral valve disease is also often caused by rheumatic fever. On the other hand, the most common cause of localized aortic stenosis is the congenital defect of the valve, in which the leaflets are damaged by turbulent blood flow, resulting in stenosis of the bicuspid valve.

Tricuspid stenosis is divided into congenital (abnormal leaflets), rheumatic, and degenerative (calcification due to aging). Degenerative changes are common in patients with diabetes or high cholesterol levels. The cause of degenerative calcification of the aortic valve is degeneration of the mitral annulus due to the normal consumption of the valve. Rheumatic aortic stenosis is associated with aortic valve regurgitation and mitral valve disease. Ultimately, aortic stenosis causes left ventricular hypertrophy. Importantly, even if there is a significant pressure difference in the aortic valve, there are few symptoms. Furthermore, this condition can persist. Even if cardiac output is maintained and symptoms do not appear, it is extremely dangerous if the systolic pressure difference is greater than 50 mmHg or if the valve area is less than 0.4 cm^2/m^2.[57]

Severe ventricular hypertrophy is caused by a decrease in compliance, an increase in diastolic pressure, and a decrease in the ventricular filling. The presence of tachycardia with reduced atrial contractility and atrial fibrillation indicates that the tolerance is further exacerbated. Patients with aortic stenosis may not have symptoms for a long time. However, when the symptoms start, they may quickly deteriorate and die within five

43) Phenytoin: Anticonvulsants and cardiac inhibitors. It is used for all types of epilepsy except small seizures and as antiarrhythmics, administered orally. It has side effects of hypotension, unconsciousness, dizziness, periodontitis, and anemia.

years. The most common symptoms are dyspnea, syncope, and angina. However, sudden death is rare in asymptomatic patients.[67, 68]

Doppler echocardiography computes the difference in pressure across the valve and facilitates the diagnosis. Because the pressure difference of aortic stenosis is likely to reach a critical level, the patient must undergo echocardiography every two years. Cardiac catheterization should be considered if the condition is severe.

Management Methods

In reality, medication has little effect. In particular, digitalis is used toward the end of the disease in which the systolic and diastolic dysfunction of the ventricles are visible. Diuretics should be treated with caution in case of severe edema as beta blockers may aggravate left ventricular dysfunction. Commissurotomy or balloon valvuloplasty provides a positive effect during the stage of increased valvular disease [Fig. 5.8]. The mortality rate is also very low for patients without symptoms. On the other hand, valvular replacement should be considered in patients with symptomatic and calcified stenosis, patients with severe obstruction, and asymptomatic patients with progressive left ventricular dysfunction.[57]

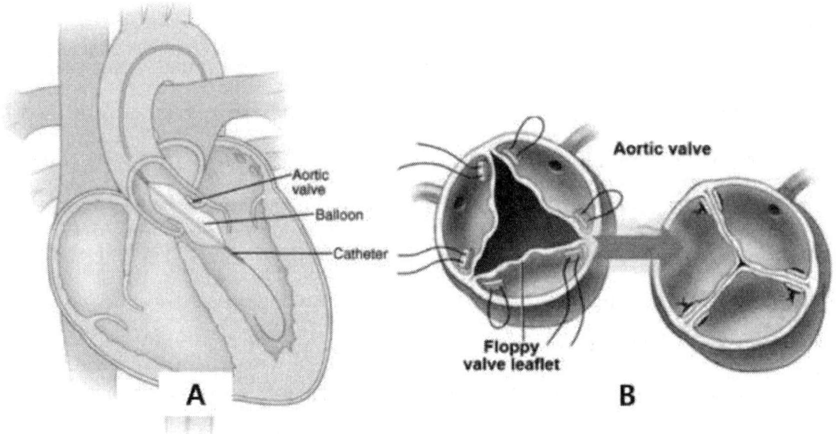

Fig. 5.8 ***A Balloon Valvuloplasty, B Commissurotomy***

Aortic Valve Regurgitation

Symptoms and Features

A common cause of aortic valve regurgitation is rheumatic fever and is associated with mitral valve disease. However, connective tissue disease and aortic arch dilatation are not common. Aortic valve regurgitation causes secondary mitral valve insufficiency by dilating the left ventricle. Initially, eccentric hypertrophy of the heart occurs as a compensatory action, which increases the diastolic volume of the left ventricle. These patients have a large heart, a good ejection fraction, a large diastolic volume, and normal diastolic pressure. However, as time goes on, the ventricles continue to expand and the left ventricular systolic function worsens. When the mitral regurgitation occurs, the left atrium is expanded, and the pressure of the left atrium and lung is increased. Because the blood flow of the coronary arteries is linearly proportional to the DBP, myocardial ischemia may occur when blood flow to the coronary arteries decreases. Myocardial ischemia occurs at the end of the disease and when exercise or nocturnal angina with bradycardia is seen. Doppler echocardiography is used to assess and diagnose the severity of the aortic valve. The end-systolic volume demonstrated by the test is a good indicator of myocardial function.

Management Methods

Digitalis is used as treatment for all patients with expanded ventricles. Vasodilators and diuretics are used in patients with left ventricular dysfunction. Patients with good left ventricular function should be evaluated by repeated GXT and Doppler echocardiography at least once every 6 months. Surgical therapy may be used in patients with progressive weakness of athletic ability even before left ventricular dysfunction becomes severe, but the prognosis for surgery is poor.[57]

Multivalvular Disease

Symptoms and Features

Multivalvular disease is caused by one or more valves and is most easily observed in patients with rheumatic valve disease or in patients with valve regurgitation due to ventricular dilatation. It is evaluated by examining general symptoms and clinical findings. However, if two valves are damaged at the same time, symptoms will appear in the more severe valve. Multivalvular disease is most commonly associated with mitral regurgitation and aortic valve regurgitation and rarely accompanied by aortic stenosis and mitral stenosis.

Valvular Disease and Exercise

The GXT for patients with valve disease should not be used often because the variables in the GXT using a treadmill have a low correlation with the degree of mitral stenosis. Rather, echocardiography with a stationary bicycle is more useful in assessing the left ventricular function of a patient during exercise [Fig. 5.9].

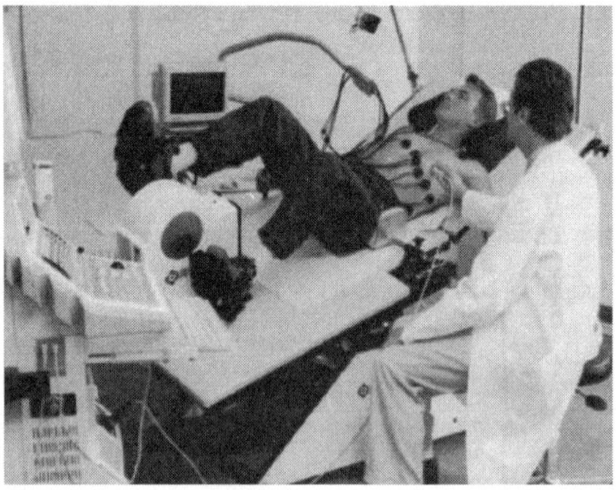

Fig. 5.9 ***Echocardiography and electrocardiography during exercise***

In general, the patient's symptoms are assessed through radiation, ECG, and echocardiography. In general, there is a difference in athletic ability between aortic valve surgery patients, mitral valve surgery patients, and mitral and aortic valve surgery patients. In other words, functional capacity gradually increases after aortic valve surgery, but the increase in functional capacity is limited in patients with mitral and aortic valve surgery. This difference in functional capacity is mainly due to differences in oxygen uptake capacity associated with arteriovenous oxygen difference and heart rate. Exercise may be useful because it alerts early risk signals to patients with mitral valve disease such as mitral stenosis. On the other hand, dyspnea during vigorous exercise means that clinical functional capacity has begun to decrease. The patient may need surgery if the dyspnea becomes severe during exercise.

Patients with mitral regurgitation should be tested to conclude whether surgery is necessary immediately after severe dyspnea occurs during intense exercise which is due to a lack of early warning of mitral stenosis. The most common cause of mitral regurgitation is mitral valve prolapse. If thallium is given to a patient with mitral valve prolapse and a graded exercise test is performed, the ST segment is more likely to be abnormal, and exercise-induced arrhythmia, chest pain, palpitations, and other abnormal changes in ECG may be evaluated. However, these changes may be false positives for

CAD. On the other hand, aerobic exercise has been reported to be useful in patients with mitral regurgitation, especially in patients without functional mitral regurgitation.[28] However, the research on these patients is very scarce and the patients are few, so more research is needed in the future.

In patients with aortic stenosis, a dangerous situation may arise during a GXT. However, it should be recalled that there is more information available from testing than there are risks. In other words, evaluation based on functional status and other non-invasive clinical evaluations are more important in patients who want to undergo aortic valve replacement. Asymptomatic patients with mild stenosis have no exercise limitations, but should consult a specialist if they develop dyspnea, syncope, fainting, or chest pain. If symptoms become severe, the patient should avoid exercising with an intensity of over 60% of $\dot{V}O_2max$ until reassessment. Patients with severe obstruction should avoid mild exercise. However, if aortic valve regurgitation does not show left ventricular dysfunction, 60% of $\dot{V}O_2max$ is possible. It should be noted that angina pectoris in patients with valvular disease occurs when there is severe regurgitation or when the disease is accompanied by CAD.[27] Overall, aerobic exercise can be prescribed for most patients with mild valve dysfunction. However, caution should be exercised in patients with prosthetic valves that have been treated with anticoagulants and patients with limited valve diameters because mechanical hemolysis may occur at the time of exercise-induced tachycardia.

The intensity of aerobic exercise for valve patients should be set to 40~80% of the target heart rate, 11~16 for RPE, or 6 or less on the dyspnea scale. Frequency and time should be 4~7 days per week and 20~60 minutes per day. For muscle strength exercise, choose 4~8 items using isokinetic or isotonic equipment, and perform 2~4 sets of 12~15 repetitions at 30~50% of maximum voluntary contraction.[47] The frequency is preferably 2~3 days per week.

Ultimately, exercise prescribers should be familiar with the tests, medications, and considerations of the exercises presented in [Table 5.34]. Based on this, the management methods presented in [Table 5.35] should be explained in detail to patients with valve disease.[3,5,22,25,83,86,88]

Table 5.34 ***Exercise test, drug, and specific considerations for valvular disease patients***

Test Item		Measurement	Recommended Stopping Point	Remarks
Aerobic Power Ability	■ Cycle (17watt/min) Ramp protocol (10~25watt/ 3min stage) ■ Treadmill (1~2METs/ 3min stage)	■ 12 lead ECG	■ Severe arrhythmia appearance ■ ST segment depression / elevation > 2 mm ■ Ischemic threshold ■ T wave inversion with ST change	■ It is useful for making exercise prescriptions and determining whether or not to perform an operation.
		■ BP	■ SBP/DBP >250/115 mmHg	
		■ RPE	■ Sudden increase of psychological fatigue	
		■ Stress echocardiography	■ The ST changes lost the specificity of mitral valve / aortic stenosis and mitral prolapse according to CAD diagnosis.	■ Determine stenosis, reflux, degree of left ventricular function, and appropriate timing of surgery.
Muscle Strength	■ Isokinetic ■ Isotonic			■ Weakness due to left work life is improved by resistance exercise.
Pharmacotherapy	■ Most cardiac medications cause changes in hemodynamic responses during exercise.			
Considerations	■ Careful observation of new symptoms (fatigue, chest pain, dyspnea and fainting) is required. ■ Acute aortic stenosis is a very dangerous situation and the patinet should be transferred directly to the emergency room.			

Table 5.35 ***Management program for valvular disease patients***

	Type	Goal	Intensity/Frequency/Time	Period
Aerobic Exercise	■ Major muscle exercise ■ Leg ergometer	■ Increase in functional ability ■ Development of muscle function ■ Improvement of daily living activities with less symptoms	■ THR 40~80% ■ RPE 11~16 ■ 4~7 days a week ■ 20~60 min/bout	■ 4~6 month
Strength Exercise	■ Isokinetic / Isotonic	■ Improvement of muscle function ■ Less than 1 hour	■ MVC 30~50% ■ 2~3 days per week ■ 4~8 items ■ Repeat 12~15 reps × 2~4 sets	■ 4~6 month
Flexibility Exercise	■ Upper / lower body ROM activity ■ Shoulder wheel exercise	■ Increase of ROM ■ Intensity: slightly uncomfortable	■ 3 days or more per week ■ Static stretching (10 to 30 seconds)	■ 4~6 month
Pharmacotherapy	■ Coumadin : No effect on heart rate or blood pressure.			
Considerations	■ High-risk patients should be closely monitored. ■ Symptoms can be improved at a rapid rate, typically starting rehabilitation from admission. ■ Generally, the patient can concentrate on upper ROM exercise. ■ Continuous ECG monitoring may be helpful for symptoms associated with valve disease.			

Hypertrophic Cardiomyopathy

Symptoms and Features

Hypertrophic cardiomyopathy shows severe hypertrophy of the ventricular septum and normal thickness of the posterior wall of the left ventricle. In other words, it is characterized by hypertrophy of the asymmetric ventricular septum. Fifty percent of patients are congenital, and some are acquired. Patients with acquired hypertrophic cardiomyopathy are less than 0.2%, which is also the cause of sudden death in young patients.

In patients with hypertrophic cardiomyopathy, the outflow tract of blood located between the enlarged frontal septum and anterior leaflets at the posterior surface of the mitral valve narrows with diastolic dysfunction. The strong and rapid flow of blood through the narrow left ventricular outflow tract induces a valve corresponding to the septum and blocks blood flow during systole. This is called the Venturi effect[44] [Fig. 5.10].

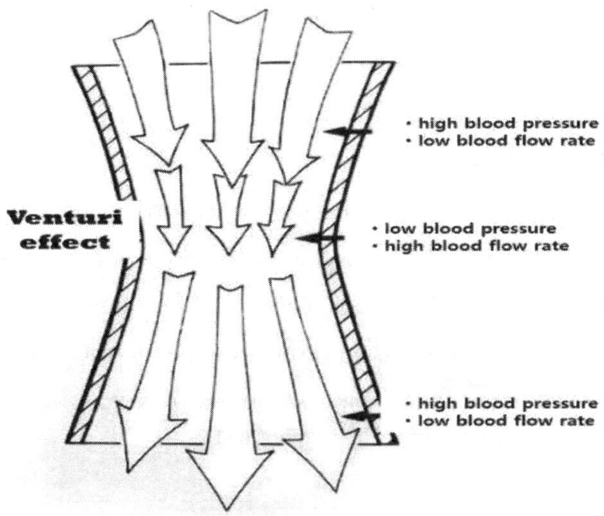

Fig. 5.10 ***Venturi effect on blood pressure***

In addition, elevated diastolic pressure and increased myocardial oxygen consumption exacerbate myocardial ischemia. These patients do not present symptoms in their daily lives, but they may develop syncope or experience sudden death during competitive sporting activities. Patients in their 30s and 40s should be tested for exercise-induced dyspnea, angina, and syncope. The history of syncope is more likely to cause sudden death in children and adolescents than adults. On ultrasonography, the septum is thicker than 15 ㎜ (normal < 11 ㎜), and the ventricular septal thickness: left ventricular posterior wall thickness ratio is 1.3~1.5:1 or more before contracting the atrium. In addition, the mitral valve that is abnormally close to the interventricular septum, mitral

44) Venturi effect: It means that the blood flowing into the relatively large blood vessels goes into the narrowed blood vessels and the blood pressure rises. It was named after the Italian physicist Giovanni Battista Venturi (1746-1822).

regurgitation, and diastolic dysfunction can be seen.[35]

Management Methods

Beta-blockers and calcium channel blockers (verapamil) are used for hypertrophic cardiomyopathy. Beta-blockers have a reduced heart rate (increased diastolic filling), reduced myocardial oxygen consumption, and an antiarrhythmic effect. Verapamil is widely used in therapy because it can improve functional ability, unlike beta-blockers. It improves diastolic filling and alleviates myocardial tension. As evidence for this, two-thirds of patients taking verapamil have been reported to have improved symptoms, including athletic performance. Ultimately, surgery should be given to patients who do not improve symptoms despite medication.[27,69,73]

Rehabilitation Exercise

The improvement in exercise capacity seen in patients taking verapamil seems to be due to a decrease in left ventricular outflow tract obstruction. Propranolol can improve athletic performance in a similar fashion, but it may weaken functional capacity in some patients. Patients who have undergone myotomy and partial myectomy due to obstructive hypertrophic cardiomyopathy have been reported to have improved cardiac output and left ventricular function in GXT.

Table 5.36 ***Controindications in patients with hypertrophic cardiomyopathy***

. Family history of sudden death
. Severe ventricular hypertrophy
. If the cardiac output is less than 40 ㎜Hg at rest
. Young patient with exercise-induced syncope

On the other hand, intense exercise should be avoided because of the danger of sudden death. In particular, patients with asymptomatic hypertrophic cardiomyopathy should regularly exercise, but it is better to avoid competitive sports and high-intensity exercise of more than 85% of $\dot{V}O_2$max. It is also preferable to perform at a RPE of 11 or less. Exercise should be contraindicated if the patient has any of the items listed in [Table 5.36]. Ultimately, exercise prescribers need to be familiar with the tests, medications, and considerations for exercise [Table 5.37] and explain the management method presented in [Table 5.38] to patients with hypertrophic cardiomyopathy in detail.[3,5,22,25,47,83,86,88]

Table 5.37 ***Exercise test, drug, and specific considerations for hypertrophic cardiomyopathy patients***

Test Item		Measurement	Recommended Stopping Point	Remarks
Aerobic Power Ability	■ Cycle (10~25watt/ 3min stage) ■ Treadmill (1~2METs/ 3min stage)	■ 12 lead ECG	■ Severe arrhythmia appearance ■ ST segment depression / elevation > 2 ㎜ ■ Ischemic threshold ■ T wave inversion with ST change	■ ECG sensitivity is low for ischemic responses.
		■ HR	■ More than 85% of maximum heart rate	
		■ BP	■ SBP/DBP >250/115 ㎜Hg ■ No change in SBP despite increased intensity	■ Maximum SBP can disappear. SBP is a left ventricular dysfunction, and may not decrease or increase.
		■ RPE	■ Sudden increase of psychological fatigue	■ RPE monitoring is highly recommended because HR observation is difficult.
		■ Radiation Nuclear Medicine ■ Stress echocardiography		■ It may be very useful in estimating ischemic heart disease.
Pharmacotherapy	■ Beta-blocker : It decrease maximal heart rate, blood pressure, and exercise capacity when mixed with non-selective drugs. ■ Vasodilator and ACE inhibitor : Generally, it does not affect heart rate during exercise, but it is sensitive to hypotension after exercise. ■ Calcium channel blocker : It may cause changes in heart rate response during exercise (Verapamil). ■ Central nervous system-active drug : Effective on heart rate and blood pressure during exercise. Pay attention to low blood pressure, dizziness, syncope. ■ Alpha blocker : It reduces SBP / DBP, but has a small effect on heart rate and oxygen intake during exercise. ■ Digitalis : Promote deformation of the above ST-T wave. Sometimes it is used to control atrial arrhythmia. ■ Nitroglycerin : Ischemic reaction may be lost or relieved.			
Considerations	■ Careful observation of new symptoms (fatigue, chest pain, dyspnea and fainting) is required. ■ It is preferable to prescribe RPE 11 range.			

Table 5.38 ***Management program for hypertrophic cardiomyopathy patients***

	Type	Goal	Intensity/Frequency/Time	Period
Aerobic Exercise	■ Major muscle exercise ■ Stand-up ergometer	■ Increase in functional ability ■ Improvement of daily life ability ■ Increased self-efficacy	■ HRR 50~85% ■ RPE 11 ■ 4~7 days a week ■ 20~60 min/bout	■ 4~6 month
Strength Exercise	■ Circuit training	■ Improvement of muscle function ■ Improvement of leisure / work ability	■ Low / Medium intensity ■ 2 days per week ■ 15~20 min/bout	■ 4~6 month
Flexibility Exercise	■ Upper / lower body ROM activity	■ Increase of ROM	■ 2~3 days per week	■ 4~6 month
Pharmacotherapy	■ Beta-blocker : It does not affect the exercise / training effects of patients with heart disease. ■ Calcium channel blocker : It does not affect the exercise / training effects of patients with heart disease.			
Considerations	■ Patients with high-risk hypertrophic cardiomyopathy should be closely monitored. ■ RPE should be used in conjunction with heart rate for intensity observation. ■ Ventricular tachyarrythmias may be caused. ■ Exercise should be prescribed in RPE 11 range.			

Arrhythmia

Symptoms and Features

The most common cause of cardiac arrhythmia in patients without heart disease is ventricular arrhythmias. Among them, supraventricular arrhythmia and conduction defects are important problems to be solved. The prevalence of premature ventricular contraction occurs in 40~70% of normal subjects. A long-term follow-up study showed that there was no significant difference between the prognosis of asymptomatic complex ectopy patients with premature ventricular contractions and tachycardia, and those with no arrhythmia. This suggests the possibility that arrhythmias may occur in normal people. On the other hand, the incidence of premature ventricular contraction in patients with CAD increases the risk of sudden death. The most important treatment to prevent sudden death is to prescribe antiarrhythmic drugs, which have efficacy but cannot prevent mortality. If non-symptomatic patients who are not at high risk of sudden death continue to take the drug, there may be a number of problems, including side effects.[57] Holter monitoring and graded exercise tests should be performed continuously to verify the effectiveness of the drug. If a graded exercise test is possible, the test can be performed even when taking the drug. All antiarrhythmics may cause hypokalemia45) and hypomagnesias,46) which may increase the risk of arrhythmias and should be used with caution in patients with ventricular systolic dysfunction.

Management Methods

The best treatment for arrhythmia is to treat the heart or metabolic condition that causes it, but sometimes it is not possible. Beta-blockers reduce heart rate and blood pressure at specific exercise intensities, and patients with abnormal left ventricular function may be at increased risk of heart failure or exercise limitations when using beta-blockers. In addition, high-intensity exercise may cause exercise-induced hypotension. Patients taking antiarrhythmics are more likely to develop arrhythmias during exercise. Furthermore, it should be kept in mind that drugs used to prevent arrhythmias can cause or worsen arrhythmias [Table 5.39, 5.40].[3,5,22,25,83,88]

---

45) Hypokalemia: An abnormally low potassium concentration in blood. It leads to various neuromuscular disorders that can cause paralysis, and abnormal ECG.

46) Hypermagnesia: Magnesium in the blood plasma is lower than normal and is characterized by hyperactivity of nerve root stimulation.

Table 5.39 ***Exercise test, drug, and specific considerations for arrhythmia patients***

Test Item		Measurement	Recommended Stopping Point	Remarks
Aerobic power ability	■ Cycle (10~25watt/ 3min stage) ■ Treadmill (1~2METs/ 3min stage)	■ 12 lead ECG	■ Severe arrhythmia appearance ■ ST segment depression / elevation > 2㎜ ■ Ischemic threshold ■ T wave inversion with ST change	■ ECG sensitivity is low for ischemic responses.
		■ HR	■ More than 85% of maximum heart rate	
		■ BP	■ SBP/DBP > 250/115 ㎜Hg	
		■ RPE	■ Sudden increase of psychological anxiety	■ Since HR observation is difficult, RPE is applied.
Pharmacotherapy	■ Beta-blocker : Decreased maximal / maximal heart rate / blood pressure and reduced exercise capacity when mixed with non-selective drugs.			
Considerations	■ Modified Bruce Protocol, which is a low-level protocol, is appropriate because the maximum exercise performance is less than 5 METs.			

Table 5.40 ***Management program for arrhythmia patients***

Type		Goal	Intensity/Frequency/Time	Period
Aerobic Exercise	■ Major muscle exercise ■ Stand-up ergometer	■ Increase in functional ability ■ Improvement of daily life ability	■ 50 to 70% of VO_2peak / HRR ■ target heart rate should be kept below ventilation threshold. ■ RPE 16 ■ 4 days a week ■ 20 to 40 minutes /bout	■ 4~6 month
Strength Exercise	■ Circuit training	■ Improvement of muscle function ■ Improvement of daily life activity ability	■ Low / Medium intensity ■ 2 days per week ■ 15 to 20 minutes/bout	■ 4~6 month
Flexibility Exercise	■ Circuit training	■ ROM increase	■ 2~3 days per week	■ 4~6 month
Pharmacotherapy	■ Beta-blocker : It does not affect the exercise / training effects of patients with heart disease.			
Considerations	■ RPE should be used in conjunction with heart rate for intensity observation. ■ Some patients may feel fatigue for a long time after exercise.			

Rehabilitation Exercise

For patients taking digitalis and diuretics, exercise can cause arrhythmias. The GXT can be used as a means of assessing the course of antiarrhythmic therapy and as a method to predict the likelihood of arrhythmias. The greatest risk of exercise is sudden death which is caused by ventricular arrhythmias and the worsening of ventricular dysfunction. Therefore, if the patient has one or more of the features listed in [Table

5.41], the risk of sudden death is high and careful observation is required.

Table 5.41 ***Types of diseases that can cause sudden death***

- Severe hypertrophic cardiomyopathy
- Severe aortic stenosis
- Severe left ventricular systolic dysfunction
- Exercise-induced complex ventricular arrhythmia
- Exercise-induced hypotension (reduced by more than 20 ㎜Hg in SBP)
- Exercise-induced angina
- Past history of ventricular fibrillation
- Patients with angina experiencing ventricular arrhythmia
- Patients with a delayed QT interval and a history of syncope

Precautions for Exercise in Heart Patients

For the first two to three months, exercise should be regularly supervised. Exercise items such as walking, jogging, swimming, indoor bicycling exercise is good. However, patients should refrain from anaerobic movements such as resistance exercise, running, and tug of war. In particular, warm-up and cool-down should be performed before and after exercise to reduce the burden on the heart due to sudden exercise. If chest pain occurs during exercise, dyspnea, dizziness, or arrhythmia, stop the exercise immediately and consult a doctor. Patients must also quit smoking. In case of the mental anxiety or within 1 hour after meals, patients should refrain from exercising. Finally, from the dynamic aspects of exercise, it is desirable to avoid movement of the head down the chest during exercise.

Patients suffering from aggravated conditions of the disease or symptoms mentioned in [Table 5.41] should not exercise. However, patients with mild or moderate symptoms may perform appropriate exercise after receiving a GXT under the supervision of a specialist. Exercise-induced syncope is common in patients with pulmonary arterial hypertension, coarctation of aorta, myocardial hypertrophy, and CAD. Ventricular arrhythmias cause syncope and sudden death in patients with hypertrophic cardiomyopathy. On the other hand, abnormal exercise-induced arrhythmias need to be corrected before starting the exercise program. If this is not possible, exercise should be performed at a level about 10 beats per minute lower than the target heart rate. Patients who cannot measure exercise intensity can also exercise with heart rate monitors. In particular, warm-up and cool-down are very important processes and should be done sufficiently.

Patients who take beta-blockers may be prescribed an exercise intensity using a target heart rate, even if their heart rate is slow during exercise. These patients are encouraged to exercise with the target heart rate to the point of anaerobic threshold. If the graded exercise test cannot be performed, a target RPE should be used to select exercises that remain lower than 16. The GXT is not sensitive, but it is the only method for assessing the likelihood of developing an exercise-induced symptom. In other words, the abnormal results in the low-intensity exercise test help to predict the risk factors, while the results in the high-intensity exercise test make it difficult to predict the risk factors. On the other hand, ventricular arrhythmia does not appear in a stable state, but frequently occurs during exercise. In particular, if the risk of arrhythmia is found on the ECG of the GXT, it means that it is more severe than itself.

In a high-intensity exercise, ventricular tachycardia can be easily observed because myocardial ischemia and catecholamine increase. Ventricular tachyarrhythmia may occur immediately after exercise because of the relatively high levels of norepinephrine and lactate-induced vasodilation during exercise. Supraventricular tachycardia is rarely caused by exercise. However, patients with lung disease or WPW syndrome (Wolff Parkinson White syndrome) or those who abuse alcohol and caffeine are more likely to develop the disease.[86] Also, exercise-induced atrial flutter and atrial fibrillation are common in patients with valvular disease, hyperthyroidism, or cardiomyopathy. Exercise can cause left and right branch blockages as a result of myocardial ischemia (which usually occurs at 125 bpm or more) or as a result of heart rate related events.

Pacemaker

Symptoms and Features

The cardiac pacemaker was first introduced about 40~50 years ago and has been used to prevent death and recurrent syncope. These days, pacemakers are the standard treatment for syncope, pre-syncope, exercise intolerance, or chronotropic intolerance. A permanent pacemaker is required and indicates signs of clinically significant bradycardia [Table 5.42].

Table 5.42 ***Types of diseases that can cause sudden death***

- Complete atrioventricular block (3° atrioventricular block)
- Mobitz Type I 2° atrioventricular block (Wenckebach)
- Mobitz Type II type 2° atrioventricular block
- Sinus pauses
- Sinus or atrial arrest
- Trifascicular blocks in fiber branch, left front fiber barrier, left rear fiber of myocardium

Clinical considerations for the transplantation of a cardiac pacemaker include the absence of other life-threatening diseases, cardiac conditions exacerbated by bradycardia, the use of medications to inhibit nerve conduction, and the absence of cerebrovascular disease aggravated by bradycardia.[46,50,78]

Patients who are implanted with a pacemaker should undergo a GXT under thorough supervision prior to the beginning of the exercise program. The heart rate of a patient with a fixed rhythm pacemaker depends on the amount of venous return and how much the stroke volume is increased. Patients who underwent surgery with a fixed rhythm pacemaker, an asynchronous pacemaker, do not increase their heart rate even after exercise. In patients with the atrioventricular node conduction blocked, the ventricular rate remains the same due to the pre-set pacemaker rate, even though the atrial pace increases with exercise. However, patients with an intermittent atrioventricular block, sick sinus syndrome, and dual chamber pacemakers experience increased heart rate during exercise. Patients who have inserted a synchronous pacemaker that can increase the ventricular rate by exercise may be prescribed exercise at the target heart rate. However, it is more desirable to prescribe exercise intensity using blood pressure rather than the Karvonen formula or the heart rate formula based on heart rate [Reference 2]. Ideally, RPE should be prescribed at an exercise intensity lower than 16. If the heart rate is not controlled by the pacemaker, the exercise intensity may be prescribed as an anaerobic threshold or slightly lower. On the other hand, high-intensity movements above 60% of the $\dot{V}O_2max$ and excessive arm and upper body movements should not be performed because they can change their position of the ventricular pacing wires.[57] The ideal aerobic exercise intensity for pacemaker patients is 40~80% of peak heart rate and 4~7 days per week for 20~60 minutes per day. Muscle strength exercises should be avoided early in the insertion of the pacemaker. Strength exercise should be carried out for 15~20 minutes with a light weight selected, preferably twice a week.

[Reference 2] Exercise load test showed resting SBP of 130 ㎜Hg and maximum SBP of 190 ㎜Hg. When the patient is to exercise 40% of the pacemaker, the target blood pressure during exercise is as follows.

$$\begin{aligned}\text{Target SBP during exercise} &= \text{\%Intensity} \times (\text{Maximum SBP - resting SBP}) + \text{resting SBP} \\ &= 0.40 \times (190 - 130) + 130 \\ &= 0.40 \times (60) + 130 \\ &= 24 + 130 \\ &= 154 \text{ ㎜Hg}\end{aligned}$$

Table 5.43 ***Exercise test, drug, and specific considerations for pacemaker patients***

Test Item		Measurement	Recommended Stopping Point	Remarks
Aerobic Power Ability	■ Cycle (10~25watt/ 3min stage) ■ Treadmill (1~2METs/ 3min stage)	■ 12 lead ECG	■ Severe arrhythmia appearance ■ ST segment depression / elevation > 2 ㎜ ■ Ischemic threshold ■ T wave inversion with ST change	■ ECG sensitivity is low for ischemic responses. ■ ICD : Implantable cardioverter defibrilators
		■ HR	■ The maximum HR should be kept below the activity rate of the ICD	
		■ BP	■ SBP/DBP >250/115 ㎜Hg ■ No change in SBP despite increased intensity	■ Maximum SBP can disappear. SBP may not decrease or increase due to left ventricular dysfunction.
		■ RPE	■ Sudden increase of psychological fatigue	■ Because HR observation is difficult, RPE application is highly recommended.
		■ Radiation ■ Stress echocardiography		■ It may be very useful in estimating ischemic heart disease.
Strength	■ Isokinetic			■ Myocardial function after pacemaker / ICD insertion is not recommended. Conduct later.
Pharmacotherapy	■ Beta-blocker : Submaximal / maximum heart rate / blood pressure reduction and reduced exercise capacity when mixed with non-selective drugs. ■ Vasodilator/ ACE inhibitor : Generally, it does not affect heart rate during exercise, but it is sensitive to hypotension after exercise. ■ Calcium channel blocker : It may cause changes in heart rate response during exercise (Verapamil). ■ Central nervous system-active drug : Effective on heart rate and blood pressure during exercise. Pay attention to low blood pressure, dizziness, syncope. ■ Alpha blocker : It reduces SBP / DBP, but has a small effect on heart rate and oxygen intake during exercise. ■ Digitalis : It promote deformation of the above ST-T wave (note the interpretation). Sometimes it is used to control atrial arrhythmia. ■ Nitroglycerin : Ischemic reaction may be lost or relieved.			
Considerations	■ Patients with an ICD inserted are at greater risk of receiving inappropriate shocks. ■ Heart rate should not be applied to the activity rate of ICD. Some patients who have inserted a tachycardia / ICD may have severe or significant left ventricular dysfunction. Therefore, it is necessary for the affected people to be aware of appropriate measures. ■ The Naughton protocol, which is a low-level protocol, is adequate because the maximum exercise performance is less than 5 METs. ■ Unbalance of ventilation / perfusion increases mollusc, and causes overflow and dyspnea.			

Table 5.44 ***Management program for pacemaker patients***

	Type	Goal	Intensity/Frequency/Time	Period
Aerobic Exercise	■ Major muscle exercise ■ Stand-up exercise	■ Increase in functional ability ■ Improvement of daily life ability ■ Increased self-efficacy	■ $\dot{V}O_2$peak 40~80% ■ Target heart rate should be maintained below ischemic threshold and ICD activity threshold. ■ 4~7 days a week ■ 20~60 min/bout	■ 4~6 month
Strength Exercise	■ Circuit training	■ Improvement of muscle function ■ Improvement of daily life activity / leisure / work ability	■ Low / Medium intensity ■ 2 days per week ■ 15~20 min/bout ■ Avoid pacemaker insertion at the beginning.	
Flexibility Exercise	■ Upper / lower body ROM activity	■ Increase of ROM	■ 2~3 days per week	
Pharmacotherapy	■ Beta-blocker : It does not affect the exercise / training effects of patients with heart disease. ■ Calcium channel blocker : It does not affect the exercise / training effects of patients with heart disease.			
Considerations	■ Upper body ROM exercise should be used for limited pacemaker and ICD insertion patients. ■ It is important to be familiar with the type and function of the pacemaker. ■ RPE should be used in conjunction with heart rate for intensity observation. ■ It is important to be familiar with ICD activity rates. ■ Ventricular tachyarrythmias may be induced. ■ Intensity tolerance may be somewhat less for pacemaker patients. ■ Some patients may feel fatigue after exercise. ■ Weight gain and increased breathing difficulty can cause decompensated heart failure.			

Ultimately, exercise prescribers should be familiar with the tests, medications, and considerations of the exercises presented in [Table 5.43]. Based on this, the management methods presented in [Table 5.44] should be explained in detail to patients with valve disease.[3,5,22,25,83,88]

Pulmonary Disease

Chronic Lung Disease (CLD) refers to a chronic obstructive pulmonary disease (COPD), cystic fibrosis (CF), and pulmonary heart disease (CP). These diseases are characterized by a poor prognosis over time, and when exacerbated, breathing difficulties become worse. The severity of dyspnea varies from patient to patient but increases with exercise intensity. In the past, pulmonary rehabilitation programs failed to provide hope to patients due to the announcement that they could not improve their functioning. Recently, however, many studies have suggested that pulmonary function rehabilitation programs are very useful and can produce positive results. This suggests that the goal of CLD should be to reduce functional impairment with exercise-based rehabilitation programs rather than to cure the disease. Most of the investigations for pulmonary rehabilitation are for COPD patients, but there are also studies on patients with airway obstruction, CF, other chronic lung diseases (airway, parenchyma, thoracic cage injury) and patients with multiple diseases. Recently, studies suggest that exercise for CLD patients improves endurance, dyspnea, and emotional support, and that exercise reduces hospitalization rates.[17,26]

Breathing exercises should include diaphragmatic breathing and mouth exercises and should be done on a regular basis. However, in patients with COPD symptoms, the ventilatory capacity is impaired and the exercise capacity is limited. There are resistive and hyperpneic training methods. The resistance method is applied as a method of breathing while overcoming the resistance which is higher than the normal oral pressure which occurs during each breath, but there is a lack of evidence showing that exercise tolerance has been increased. Respiratory hyperventilation uses a specially designed rebreathing device. This method can improve maximum sustained ventilation (MSV)[47] and exercise capacity, which is interpreted as a result of increasing the enzymes required for the aerobic metabolism of the diaphragm and improving the function of the inspiratory muscle.[76] The most effective way to improve the physical fitness of patients with CLD is to combine proper nutrition and regular professional exercise.

Table 5.45* *General guidelines for patients with lung disease

- Balanced nutrition / stress reduction
- Pneumococcal vaccine once every six years
- Influenza vaccination every fall
- Bronchial hygiene therapy for mucus secretion
- Breathing training to improve diaphragm and breathing pattern
- Oxygen therapy for patients with hypoxia
- Treatment of congestive heart failure
- Psychosocial treatment, including professional rehabilitation

Breathing exercises should include diaphragmatic breathing and mouth exercises and should be done on a regular basis. However, in patients with COPD symptoms, the ventilatory capacity is impaired and the exercise capacity is limited. There are resistive and hyperpneic training methods. The resistance method is applied as a method of

47) MSV: The maximum amount of ventilation that can maintain a constant state of arterial CO_2 for 15 minutes.

breathing while overcoming the resistance which is higher than the normal oral pressure which occurs during each breath, but there is a lack of evidence showing that exercise tolerance has been increased. Respiratory hyperventilation uses a specially designed rebreathing device. This method can improve MSV and exercise capacity, which is interpreted as a result of increasing the enzymes required for the aerobic metabolism of the diaphragm and improving the function of the inspiratory muscle. The most effective way to improve the physical fitness of patients with CLD is to combine proper nutrition and regular professional exercise.

Respiratory training can improve the respiratory muscles and lung function of respiratory patients. However, if you have difficulty breathing even if you are walking slowly or a short distance, you should exercise in conjunction with medication. However, because the drug may suddenly increase the heart rate, intermittent exercise should be performed after 10 minutes of preparatory exercise with bare hand gymnastics and walking. In other words, respiratory disease patients cannot measure the maximum heart rate or $\dot{V}O_2max$, so a RPE range from 11~13 is used and performed 3~7 days a week, once or twice a day. At this time, the exercise duration should be 30 minutes.[17] For reference, intermittent exercise refers to a type of walking for 5 minutes, followed by resting for 1 minute and then walking for 5 minutes. After conditions are improved, it can increase to 10 minutes of exercise, 2 minutes of rest, and 10 minutes of exercise. However, if this method is somewhat unfamiliar or complicated, it is advisable to continue the exercise just before the point where breathing becomes difficult, rest, and then repeat once or twice.

In patients with relatively low pulmonary dysfunction or in patients who do not feel dyspnea when walking at normal speed, intermittent exercise may be repeated 5~6 times to reduce the number of airway obstacles caused by exercise. In order to improve the effectiveness of the treatment, rehabilitation training should be provided for about five days a week.

Guidelines for Management of Patients with Pulmonary Disease

The best way for patients with pulmonary disease such as COPD, chronic bronchitis, emphysema, asthma is breathing exercises. However, since lung capacity and FEV_1 are less than 70% of that of a normal person due to chronicity, the patient does not exercise forcibly. The exercise goals of respiratory disease patients are improvement of respiratory muscle and increased lung function, and general management methods are as shown in [Table 5.45].

Chronic Obstructive Pulmonary Disease

Chronic obstructive pulmonary disease (COPD) is a pathologic condition with chronic airflow limitation regardless of the airway hyperreactivity48) [Fig. 5.11]. Chronic obstructive airway obstruction should be diagnosed before the diagnosis of chronic obstructive pulmonary disease. COPD is caused by chronic bronchitis and emphysema. In patients with COPD, the residual volume of the lung is higher than normal immediately after intense exhalation. Increased functional residual capacity (FRC) and residual volume (RV) cause an exercise-induced tachypnea49) and increase the amount of air clogged which causes hyperinflation.[9,76] On the other hand, when the lungs expand, the diaphragm moves down and the pressure increases as the air moves, and the ability of the diaphragm to generate pressure decreases. Treatment of COPD includes bronchodilators, antibiotics, air purification, and adequate nutrition.

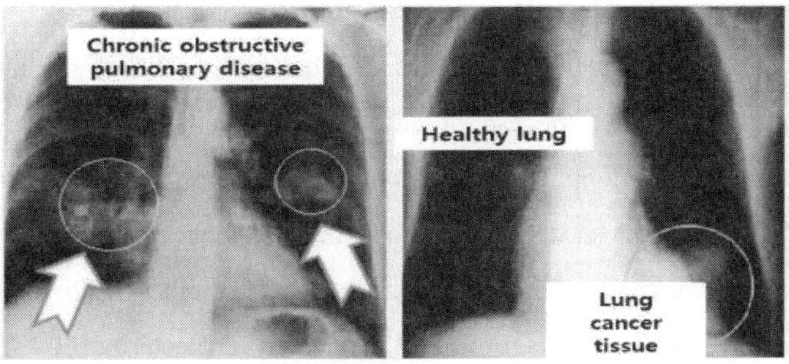

Fig. 5.11 *COPD status*

Ipratropium bromide, a drug for COPD, is known to be the most effective bronchodilator for treatment and should be taken regularly. However, in patients with reversible bronchospasm, inhalation therapy with beta-2 agonists may be effective, if necessary. When taking theophylline50) at bedtime, serum theophylline levels are normalized between 2 and 4 am, the time that airway obstruction worsens. Additionally, prednisone51) is not as effective as theophylline, but it increases the forced expiratory volume in 1 second (FEV_1) by about 10%.

---

48) Hyperreactivity: Abnormal increase in reactivity to stimulation.
49) Tachypnea: A state in which breaths excessively become rapid and shallow.
50) Theophylline: For the purpose of bronchodilation, it is used for the treatment of bronchial asthma, chronic bronchitis and bronchospasm.
51) Prednisone: White crystalline powder, administered orally for the purpose of treating inflammation.

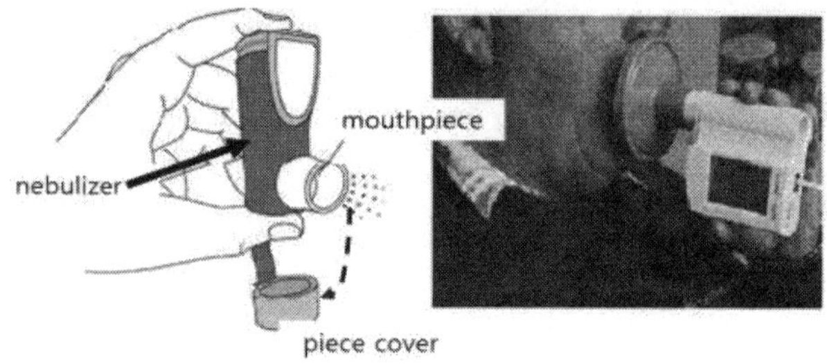

Fig. 5.12 ***Use of Inhaler***

Patients who do not improve their function after taking the maximum amount of bronchodilator should use prednisone (40 mg / 2 weeks) to see if there is any change in FEV_1. If FEV_1 is improved by more than 15% after using prednisone, it is effective to inhale 1 mg of corticosteroid[52] daily. This amount has the effect of 20 puffs of beclomethasone[53], 10 puffs of triamcinolone[54]. Continuous prednisone therapy is only given to patients in which the drugs are effective [Fig. 5.12].

The efficacy of antibiotics in the course of worsening COPD is unknown. Recently, the tendency is to prohibit the use of antibiotics when the symptoms worsen. When symptoms begin to deteriorate, treatment with trimethoprim[55], sulfamethoxazole[56], or doxycycline[57] is recommended. Physiotherapy of the thorax is especially necessary for patients with high secretions or bronchiectasis. On the other hand, cachexia[58] may appear in patients with end-stage COPD, which is characterized by higher energy consumption and muscle with visceral protein burning at rest than normal. That is, when the cachexia state is reached, body weight is extremely reduced. A rehabilitation program with proper nutrition and weight loading exercise is an essential way to prevent weight loss and maintain fitness.

Cor Pulmonale

The presence of right ventricular dysfunction means that the prognosis of COPD patients

---

52) Corticosteroid: Steroids produced by the adrenal cortex.
53) Beclomethasone: Used as a spray for bronchial asthma, logically for skin diseases.
54) Triamcinolone: Adrenocortical steroid, present in the form of white crystalline powder, used as an anti-inflammatory agent.
55) Trimethoprim: Antibacterial agents similar to pyrimethamine that is an anti-malarial agent.
56) Sulfamethoxazole: Used as an antimicrobial in the prevention and treatment of acute urinary tract infections, pyoderma, and soft tissue infections.
57) Doxycycline: Light yellow crystalline powder which is effective against a wide range of gram positive and gram negative bacteria.
58) Cochaexia: As a constitutional disorder, refers to malnutrition or unhealthiness of the whole body.

is poor. The most effective treatment for patients with cor pulmonale (CP) is to treat the symptoms of the lungs depending on the cause. Specifically, diuretics are effective for patients with severe edema. Furosemide[59)] may be used selectively for hyponatremia[60)]. Taking furosemide and thiazide diuretic together has a greater effect and helps to alleviate the calcium reduction associated with furosemide. Digitalis[61)] is not used for CP patients. The reason is that it does not improve the function of the right ventricle and shrinks the arterial blood vessels, increasing the risk of arrhythmia as well as pulmonary vascular resistance. Patients with chronic lung disease may have multifocal atrial tachycardia and atrial fibrillation. Quinidine[62)] or lidocaine[63)] is ineffective, and verapamil[64)] or amiodarone[65)] is recommended as an arrhythmia remedy. Diltiazem[66)] is useful for patients with pulmonary hypertension. For effective treatment, it is necessary to inject diltiazem after right-side cardiac catheterization.[67)][57] Patients with improved status are treated orally, which is proportional to intravenous tolerance for maximum benefit. Most patients with pulmonary hypertension according to CLD cannot be improved with nifedipin[68)]. It is not desirable to administer pulmonary vasodilators without oxygen therapy to patients with hypoxia.

Lung Disease and Exercise

Studies evaluating the effects of exercise programs on COPD patients have demonstrated improved exercise tolerance after only 3~4 weeks. Improvement in exercise tolerance depends on various factors, such as the severity of the disease. The lung rehabilitation program consists of educational programs and exercise programs that include patient education, information on the pulmonary disease, treatment methods, and coping strategies. Exercise programs are the most important part of the lung rehabilitation program, and all lung patients can benefit from exercise as listed in [Table 5.46].

---

59) Furosemide: It is a powerful, fast-acting, short-acting type diuretic and used as a treatment for hypertension.
60) Hyponatremia: The production of antidiuretic hormone increases secondary to chronic pulmonary diseases.
61) Digitalis: It is a cardiotonic agent for increasing myocardial contractility and is used as a conduction system inhibitor to reduce heart rate.
62) Quinidine: A treatment for atrial fibrillation.
63) Lidocaine: Local anesthetics.
64) Verapamil: It is a coronary vasodilator and is used for the treatment and prevention of angina.
65) Amiodarone: Cardiac vasodilators and antiarrhythmics.
66) Diltiazem: Coronary vasodilators and a treatment for angina pectoris.
67) Right-side cardiac catheterization: A method of inserting a catheter into the heart through the veins of the arms and legs.
68) Nifedipine: As a coronary vasodilator, it is used as a treatment for coronary circulation disturbance and angina pectoris.

Table 5.46 ***Effects of exercise therapy for patients with pulmonary disease***

- Increased skeletal muscle tolerance and muscle strength
- 6% reduction in ventilation rate per minute
- 30% reduction in dyspnea level
- 17% reduction in lactate levels for exercise load
- Increased motivation for exercise
- Improvement of ventilatory muscle function and exercise performance

These benefits are seen in all patients with mild, moderate, and severe lung disease. The magnitude of improvement does not depend on the degree of lung injury. It is also possible to do at home. However, it is recommended to conduct it under the supervision of an expert for various tests and safety. In fact, most lung disease patients are afraid of exercise. Patients are trying to avoid all types of exercise because of the dyspnea that can occur during exercise. However, by exercising under the supervision of a specialist, the fear and resistance to exercise can be reduced. In particular, experiencing the effects of exercise greatly encourages the patient's attitude toward exercise therapy.

Pulmonary Disease and GXT

All CLD patients should receive a 'symptom-limited GXT' before participating in the exercise program [see Appendix B]. If gas measurement equipment is not available, it may be possible to measure oxygen saturation before and after exercise and cope with a cardiac stress test, including spirometry. The advantages of such cardiopulmonary exercise tests are shown in [Table 5.47].

Table 5.47 ***Advantages of cardiopulmonary test***

- Detection and intervention of exercise-induced hypoxia
- Detection and intervention of exercise-induced bronchial spasm
- Detection of exercise-induced cardiac arrhythmia/other cardiovascular diseases
- Calculation of anaerobic threshold and prescription of intensity
- Determine whether oxygen supplementation is necessary

In general, patients with FEV_1 of less than 50% and requiring oxygen supplementation during exercise should have an arterial oxygen partial pressure (PaO_2) of less than 55 mm Hg or arterial oxygen saturation (SaO_2) of less than 85%. The maximum respiratory ability of CLD patients with severe symptoms can be obtained at a level close to the maximum voluntary ventilation (MVV), but the functional capacity of the heart is relatively low. In healthy people, the opposite situation arises. In addition, the demand for ventilation during exercise increases abnormally in patients with CLD, suggesting that the amount of oxygen required for a given exercise load should be higher than normal. This means that the ratio of tidal volume (VT) to dead space volume (VD) of the patients is increased, and the efficiency of gas exchange is reduced due to the ventilation equivalents ($\dot{V}E/\dot{V}CO_2$ and $\dot{V}E/\dot{V}O_2$).[14]

Lung Disease and Exercise Prescription

Exercise intensity prescribed to pulmonary patients may be established through graded exercise test data, but there is no general standard for exercise intensity. The following points should be noted when prescribing exercise intensity using graded exercise test data.

First, when using the data of the graded exercise test for exercise prescription, the heart rate corresponding to 40~50% of $\dot{V}O_2max$ is set as the target heart rate. This exercise intensity is the recommended minimum exercise intensity for healthy adults, minimizing the risk of injury and helping to control the conditions of lung disease. However, it is not appropriate for patients with pulmonary disease with reduced MVV. Second, the minute ventilation volume should be less than 80% of the maximum ventilation in order to prescribe a heart rate consistent with the ventilation threshold. Patients with severe COPD do not reach anaerobic threshold (AT) in the graded exercise test. However, if the patient is able to reach the AT, it is advisable to prescribe the heart rate at that point as their exercise intensity or prescribe less than 80% of the maximum ventilation capacity. Third, exercise intensity should be set to a heart rate corresponding to 80% of maximal work for severe lung disease patients. Patients with moderate to severe lung disease can maintain the rate of MVV. However, patients with mild lung disease who have cardiovascular limitations may not be able to do so. In other words, these patients cannot continue their exercise at an intensity above the AT level. Fourth, if the lung disease is mild and the GXT cannot be performed, exercise intensity should be set using the dyspnea scale or RPE. The 3~6 on the dyspnea scale in normal individuals are consistent with 50~85% of $\dot{V}O_2max$. This intensity seems appropriate, but patients with severe symptoms or fear of exercise may also develop dyspnea at a very low intensity. Fifth, the proper type of exercise is a large muscle group oriented exercise. Exercise with lower extremity muscles consumes more ventilation than upper body exercises, but it is not contraindicated.[4,10]

Table 5.48 ***Exercise test, drug, and specific considerations for lung disease patients***

Test Item		Measurement	Recommended Stopping Point	Remarks
Aerobic Power Ability	■ Cycle (10, 15, 20 watt/min) ■ Cycle Ramp protocol (10~25 watt/3min stage) ■ Treadmill (1~2METs/stage)	■ 12 lead ECG	■ Severe arrhythmia appearance ■ ST segment depression / elevation > 2 ㎜ ■ Ischemic threshold ■ T wave inversion with ST change	■ Patients with COPD are more likely to have CAD.
		■ BP	■ SBP/DBP >250/115 ㎜Hg	
		■ RPE ■ Dyspnea scale	■ Sudden increase in psychological anxiety	
		■ Arterial oxygen partial pressure		■ Pulse Oximetry
		■ Gas analysis	■ Maximum ventilation ■ Peak oxygen uptake	■ Breathing pattern analysis can also help.
		■ Blood lactate concentration	■ Lactate threshold and ventilation threshold	■ Lactic acid acidosis limits exercise capacity.
Endurance/ Strength	■ 6-min walk ■ Isokinetic ■ Isotonic	■ Distance ■ Maximum number of iterations ■ Peak torque ■ 1RM	■ Time	■ It is useful for measuring the degree of improvement of the adaptation step. ■ The angular velocity for comparison of peak torque before and after training should be constant.
Flexibility	■ Sit-and-reach	■ Hip, hamstring, lumbar flexion	■ An unbearable trigger point	
Neuromuscle	■ Gait analysis ■ Balance analysis			■ Human body mechanics and coordination ability and efficiency inspection
Functional ability	■ Squat ■ Climbing stairs ■ Raise something			
Pharmacotherapy	■ All of the drugs listed below, despite side effects, can improve exercise capacity with bronchodilation, relief of congestive heart failure, and antipsychotic effects. ■ Methylxanthines : It may induce tachycardia, arrhythmia, and increase the level of dyspnea. ■ Sympathomimetic bronchodilators : It may cause tachycardia. ■ Loop and thiazide diuretics : Hypokalemia can lead to arrhythmias and heart failure. ■ Antidepressants : It may cause tachycardia during rest and exercise.			
Considerations	■ The risk of CAD is high. Exacerbated hypoxia during exercise can cause angina and arrhythmia. ■ It is important to observe 12 lead ECG, blood pressure and oxygen saturation. ■ Measurements of respiration, especially the maximum voluntary ventilation, may help to determine the extent of ventilation capacity. ■ Patients with pulmonary disease usually show deteriorated symptoms early in the morning, so it is advisable to perform an exercise test between 10 am and 11 am or between 2 pm and 4 pm. ■ Drugs should be administered after the best efforts are made for the purpose of exercise prescription. ■ Patients may get more dyspnea when lifting heavy objects.			

The frequency and intensity of exercise need to be adjusted according to the individual's condition. All patients should be given breathing training to reduce the respiratory rate, increase tidal volume and oxygen uptake, and adjust breathing sensation [see Appendix B]. Ultimately, exercise prescribers should be familiar with the tests, medications, and considerations of the exercises presented in [Table 5.48]. Based on this, the management methods presented in [Table 5.49] should be explained in detail to patients with lung disease.[3,5,22,25,66,83,88]

Table 5.49 ***Management program for lung disease patients***

Type		Goal	Intensity/Frequency/Time	Period
Aerobic/ Endurance Exercise	■ Major muscle exercises ■ Stand-up ergometer ■ Walking ■ Swimming	■ Increase in peak oxygen uptake ■ Increase in lactate / ventilation threshold ■ Decrease in dyspnea ■ Increase in efficient breathing pattern ■ Improvement of daily living activities	■ RPE 11~13 ■ Dyspnea scale ■ 3~7 day per week × 1~2 time per day ■ 30 min/bout (intermittent manner) ■ Emphasize longer time	■ 2~3 month
Strength Exercise	■ Free weight ■ Isotonic equipment ■ Isokinetic equipment	■ Increase in the maximum number of iterations ■ Increase in isokinetic torque / workload ■ Increase in lean body mass	■ Low intensity, high repetitions ■ 2~3 day per week	■ 2~3 month
Flexibility Exercise	■ Stretching	■ Increase of ROM	■ 3 days per week	
Neuromuscular Exercise	■ Walking, balancing exercise ■ Respiratory exercise	■ Improvement of walking and balancing ■ Improvement of respiratory muscle efficiency	■ Every day	
Functional Exercise	■ Activity type application and increase in daily life	■ Increase daily activities ■ Return to work ■ Improve the quality of life ■ Recreation / Fun	■ Every day	
Pharmacotherapy	■ Corticosteroids : Psychological anxiety / disability can be solved. ■ See pharmacotherapy during testing.			
Considerations	■ RPE and dyspnea scales are recommended methods for observing strength. Many patients can not reach their heart rate during training, but they can show a degree of psychological improvement. ■ CAD, peripheral arterial disease, and musculoskeletal problems (eg, arthritis and osteoporosis) are common disorders in patients with COPD. ■ Muscular disorders (including respiratory muscles) can be caused by corticosteroids, leading to muscle atrophy. ■ It is advisable to exercise at 10 to 11 am or 2 to 4 pm. ■ Do not exercise in a hot and humid environment. ■ Supplementary injection of oxygen should be adjusted so that the saturated oxygen concentration remains above 90%. ■ Anxiety, depression or panic are commonly caused by dyspnea and physical disability.			

Cystic Fibrosis

Symptoms and Features

Cystic fibrosis (CF) is a common life-threatening genetic disorder. Until recently, patients with this disease were rarely able to live to adulthood. However, nowadays, mortality is decreasing and adults account for 34% of all patients. CF is a disease caused by a defect in the production or transport of a protein called cystic fibrosis transmembrane conductance regulator (CFTR) due to malformations on chromosome 7. The CFTR protein is produced in the cytoplasm of the epithelial cells and is transported into the cell through the Golgi body to regulate sodium and other chloride channels. 70% of CF patients lack amino acids (phenylalanine) in #508. This mutated CF patient is capable of producing CFTR but is characterized by a defect in transport through the cytoplasm. CF affects whole body organs such as sinuses, pancreas, liver and sweat parenchyma, and 95% of male patients are infertile due to loss of left and right vas deferens. The biggest problem with CF patients is that lung disease progressively worsens. Due to electrolyte transport defects, the saline concentration of the airway mucus increases and electrolyte abnormalities occur, impairing the function of normal bacteria in the airways. That is, the ability to wash microorganisms is decreased, and metastatic growth such as staphylococcus occurs. Neutrophils reduce mucus production, destroy airway fibers, and migrate to infected areas where toxins are released in large quantities. DNA released by degraded neutrophils further increases the viscosity of the mucus. Similar results were reported that patients with pulmonary disease had a negative correlation with FEV_1, either with or without chronic excretion, due to increased sputum cell (neutrophil) components [Fig. 5.13].[62]

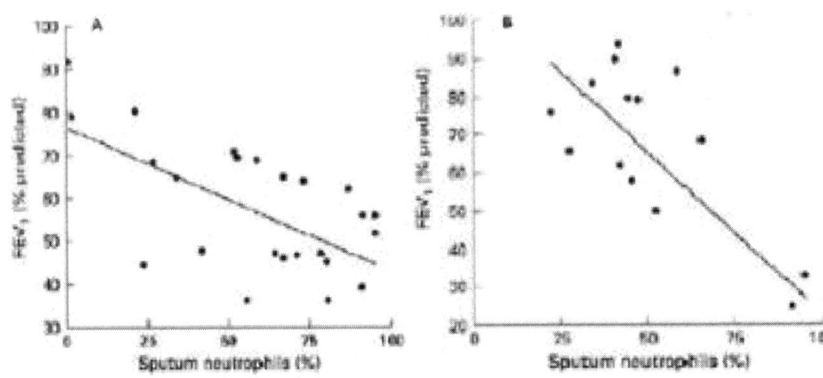

Fig. 5.13 ***Correlations between FEV_1 and sputum neutrophil cells***

Table 5.50 ***Exercise test, drug, and specific considerations for cystic fibrosis patients***

<table>
<tr><th></th><th>Test Item</th><th>Measurement</th><th>Recommended Stopping Point</th><th>Remarks</th></tr>
<tr><td rowspan="5">Aerobic Power Ability</td><td rowspan="5">■ Cycle
① Ramp protocol 10~15W/min
② 25W/ 3min

■ Treadmill (1~2METs/ 3min stage)
① Modified Balke
② Modified Bruce protocol recommended</td><td>■ 12 lead ECG
■ HR</td><td>■ Severe arrhythmia appearance
■ ST segment depression / elevation > 2 ㎜
■ Ischemic threshold
■ T wave inversion with ST change</td><td>■ The maximum heart rate may be less than the formula by age.
■ Patients with end-stage CF may have normal on ECG, but pulmonary heart disease.l</td></tr>
<tr><td>■ BP</td><td>■ Hypertensive reaction</td><td>■ Corticosteroids increase blood pressure.</td></tr>
<tr><td>■ Arterial SaO_2</td><td>■ When SaO_2 < 80% occurs</td><td>■ A FEV_1 of less than 50% indicates a reduced risk of arterial O_2 saturation or CO_2 congestion.</td></tr>
<tr><td>■ Gas analysis</td><td>■ Peak ventilation
■ Peak oxygen uptake
■ Carbon dioxide amount at the end of one ventilation</td><td></td></tr>
<tr><td>■ Spirometry</td><td>■ FVC
■ FEV_1
■ Maximum mid-expiratory flow rate</td><td>■ See also MVV.</td></tr>
<tr><td>Anaerobic Ability</td><td>■ Wingate protocol</td><td>■ Peak/average power ability
■ Fatigue degree</td><td>■ 30 second</td><td>■ Nutritional status may also be considered.</td></tr>
<tr><td>Endurance</td><td>■ 6-min walk</td><td>■ Distance
■ HR, SaO_2</td><td>■ 6 minute</td><td>■ Applied to patients with very poor exercise tolerance.</td></tr>
<tr><td>Pharmacotherapy</td><td colspan="4">■ Beta2 agonist and ipratropium bromide : It has bronchodilating effect, but it also causes tachycardia.
■ Corticosteroids : Although airway inflammation and cramps are reduced, steroids may cause myopathy, diabetes, and hypertension.
■ Sodium cromolyn : It minimize and prevent exercise-induced bronchospasm.
■ Theophylline : Although bronchodilation is effective, it can lead to tachycardia, ectopic response of the ventricles, and tachypnea.
■ Supplemental oxygen : Preventing de-saturation, reducing heart rate and ventilation, but also inducing hypoventilation.
■ Intravenous aminoglycosides : It causes dizziness and irregular walking by inducing hearing and vestibular toxicity.</td></tr>
<tr><td>Considerations</td><td colspan="4">■ It can be applied to some patients by application of equipment.
■ Supplementary oxygen supply is applied to CF patients with hypoxia.
■ Bronchial expansion therapy may help.</td></tr>
</table>

Table 5.51 ***Management program for cystic fibrosis patients***

	Type	Goal	Intensity/Frequency/Time	Period
Aerobic/ Endurance Exercise	▪ Major muscle exercises ▪ Stand-up ergometer ▪ Walking / jogging ▪ Swimming ▪ Rowing	▪ Increase in peak oxygen uptake ▪ Increase in peak power/ endurance ▪ Reduction of ventilation, HR and RPE ▪ Increased oxygen saturation ▪ Increase of respiratory muscle endurance ▪ Promoting mucus-clearance	▪ Karvonen 60~85% ▪ 3~4 d per week ▪ 10 min/bout (Increase gradually to 20~30 minutes) ▪ Using RPE and dyspnea scale ▪ Emphasize longer time	
Strength Exercise	▪ Major muscle exercises	▪ Increased strength and muscle endurance ▪ Reduction of steroid-induced depression and muscular dysfunction ▪ Reduction of airway trap by upper body workout	▪ Begin with 10 times × 3 sets at low load and gradually increase the number of repetition.	
Functional Exercise	▪ Activity type application and increase in daily life	▪ Increase in daily activities ▪ Increase in functional ability	▪ Based on clinical experience	
Pharmacotherapy	▪ Bronchodilators : It provides the effect of airway expansion before drug administration. ▪ Steroids : It can cause myopathy, diabetes and hypertension. ▪ Supplemental oxygen : It increases oxygen saturation in the arteries to increase the effect of exercise training and alleviate heart rate and ventilation (VE). However, it also causes CO_2 retention.			
Considerations	▪ For small-sized patients and young children, equipment should be modified and applied. ▪ Patients with reactive airways may also inhale Beta2 agonist or sodium cromolyn. ▪ Supplemental oxygen is applied to patients with hypoxia (SaO_2 <91%) at rest or during exercise. ▪ Some patients have complained of pain in the bones and joints (primarily the knee joint) due to hypertrophic pulmonary osteoarthropathy. ▪ Physical therapy and exercise on the chest can increase mucus clearance. ▪ The intensity should be reduced while the lung infection worsens. ▪ Increase water and salt intake during prolonged exercise or in hot weather.			

Management Methods

CF patients can be treated with antibiotics, bronchodilators, airway remodeling, and diet. Use of antibiotics in a timely manner in the vein and inhalation of tobramycin once every two months for a short period of time will be helpful in treatment. Oral bronchodilators are effective in patients with excessive airway hyper-responsiveness. Daily inhalation of pulmozyme to clean the airways and frequent physical treatment of the chest is a good method for patients with excessive secretions or bronchiectasis. There are two causes of weight loss in CF patients. First, cachexia is caused by chronic respiratory infection. Second, there is poor absorption of nutrients due to dysfunction of the pancreas. These patients require high-calorie, vitamin supplementation, and doses of pancreatic enzymes. If the pancreatic insufficiency worsens, it may progress to Type 1 DM and require further treatment.

In the sweat of CF patients, more sodium is detected than normal, and more sodium is lost during exercise.[62] This is not a big problem, but depending on the patient, an additional intake of salinity may be required, and the amount lost may need to be replenished over several hours. Water lost during or immediately after exercise should be replenished. [Table 5.50 and 5.51] shows specific details of exercise tests, drugs, and considerations in patients with cystic fibrosis.[3,5,22,25,62,83,88]

Asthma

Symptoms and Features

Asthma is a disorder characterized by bronchial hyperalgesia, which causes inflammation in the airway mucosa due to various stimuli, causing airway obstruction by contracting the bronchial smooth muscle. Specifically, asthma refers to a condition in which cellular components such as mast cells, eosinophils, T-lymphocytes, macrophages, neutrophils, and epithelial cells in the airways cause chronic inflammatory disorders.[64,66] People who are sensitive to these inflammations experience wheezing[69], dyspnea, periodic chest pain, and coughing at night and early morning. Symptoms are associated with airflow obstruction, which can be restored naturally or by treatment.[26] Inflammation may also be hypersensitive to a variety of stimuli. The clinical characteristics of asthma symptoms and pulmonary function are shown in [Table 5.52].

Table 5.52 ***Classification of asthmatic patients: clinical characteristics before treatment***

	Symptoms	Nighttime Symptoms	Lung Function
Stage 1 Mild / Intermittent	▪ Symptoms of less than 2 week	▪ < 2 month	▪ FEV_1 or PEF ≥ 80% (estimated) ▪ PEF variability < 20%
Stage 2 Mild / Persistent	▪ Symptoms of 1 time/d for more than 2 week	▪ > 2 month	▪ FEV_1 or PEF ≥ 80% (estimated) ▪ PEF variability < 20~30%
Stage 3 Moderate / Persistent	▪ Symptoms appear daily ▪ Fast acting β2 agonist daily inhalation ▪ Symptom worse affects activity ▪ Symptoms worsening ≥ 2 week or all day long	▪ > 1 week	▪ FEV_1 or PEF > 60 ~ < 80% ▪ Estimated PEF variability > 30%
Stage 4 Severe / Persistent	▪ Ongoing symptoms ▪ Limitation of physical activity ▪ Worsening of frequent symptoms	▪ Frequently occur	▪ FEV_1 or PEF ≤ 60% (estimated) ▪ PEF variability > 30%

69) Wheezing: It is a whistling sound while breathing. It occurs when bronchial stenosis or other lesions are present.

Management Methods

The purpose of the treatment and the patient's behavioral guidelines are shown in [Table 5.53]. Patients with asthma who are constantly exposed to allergies should be tested for signs of allergenic factors. Many asthmatics experience allergies to food. Patients with allergies to certain foods experience asthma for several hours after ingestion, but they do not recognize that they are related to the food. In addition, the role of antileukotrienes is unclear, but it is effective for aspirin-sensitive asthmatics and can reduce the dose of corticosteroids. Most patients with exercise-induced asthma are sensitive to cold, dry weather. In fact, asthma due to hyperventilation can happen to anyone, which is associated with the loss of respiratory heat due to cold weather. The dry air we breathe is hydrated by the moisture in the respiratory tract and warm-up before it enters the lungs. This air again comes out with water vapor at the time of exhalation. Asthma can also be found outdoors using a portable peak flow meter. A 12.5% decrease in peak flow during or after exercise is indicative of exercise-induced asthma.

Table 5.53 ***Purpose of treatment for asthmatic patients***[64]

Purpose of Treatment	Guidelines for Achieving Goals
▪ Preventing chronic and unpredictable symptoms. ▪ Maintain normal lung function. ▪ Maintaining normal physical activity including exercise and physical activity. ▪ Prevention of worsening asthma and minimization of emergency room and hospitalization. ▪ Adequate pharmacotherapy with little or no side effects. ▪ Treatment to meet patient and family's demand.	▪ Changes in the environment: Avoid occupational factors that induce asthma and airway stimulants that cause allergy. ▪ Records management: Record the extent of symptoms and the degree of asthma that appears in the morning / evening. ▪ Five things that aggravate asthma: rhinitis / sinusitis, gastroesophageal reflux, aspirin, and corticosteroids should be managed for side effects and viral infections.

In many studies, exercise-induced asthma has been proven to be preventable by the use of salmeterol, but appears to be insufficient to control it. To treat exercise-induced asthma, it is best to exercise in a warm and humid environment whenever possible and avoiding the causes of allergies. The goal of treatment is to allow the patient to participate in exercise without experiencing allergic symptoms. The most effective drugs to prevent exercise-induced asthma are salmeterol and short-acting beta-2 agonists.

Parasympatholytics[70], atropine[71], cromolyn[72], and calcium channel blockers also

70) Parasympatholytics: Drugs that counter parasympathetic nerve impulses.

71) Atropine: It is used as an anticholinergic agent to relax smooth muscle of various organs. Vagus nerve blocker is also used as a treatment for Parkinsonian syndrome.

72) Cromolyn: Cromolyn sodium, used to prevent bronchial asthma.

prevent exercise-induced asthma, but are less effective. Stepwise drug therapy for asthma patients is shown in [Table 5.54].

Table 5.54 ***Gradual pharmacotherapy for asthmatic patients***[64]

Stage	Treatment Period	Efficacy of Pharmacotherapy
Stage 1 Mild / Intermittent	■ Long-term control: None ■ Short-term stability: fast-acting β2 agonist inhalation	-
Stage 2 Mild / Persistent	■ Long-term control: Inhalation of corticosteroids in case of over 5 years old ■ Short-term stability: fast-acting β2 agonist inhalation	■ Cromolyn and nedocromil are alternative anti-inflammatory agents, but not as effective as corticosteroids.
Stage 3 Moderate / Persistent	■ Long-term control: Corticosteroids Inhalation or long-acting β2 agonist Inhalation ■ Short-term control: fast-acting β2 agonist inhalation	■ Double corticosteroids increase inhalation / specialist consultation / Theophylline is an alternative long-term bronchodilator, or salmeterol is more effective.
Stage 4 Severe / Persistent	■ Long-term control: Corticosteroids Inhalation or long-acting β2 agonist Inhalation ■ Short-term control: fast-acting β2 agonist inhalation	■ Add prednison / consultation / ■ Consider using Salmeterol and Theophylline.

Rehabilitation Exercise

There are two approaches to exercise prescription for exercise-induced asthma. The first is to prescribe an exercise intensity that does not cause asthma. If a conflicting exercise is prescribed, the patient will not be able to participate in any sports because of the limited activities. Low-intensity items that do not cause bronchospasm include short intermittent athletic activities such as swimming in a warm, humid environment and weight loading exercises. Jogging outdoors in cold weather may cause exercise-induced asthma. A 10 to 15-minute exercise at a relatively low intensity (i.e., a heart rate of 40 to 50% of $\dot{V}O_2max$, or an exercise of less than 2 on the dyspnea scale) reduces asthma symptoms. Exercise intensity in the preparation phase should be low enough for the patient to breathe comfortably through the nose. When the asthmatic patient exercises, bronchial contraction reaction occurs, so it is desirable to use stationary bicycle riding or walking with a constant load. In particular, swimming, mentioned above, offers the advantage of minimizing bronchoconstriction because it provides a humid environment.[76] If the asthmatic patient first starts exercising in the pool, the intermittent walking exercise performed in the water is effective. After walking 25 meters, the patient should take a rest for 1 minute and walk again for 5 minutes. This method should be repeated 4~5 times. However, if asthma symptoms are severe, one should inhale the bronchodilator before and after exercise and gradually exercise step by step. Drinking lukewarm water during exercise helps prevent symptoms. If the patient has to exercise in cold weather outdoors, it is better to wear a mask.

A second way to prevent exercise-induced asthma is to take β-adrenergic agonists before exercise. Exercise-induced asthma can be prevented by taking a long-acting bronchodilator, such as salmeterol 2 puffs twice a day. In addition, it is helpful to take 2~6 puffs of albuterol or β-adrenergic agonists 15 minutes before exercise. This allows the patient to participate in moderate to high-intensity exercise. When β-agonists are taken immediately before exercise, heart rate may rise rapidly, so exercise intensity should be prescribed using the dyspnea scale and the patient's condition should be monitored continuously. If the symptoms of patients with severe exercise-induced asthma are properly controlled, they can participate in an intense physical activity. However, if management is difficult, exercise should not be done to prevent exercise-induced asthma.

Guidelines for Weight Loading Exercise in Patients with Pulmonary Disease

Levels of oxygen saturation are very important when patients with pulmonary disease begin a strength training exercise for the first time. Patients who had a forced expiratory volume in 1 second (FEV_1) declining to less than 50%, had an arterial oxygen saturation (PaO_2) of less than 55 ㎜Hg and an arterial oxygen saturation (SaO_2) of less than 85%. In these patients, it is desirable to avoid strength training exercises if there is no additional oxygen supplement. Other contraindications are shown in [Table 5.55].

Table 5.55 ***Contraindications for resistance exercise***

① Congestive heart failure
② Uncontrolled arrhythmia
③ Severe valvular disease
④ Aerobic capacity less than 5 METs

When setting the intensity of the exercise, it is better to choose a weight based on the individual's ability rather than selecting a random weight. That is, 1RM is calculated. Using m1RM rather than the usual method for the calculation of 1RM is a safer method for lung disease patients [Table 5.56]. If 1RM is calculated, repeat 1 or 2 sets with a weight that can be lifted 10~15 times at an early stage. If the patient is able to lift this weight 15 times comfortably, adjust the weight so that 10 repetitions can be completed. In other words, a 30~50% load of 1RM is recommended at the beginning of training, but the load must be gradually increased to 60~80% in order to be fully effective. On the other hand, the prescribed program should be careful not to exceed 3~6 on the dyspnea scale.

Table 5.56 ***Example of modified 1RM measurement***

① Formula: 100 - (number of repetitions × 2)] = % 1RM
② If a patient with lung disease lifted 40 lbs 10 times,
③ Using the formula, {100 - (10 × 2)} = %1RM
④ 100 - 20 = 80%
⑤ That means 40 lbs is 80% of 1RM.
⑥ {40lb / 0.80} = 50 lbs becomes 1RM.

※ Initially, 30~50% of the 1RM is compatible with the weight of 15~25 lbs.

Arthritis

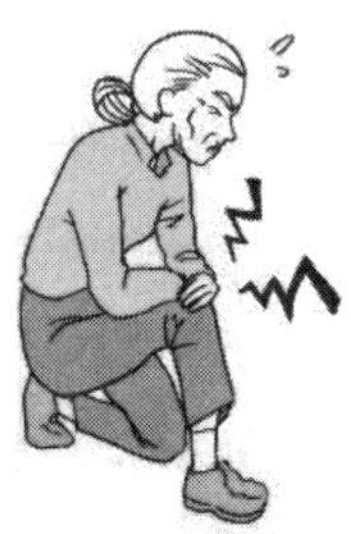

Arthritis refers to all inflammation of the joints, and Hippocrates referred to it as a "bad liquid substance that causes illness." Inflammation, which usually occurs in the joints, is temporary, but sometimes leads to permanent disability. The most common types of arthritis are degenerative arthritis and rheumatoid arthritis. The former is accompanied by gradual and reversible degeneration of articular cartilage surface, and the latter is characterized by inflammation of the bursa with abnormality of the autoimmune system. Both diseases are characterized by inflammation accompanied by pain, edema in the joints, and restricted ROM. Patients with rheumatoid arthritis typically experience throbbing pain, and patients with degenerative arthritis experience persistent discomfort. Medications for patients with rheumatoid arthritis include analgesics, glucocorticoid,73) and nonsteroidal anti-inflammatory drug (including immunosuppressive drug).[79]

There is little evidence that exercise increases OA, but rather the theory that it is beneficial to patients with arthritis is supported. However, caution should be exercised in

73) Glucocorticoid: A generic term for corticoid substances that inhibit gluconeogenesis. It increases liver glycogen and blood glucose levels.

patients with rheumatoid arthritis because exercise may not be performed properly or acute pain may exacerbate arthritis. Patients with arthritis should have an exercise program that enhances joint ROM and increases muscle strength. The type of exercise should be consulted with experts to choose the one that will maximize muscle strength, flexibility and endurance without worsening the patient's symptoms.

Degenerative Arthritis

Symptoms and Features

Osteoarthritis (OA) is the most common cause of joint disease, and the cause was unknown until now. However, it is divided into primary arthritis where degenerative changes occur in the normal articular cartilage without any specific cause, and secondary arthritis in which joint cartilage degeneration occurs due to aging, heredity, obesity, abuse and trauma, joint deformation and pain. Characteristically, OA can occur in all joints, but it usually occurs in the knee, hip, spine joint, and fingers, which have a high rate of activity and utilization or weight bearing.

Management Methods

The exercise goal for OA patients is to control and alleviate pain and reduce the dysfunction of the joints. Therefore, drug therapy or surgery should be performed first. The main objectives of exercise are weight loss and muscle strength. Among these, weight bearing exercise for strengthening muscles is very important for patients with arthritis, but there are some considerations. First, patients with arthritis need to make various changes in the type of exercise and the stimulated joint area when performing weight bearing exercise. Second, if patients have flare-ups in the joints, they should not exercise until they can endure the discomfort. Third, 1RM should be measured with a maximum muscle function test for weight bearing exercise. At this time, it is not advisable to perform an isometric test, which is recommended for testing the strength of the joint in a fixed state. However, if a patient with arthritis is accompanied by cardiovascular disease such as hypertension, an isokinetic test is more preferable. In particular, if a patient has symptoms or illnesses as shown in [Table 5.57], it is preferable not to perform a 1RM measurement or weight load exercise.

Fig. 5.57 ***Contraindication for resistance exercise***

① Congestive heart failure
② Uncontrolled arrhythmia
③ Severe valvular disease
④ Aerobic capacity less than 5MET

Methods for prescribing exercise intensity include barbells, dumbbells, weight machines, hand weights, and elastic bands. This should be prescribed in consideration of the patient's condition, and the intensity of exercise should not exceed the awareness level of 11 (usually) - 16 (hard to hard). [Table 5.58] shows the step-by-step rehabilitation treatment methods for OA patients.

Fig 5.58 ***Stages of rehabilitation for degenerative knee patients***

Stage	Practice Rehabilitation Exercise
Stage 1	■ Passive rotation exercise . Lightly push the patella toward left, right, up and down for two to three minutes with both hands. . After pushing, rotate lightly to the left and right. ※ Capsaicin including mentol contents are more effective.
Stage 2	■ Leg stretching . Apply various postures for the flexibility of the quadriceps and hamstring. . Do not bend the joint until the point of enduring the pain. . Flexibility exercises are carried out within the tolerance range.
Stage 3	■ Active rotation exercise . Recumbent cycle : To lose weight 200 ~ 300 ㎉ per day consumption. . UBX cycle : To consume 50 ~ 100 ㎉ per day. ※ Practice until reaching ideal weight / Minimize the burden of joints when losing weight.
Stage 4	■ Femoral muscle strengthening . Practice often regardless of time and place. . {During one exercise (10 seconds of contraction / 10 seconds of relaxation)} × 10 times. 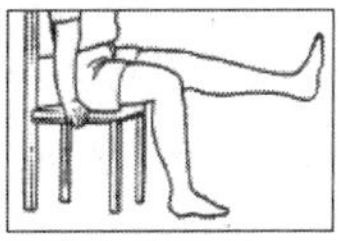 Quadriceps 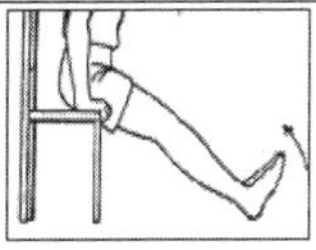 Hamstrings
Stage 5	■ 8 week training program with isokinetic equipment . Week 0 : In isokinetic mode, examine the patient's ROM and peak torque / average power / total work. . Week 1~2 : The CPM exercise is applied for two weeks in order to increase the limited ROM. During the last 3 days of Week 2, CPM mode is used to train concentric/eccentric muscle contraction. . Week 3~4 : Perform a five-step program (60°/sec→90°/sec→120°/sec→150°/sec→180°/sec) 10 times at medium speed (60°/sec~180°/sec). In the fourth week, 10 times in reverse (180°/sec→150°/sec→120°/sec→90°/sec→60°/sec). . Week 5~6 : To increase muscle strength. perform a three-step program (60°/sec→ 50°/sec→ 40°/sec) 10 times at low speed (60°/sec or less). In the sixth week, 10 times in reverse (40°/sec→ 50°/sec→ 60°/sec). . Week 7~8 : To increase muscle strength. perform a three-step program (180°/sec→ 210°/sec→ 240°/ sec) 10 times at high speed (180°/sec or more). In the eight week, 10 times in reverse (240°/sec→ 210°/sec→ 180°/sec).
Stage 6	■ Icing and massage . When the muscle strengthening exercise is over, icing is performed for 2 to 5 min. ※ Minimize inflammation and reduce pain.

Changes in Pain and Myofunction after Treatment

As shown in [Table 5.28], the management guidelines for OA patients should be modified and applied on a daily basis to the patient's pain and condition. In addition, OA maximizes the therapeutic effect when combined treatment is performed for 36 weeks as shown in [Table 5.58]. In fact, the most important factor in OA therapy is the movement of the joints. However, in general, patients do not move if they have pain, resulting in a continuous decline in myofunction around the joints. In other words, if symptoms of OA appear at all, it is important to make muscles, ligaments, tendons and bones strong through regular exercise from the beginning. Patients whose OA has already begun, can feel the relief of flexion, extension, and the improvement of symptoms when rehabilitation centered on the quadriceps is performed. This report can be verified as a result of an experiment using [Table 5.59] as a program. The degree of pain in the experimental group (measured by Taylor's pain scale[74]) was 3.50 (± 0.52) before the experiment, which was 'very severe' and 'severe', but as a result of continuous rehabilitation exercise, it decreased to 2.80 (± 0.63) after 12 weeks and to 1.70 (± 0.67) after 36 weeks. That is, when the rehabilitation exercise was performed for 36 weeks, the pain level improved to 'painless or light' or 'normal'. In the control group without rehabilitation, the pain level before the experiment was 3.40 (± 0.51). The pain level decreased to 3.70 (± 0.48) after 12 weeks and to 3.90 (± 0.73) after 36 weeks. In other words, these results show that OA-induced pain can be reduced by medication, and that it can lead to effects similar to those of medical treatment if a continuous rehabilitation exercise is performed.

The changes in the myofunctional variables were similar to the degree of pain described above. Specifically, the peak torque of the experimental group at an angular velocity of 60°/sec was increased in the right flexor and extensor muscles. All of the control group showed a statistically significant difference in the alternation effect. That is, in the experimental group, 36 weeks of rehabilitation were observed to maintain or increase myofunction. However, in the control group who did not perform rehabilitation treatment, it could be interpreted as a worsening of OA because of decreased myofunction. This tendency was similar to the average power expressed at 180°/sec and the total daily dose expressed at 240°/sec. In addition, many previous studies have confirmed that deteriorating OA was due to a sedentary occupation. Ultimately, the combination of strength training for quadriceps muscle strengthening, and aerobic training

74) The pain scale developed by Taylor et al. (1981) was modified and measured. The scale consists of mild (1), moderate (2), severe (3), very severe (4), and unbearable (5).

for body weight reductions, reduced the pain in OA patients and favorably changed body composition. These results are very similar to the results of a 12-week home rehabilitation program that increased isokinetic muscle function in OA patients by 16%, 27%, and 42% per month.

Table 5.59 ***Combination rehabilitation treatment program for degenerative arthritis***[43]

Items		Step Ⅰ (0~12 week)	Step Ⅱ (13~24 week)	Step Ⅲ (25~36 week)
Exercise Therapy	① Warm up*	10 min	10 min	10 min
	② Stationary bicycle†	15 min	20 min	25 min
	③ Isometric femoral exercise‡	5 times(15 min)	8 times (18 min)	10 times (21 min)
	④ Aquatic exercise§	-	1 set (17 min)	2 sets (34 min)
	⑤ Cool down*	10 min	10 min	10 min
Physical Therapy‖	⑥ Icing	5~10 min	10~12 min	12~15 min
	⑦ TENS	8~10 min	10~12 min	12~15 min
	⑧ Ultrasonic wave	2~3 min	3~5 min	5~8 min
Total Treatment Time		≒65~73 min	≒98~104 min	≒129~138 min

*Conduct stretching flexibly without pain and hyperflexion. †Exercise for weight loss: Adjust the knee angle from 120° to 150° to exercise at 60% of VO_2max. ‡Quadriceps muscle strengthening exercises: 10 seconds of contraction at 15°, 10°, 5° / 10 seconds rest. §Weight loss and ROM improvement exercise (Forward/ Backward walking 8 min, Crossover stepping 4 min, Straight arm pull 5 min). ‖Minimization of pain and inflammation using icing, TENS(transcutaneous electrical nerve stimulation) and ultrasound.

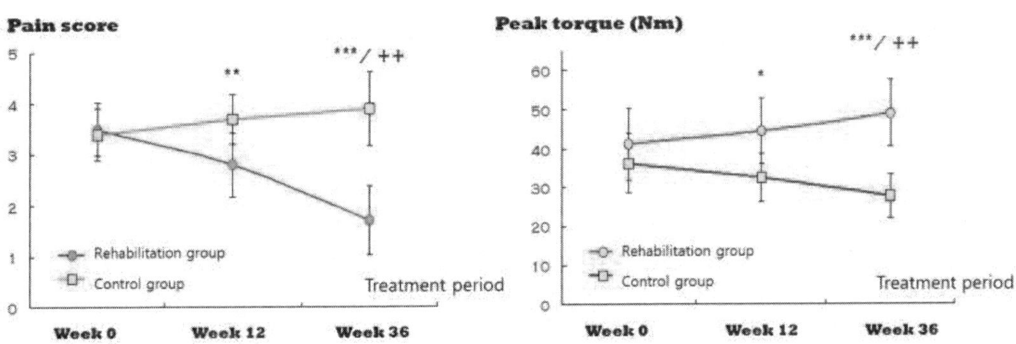

Fig 5.14 ***Changes in pain level and peak torque after 36 weeks of rehabilitation***

** Time difference: ** P<.01, *** P<.001, + Group difference: ++ P<.01*

Rheumatoid Arthritis

Symptoms and Features

Rheumatoid arthritis (RA) is an abnormally excessive immune function that causes joint destruction. Although the cause is unclear, extrinsic factors such as viruses, bacteria, and

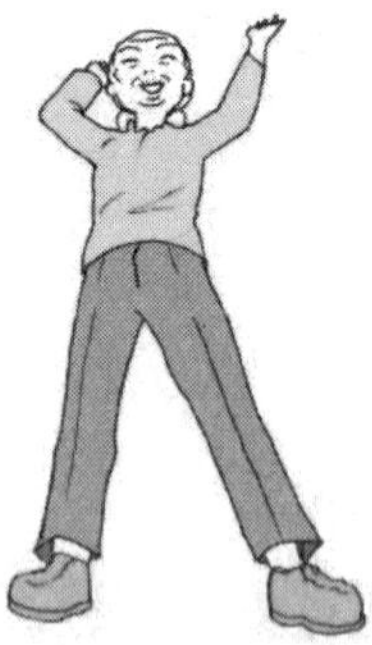

endogenous factors related to immune response are thought to cause complex lesions. Symptoms include fatigue, weakness, loss of appetite, arthralgia, inflammation of joint synovium, swelling of joints, soreness, burning, and stiffness. It affects small joints such as hands, fingers, feet, and toes, which occur symmetrically on both sides of the limb. If it continues, it will damage various parts such as vasculitis, pneumonia, pericarditis by excessive immune reaction.[79]

Management Methods

Treatment for RA is primarily to relieve pain and prevent deterioration of physical function. Typical therapies include medication, exercises that strengthen the cartilage of the joints, ligaments and muscles around the joints, and calcium accumulation in the bones. In severe cases, surgical treatment is performed.

Table 5.60 ***Classification of patients with rheumatoid arthritis***

Classification	Functional Ability
Type1	Patients who can perform daily life without difficulty
Type2	Moderate limitation: Patients who are uncomfortable but can perform a limited normal life
Type3	Severe limitations: Patients whose function is limited and do not perform their daily tasks or self-management completely
Type4	Patients who can only be active on a bed or wheelchair because their activities are almost impossible

Arthritis Impact Measurement Scale (AIMS)

Items	Survey Contents
1	When walking around the neighborhood, do you need someone else's help because of your health problems?
2	Can you use a public car (bus or taxi)?
3	Should you stay home all day for health problems?
4	Do you have to sit on a bed or a chair all day for health problems?
5	Can not you participate in running / heavy objects / hard workouts?
6	Can not you walk a long distance or jump over stairs because of your health problems?
7	Can not you bend or stretch your body due to health problems?
8	Can you walk a block or a stair climb due to a health problem?
9	Can you walk without a person, dog, splint, artificial leg or splint who can help?
10	Can not you write easily with a fan or pencil?
11	Can not you put buttons on my clothes?
12	Can not you lock the door easily?
13	Can not you wear shoes?
14	Can not you get canned easily?
15	If you have a car, can not you go shopping in a store or supermarket?
16	Can not you prepare food in the kitchen?
17	Can not you clean my house with a cleaning tool?

Patients with RA can be classified according to the measurement on the osteoarthritis scale provided in [Table 5.60], which are classified according to functional ability. Patients include: Type 1 Patients who can perform daily life without difficulty, Type 2 Patients who are uncomfortable but whose activities are limited in normal life and in more than one joint, Type 3 Patients who are somewhat limited in function and cannot perform their daily tasks easily, and Type 4 Patients who can only perform limited activities in bed or wheelchair because their activities are almost impossible to do. However, their functional capacity may be impossible to test by an exercise test. Currently, a '6-minute walk' can also be used to evaluate aerobic endurance capabilities. However, it is generally desirable to carry out the 6-minute walk mainly for women. It is advisable to consider exercise time, etc. by referring to the evaluation table in [Table 5.61].

Table 5.61 ***6-minute walk evaluation***

6-minute walk (yards)	Age			
	Under 30	30~39	40~49	50~59
Very poor	< 660	< 621	< 587	< 557
Poor	660 ~ 720	621 ~ 681	587 ~ 647	557 ~ 609
Fair	721 ~ 782	682 ~ 754	648 ~ 720	610 ~ 674
Good	783 ~ 880	755 ~ 845	721 ~ 812	675 ~ 754
Excellent	≥ 881	≥ 846	≥ 813	≥ 755

In the Arthritis impact measurement scale (AIMS) form, patients with type 1 or type 3 RA have a suitable walking and cycle ergometer. Bicycling should be done at 60~80% of maximum heart rate or 40~60% of maximum oxygen intake for 30 minutes. Walking should be done for 15 minutes at a comfortable breathing rate early, and should be increased to 30~60 minutes when adapting. On the other hand, patients with type 4 initially perform the passive ROM exercises, and help them to adjust to active and progressive movements. Particularly, for these kind of patients, it is good to exercise the joints of the whole body by water exercises after adaptation of the cycle ergometer and the upper bike which do not give impact while keeping the heart rate constant. As with OA patients, daily exercise of joint range is performed manually and actively. However, patients with RA can usually take analgesic anti-inflammatory drugs, so they do not feel pain.

Table 5.62 ***Exercise test, drug, and specific considerations for arthritis patients***

	Test Item	Measurement	Recommended Stopping Point	Remarks
Myofunction	▪ Isokinetic (90~120 ° /sec) ▪ Isometric knee extensor		▪ Extension strength of the knee exceeds 20~30% per weight ▪ At power output of 70 kg	▪ The test is limited to the affected joint or painful area.
Endurance	▪ 6-min walk ▪ Fatigue / exhaustion time	▪ Distance, HR, RPE ▪ Exhaustion time : MVC 75% or peak torque	▪ 6 minute ▪ Fatigue	
Flexibility	▪ Goniometer	▪ Muscle-joint imbalance or asymmetry		▪ It helps in setting exercise goals during exercise counseling.
Neuromuscle	▪ Gait analysis ▪ Balance analysis			
Functional Ability	▪ 50-feet walk ▪ Squat ▪ Standing time ▪ Muscle-joint questionnaire	▪ Observation of symmetry	▪ Arthritis Impact Measurement Scale	▪ Standing time applies to very fragile or unstable patients.
Pharmacotherapy	▪ Non-steroidal antiimflammatory drugs : It may cause anemia due to gastrointestinal bleeding. ▪ Rheumatoid arthritis-remitting drugs : It may cause secondary organ damage including myopathy. ▪ Oral corticosteroids : May cause myopathy due to gastrointestinal bleeding, upper body obesity, osteoporosis, anemia.			
Considerations	▪ Pain and swelling may reduce exercise performance. ▪ Patients with unstable joint conditions should avoid vigorous, high-repetition exercises. ▪ Some joint diseases affect the cardiopulmonary system and reduce exercise performance. ▪ If arthritis is involved in the spine, it may cause radiculopathy. ▪ In the case of RA patients, the morning stiffness is frequent, so morning exercise is not good. ▪ For the kock-knee patient, the foot should be fixed with a strap as the foot is easily removed from the bicycle pedal.			

Ultimately, exercise prescribers should be familiar with the methods of exercise testing for patients with arthritis (OA and RA), medications being administered, and special considerations, as shown in [Table 5.62]. Patients must be told in detail. The specific management program is summarized in [Table 5.63].[3,5,13,22,25,79,83,88]

Table 5.63 ***Management program for arthritis patients***

Type		Goal	Intensity/Frequency/Time	Period
Aerobic/ Endurance Exercise	■ Major muscle exercises ■ Stand-up ergometer ■ Walking / jogging ■ Aquarobics ■ Rowing	■ Increase in maximal oxygen uptake ■ Increase in peak power / endurance	■ HR peak 60~80% ■ VO_2max 40~60% ■ RPE 11~16 ■ 3~5 days per week ■ 5~10 min/bout (gradually increase to 30 min) ■ Emphasize longer time	■ 3~6 month
Strength Exercise	■ Free weight, weight machine, circuit training by isometric exercise or elastic band	■ Increase in MVC ■ Increase in peak torque and power	■ Set MVC% and to the point of pain tolerance ■ Repeat 2 ~ 3 times in the beginning (gradually increase to 10 ~ 12 times) ■ 2~3 days per week	
Flexibility Exercise	■ Stretching	■ Relieve pain, increase ROM ■ Decrease in rigidity	■ 1~2 times daily exercise	
Neuromuscular Exercise		■ Improve walking and balancing	■ Everyday	
Functional Exercise	■ Activity type application and increase in daily life	■ Increase daily activities ■ Return to work ■ Improve the quality of life	■ Everyday	
Pharmacotherapy	■ Steroids : It may cause stress fractures. ■ See pharmacotherapy for exercise testing.			
Considerations	■ Avoid the hyperextension stretching about unstable joints. ■ High repetitions, high load and high impact exercises are contraindications. ■ Depression is a disability that can lead to changes in the type of life and a pleasant program should be provided.			

Osteoporosis

Symptoms and Features

Osteoporosis is a disease that increases bone fragility and increases the risk of fracture due to low bone mass and the microscopic structural deterioration of the bone tissue. Specifically, 99% of human bones are made up of calcium. When the aging process starts, calcium exits the bone and becomes like a sponge. This is called osteoporosis. In other words, osteoporosis is a progressive process of bone destruction or resorption, in whcih calcium is released into the blood by osteoclast.

Osteoporosis is thought to be dangerous because once it is triggered, bones can easily fracture, even with a small impact. Furthermore, the fractured bone will not heal well. Symptoms include severe fatigue and pain in the thoracic and lumbar spine. In particular, if severe pain occurs when a specific operation is performed, it is a state of fatigue fracture, so it requires immediate inspection.

Both men and women have the risk of fractures due to osteoporosis, but they are especially common among women. In North America, one in three elderly women aged 70 or older experienced a vertebral fracture. One in three elderly women aged 85 or older reported having experienced a hip fracture.[10,30] This hip joint fracture has been reported by about one out of six elderly men aged 85 or older, suggesting that women are twice as likely to fracture due to osteoporosis than men [Fig. 5.15]. Factors affecting fracture risk include skeletal vulnerability, frequency and severity of falls, and tissue mass around the bone. Therefore, in order to prevent fractures due to osteoporosis, it is necessary to focus on increasing bone nutrients and structural properties, preventing falls, and increasing total fat mass.

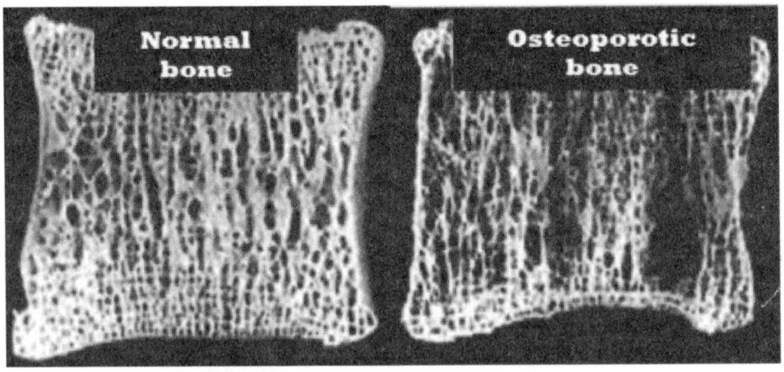

Fig. 5.15 *Normal and osteoporotic bone*

Diagnosis of osteoporosis is based on clinical history and bone scan. Measurement of bone density (BMD) is a useful method for assessing the risk of fracture. For example, if bone density falls below 10%, the risk of fracture is doubled. On the other hand, the measurement of bone density using Dexa is interpreted in comparison with the normal mean value among age, sex and race. Clinically, T-score is mainly used. This is the difference between the measured bone density level and the mean theoretic value of the peak bone mass (a value obtained under the assumption that the long-term bone density is lost at a constant rate in an adult who is not treated for osteoporosis) divided by the standard deviation. This can be useful in assessing the risk of fracture. The range of bone density levels currently used, osteopenia and osteoporosis, are shown in [Table 5.64].

Table 5.64 ***Levels of bone mineral density according to T-scores' measurement***

	Normal	Osteopenia	Osteoporosis
T-score	-1.0 or less	-1.0 ~ -2.5	-2.5 or more

T-score = (Measured value - mean value of young group) ÷ standard deviation

Management Methods

General Guidelines

Many diseases and medications are known to cause osteoporosis, but most of the causes are still unclear. In general, osteoporotic fractures occur mainly in the trabecular bone, such as vertebrae, ribs, distal forearm, and proximal femur. In the elderly, the initial bone mass is determined by degenerative bone loss and the peck bone mass (trigenerian amount of bone mass). Congenital factors, dietary intake, hormones, physical activity, lifestyle factors, medications and other diseases should be considered to maintain peck bone mass. Estrogen administration is ideal for people with hypoestrogenemia. Calcium intake is not beneficial to the human body when consumed in excess, and may adversely affect health. An intake of about the threshold level of 1,000~1,500 ㎎/day is desirable. Recently, however, many studies have been conducted on the optimum level of calcium intake. Therefore, more accurate measurements are expected.[13] In addition, mechanical load exercises can have a positive impact on the bone, which can be of great help to the patient.

Management for Elderly Women

The diet and exercise needed to prevent bone loss in elderly women also reduces the chance of osteoporosis in later years for middle-aged or younger women. It is essential to have a calcium-rich diet for pregnant and lactating women, as well as women in their youth and mid-20s who need 1,200 ㎎ of calcium daily. However, 1,000 ㎎ per day is enough for women who have not entered menopause. It is advisable to increase the daily calcium intake to 1,500 ㎎ for the elderly over 65 years, pregnant or lactating women, or women without estrogen treatment after menopause.

Dairy products rich in vitamin D are the most important source of calcium intake in the diet. Also, green plants, nuts, and seafood are important sources of calcium-rich ingredients and must be considered when constructing a diet. On the other hand, one cup of skim milk contains 300 ㎎ of calcium, and drinking 3.3 cups results in 1,000 ㎎ of calcium. Women who do not consume milk or do not get enough calcium for other reasons must take other supplements. On the other hand, sugary foods such as soft drinks, candy, and confectionary should be avoided to prevent inhibiting bone formation. Estrogen treatment is necessary for women with rapid bone loss after menopause because the amount of estrogen supplied is extremely low. Estrogen prevents bone loss, improves calcium intake, and increases the effect of exercise for the bones.[30]

Osteoporosis is the most significant health problem in healthy elderly women after menopause. That is, the higher the age, the greater the prevalence of osteoporosis and fractures in women. In fact, estrogen treatment can prevent osteoporosis and CAD, but it can cause endometrial carcinoma in the first 5 years and the risk is about 6 times greater. On the other hand, the risk increases by 15 times when taken over a long period of time. Estrogen also increases the risk of breast cancer. For example, women who received estrogen therapy for 10 years or more had 45% more breast cancer deaths compared to women who did not. Therefore, women with a low risk of heart disease need to ask their specialists whether estrogen affects uterine cancer and breast cancer and if not, the degree of osteoporosis. However, supplements of progesterone on the last 12 days of estrogen therapy can lower the risk of endometrial hyperplasia and uterine cancer. Meanwhile, tamoxifen and raloxifen, estrogen replacement drugs, have been used as anticancer drugs in the past. Tamoxifen can prevent osteoporosis and protect breast cancer to a certain extent, but it cannot prevent heart disease. Raloxifene can prevent osteoporosis and reduce the risk of breast cancer, but unlike tamoxifen, it affects cardiovascularity positively. Recently, alendronate, which is in the limelight, can promote bone growth without causing cancer, but it has been reported that it cannot help the cardiovascular system like estrogen or raloxifene. Alendronate inhibits bone resorption and normalizes bone turnover rate. 10 ㎎ is effective as 20 ㎎ and has an effect greater than 5 ㎎.[13]

Calcium and vitamin D supplements are the most effective way to lower the risk of osteoporosis and cardiovascular disease when combined with exercise. Daily doses of 1,000 ㎎ of calcium and 500~800 ㎎ of vitamin D3 do not increase calcium excretion into the urine and do not cause hypercalemia. In addition, this supplement is said to reduce fracture of femur, which is common in older women, and to maintain bone density levels in patients with lumbar spine treated with small amounts of corticosteroids.

Rehabilitation Exercise

Numerous human and animal studies have shown that exercise affects bone components and mechanical properties positively. High-intensity exercise, however, may delay bone growth and cause fatigue fractures. The load bearing of the bone to the load reflects bone matrix, such as bone density and spatial distribution of bone tissue. These bone tensions can all be developed and are maintained through partial daily exercise.

Although functional load through physical activity positively affects the bone mass in the human body,[37] it has not been suggested in the past that the type of exercise program stimulates bone formation or the improvement of bone mass after increasing physical activity.[43] In recent years, however, several studies have shown that there are various results depending on age, hormone status, nutrition, and exercise. Some similar studies have shown that athletes have higher bone mass and strength than the sedentary. More specifically, running athletes and weightlifters among athletes are reported to have stronger bones than swimming athletes. It is reported that exercise stimuli performed on the ground give more stimulation than those performed in the water.

Table 5.65 ***Exercise program for the elderly***

Item	Type	Period (week)			Remarks
		0~8	9~24	25~54	
Warm-up	Standing stretching	10 min	10 min	10 min	**Sequence of weight bearing:** Leg-press, Shoulder-dumbbell, Leg-extension, Leg-curl, Arm-curl, Back-extension, Abdominal-crunch, Torso
Workout	Stationary bicycle	20 min	25 min	30 min	
	Walking on a treadmill	20 min	25 min	30 min	
	Weight bearing exercise	10 reps × 2set	12 reps × 2set	15 reps × 2set	
Cool-down	Stretching in a lying position	20 min	20 min	20 min	

In fact, regular weight-bearing exercise should be emphasized to improve and maintain bone mass. This is important for men and women of all ages, but is especially important for older people who have not been exercising. In one study, a total of 93 elderly people (43 males, 50 females) participated in the exercise program shown in [Table 5.65] for 5 days per week (group A, 14 males and 14 females), group participating 2~3 days per week (group B, 14 males and 17 females), group participating 1 day per week (Group C, 8 males, 13 females), and group not participating in exercise (group D, 7 males, 6 females), and the bone density level of the human body was examined. Results showed that for group A, which participated in exercise for 5 days or more per week, had a bone density of the legs measuring 1.58 g/㎠ and 1.17 g/㎠ for male and female, respectively. There were statistically significant differences. The bone density of the spine was also higher in group A than in the three other groups: 1.7 g/㎠ and 1.16 g/㎠ for male and female, respectively.[42] There was also a statistically significant difference [Fig. 5.16].

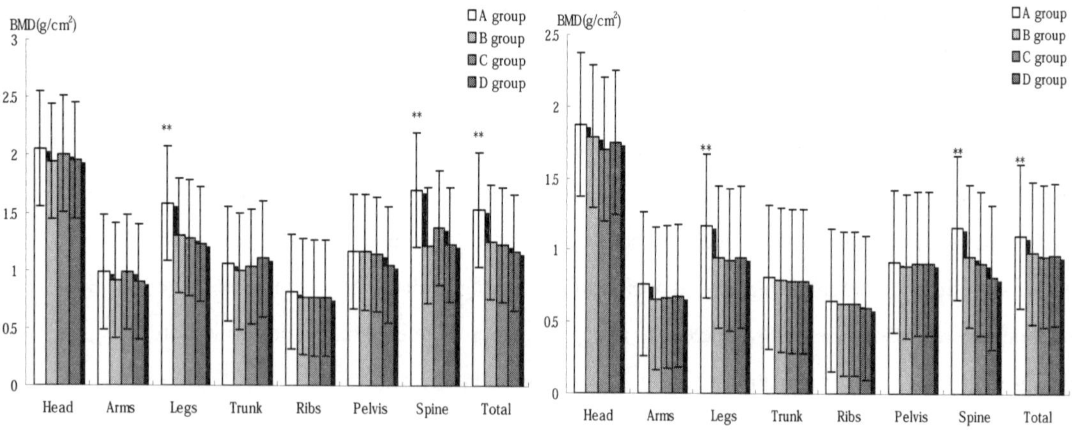

Fig. 5.16 Comparison of BMD after 1 year of exercise program

*(Results of male(left)/ female(right) group), **: P<.01*

These results were consistent with the fact that the BMD levels after regular exercise were 3.8% higher than the BMD of the control group.[77] In addition, it was also consistent that the regular running increased the lumbar spine BMD of women over 50 years from 9.2% to 35% compared with that of the non-exercise group.[20]

In addition to weight-bearing exercise, which is effective for osteoporosis, walking, quick paces, swimming and underwater walking are among the most popular sports for osteoporosis. Exercise intensity should be performed at a relatively low or moderate intensity of about 40~70% of the maximum heart rate. Exercise time should be between 30~60 minutes, 3~5 days a week. Particularly, it is effective to carry out full weight-bearing exercises after becoming comfortable performing push-ups, sit-ups, squats, and using weights first. Exercise intensity should be set at 75% of 1RM, and two sets should be performed at a weight that can be lifted eight to twelve times. There is a report that positive effect is obtained when this exercise is performed for 2 days per week for 2~3 months.[10] In addition, 70% of 1RM was performed twice a week for 6 months, and it was reported that bone density levels of lumbar spine and femoral head were preserved.

Table 5.66 ***Exercise test, drug, and specific considerations for osteoporotic patients***

<table>
<tr><th colspan="2">Test Etem</th><th>Measurement</th><th>Recommended Stopping Point</th><th>Remarks</th></tr>
<tr><td rowspan="3">Aerobic Power Ability</td><td rowspan="3">■ Cycle (5~20 watt/min) Ramp protocol (10~25 watt/ 3min stage)
■ Treadmill (1~2METs/ stage)</td><td>■ 12 lead ECG
■ HR
■ METs</td><td>■ Severe arrhythmia appearance
■ ST segment depression / elevation > 2 ㎜
■ Ischemic threshold
■ T wave inversion with ST change
■ HR and MET are useful for creating exercise programs.</td><td>■ Most people with osteoporosis have a high risk of CAD.</td></tr>
<tr><td>■ BP</td><td>■ SBP/DBP >250/115 ㎜Hg</td><td></td></tr>
<tr><td>■ RPE</td><td>■ An extreme fatigue point</td><td>■ Useful for patients with difficult HR measurements.</td></tr>
<tr><td>Myofunction</td><td>■ Weight machine</td><td>■ 1~10RM</td><td>■ Pain
■ Fatigue</td><td>■ Useful when setting exercise intensity.
■ Decreased muscle strength in postmenopausal older women is associated with osteoporosis.</td></tr>
<tr><td>Neuromuscle</td><td>■ Gait analysis
■ Balance</td><td>■ Observation
■ Time
■ Force plate
■ Balance scale(Berg)</td><td>■ Pain
■ Fatigue</td><td>■ For patients with severe symptoms.</td></tr>
<tr><td>Functional Ability</td><td>■ 6-min walk
■ Walking speed
■ Sitting-rising</td><td>■ Distance
■ Speed
■ Grasp the degree of performance that the patient can stand up without using the arm</td><td>■ Pain
■ Fatigue</td><td>■ The sitting rising test provides useful information as a strength assessment, and in particular, estimates the state of muscles and ligaments around the hip.</td></tr>
<tr><td>Postural Examination</td><td>■ Check for kyphosis</td><td>■ Flexicurve</td><td></td><td></td></tr>
<tr><td>Pharmacotherapy</td><td colspan="4">■ Drugs such as diuretics, antihypertensives, anti-anginal drugs, antiarrhythmics, psychostimulants, insulin and anticoagulants are investigated.</td></tr>
<tr><td>Considerations</td><td colspan="4">■ Neuromuscular and functional performance tests should be performed by experienced clinicians.
■ Orthopedic considerations: Patients with severe kyphosis also have changes in the center of gravity, affecting walking and balance.
■ Pulmonary functional considerations: Severe kyphosis affects the thoracic structure and may affect respiratory muscles.
■ Neurosensory considerations: Severe kyphosis may prevent the patient from performing treadmill walking.
■ Muscle problems: Patients complaining of chronic back pain due to complex vertebral fractures are susceptible to lumbar extensor weakness.
■ Psychological problems: Anxiety about falls may cause the test to stop before it is desirable to perform a cycle test.</td></tr>
</table>

However, weight-bearing exercise should be performed carefully and focus on muscle development, not muscle endurance. Ultimately, exercise prescribers should be familiar with the exercise tests, ophthalmic drugs and special considerations for osteoporosis patients listed in [Table 5.66]. It is important to inform everything to the patient in detail. The specific management program is shown in [Table 5.67].[3,5,10,20,22,25,83,88]

Table 5.67 ***Management program for osteoporotic patients***

	Type	Goal	Intensity/Frequency/Time	Period
Aerobic Exercise	▪ Cycling ▪ Walking ▪ Swimming	▪ Increase and maintain power	▪ HR peak 40~70% ▪ METs 40~70% ▪ 3~5 days per week ▪ 30~60 min/bout	▪ 2~6 mon ▪ BMD changes occur between 9 and 24 mon.
Strength Exercise	▪ Dumbbell ▪ Weight machine ▪ Floor calisthenics	▪ Increase muscle strength of whole body ▪ Emphasize the development of hip flexior / extensior and lumbar extensior	▪ 1RM 75%, 8~12 times ▪ 8 to 10 times × 2 sets ▪ 2 to 3 days per week × 20 to 40 minutes	▪ 6 mon or more
Flexibility Exercise	▪ Stretching ▪ Chair gymnastics	▪ Increase and maintain ROM ▪ In particular, pectoralis	▪ 5~7 days a week	
Functional Exercise	▪ Application of activity type of everyday life ▪ Brisk walking ▪ Sitting-rising on a chair ▪ Balancing exercise	▪ Increase daily activities ▪ Improved balance ▪ Reduced risk of falling	▪ 3~5 days a week ▪ 2~3 days per week	▪ 2~6 wk
Pharmacotherapy	▪ Estrogen and bisphosphonates : Experience with nausea and diarrhea can also affect exercise programs and motivation.			
Considerations	▪ Aerobic power capability : All forms of exercise should minimize the forward flexion. ▪ Time planning: At least 9 to 12 months is required for long-term preservation of bone mass. ▪ Orthopedic Problems: Patients with severe kyphosis are restricted to stationary bicycles or independent walking. Also, keeping the spine bent for a long time doubles the risk of vertebral fracture. ▪ Heart problems: Most osteoporosis patients are older than 50 years old, and are likely to have CAD. Therefore, prescribers need to closely observe changes in myocardial ischemia. ▪ Muscle Problems: Patients with vertebral fractures are more likely to have weak muscles of lumbar extension muscles, so it is advisable to perform slowly with low intensity to strengthen lumbar extension muscles. ▪ Psychological problems: Provide a safe environment to prevent anxiety and actual falls.			

Lower Back Pain

Symptoms and Features

Lower back pain (LBP) is a common disease that affects about 80% of the world's population. It is not a characteristic term for any disease, but it refers to the pain syndrome in the lower lumbar region, that is, the range from the L2 ending of the spinal nerve to the sacroiliac joint. Lower back pain can be distinguished by precise diagnosing methods such as CT, MRI and neuromuscular test. The types of lesions include sprain of lumbar spine, lumbar herniated intervertebral disc, sciatica, ankylosing spondylitis, spondylolysis, spondylolisthesis, etc. In some cases, there is no specific type.[41] The main symptoms vary depending on the cause. The main symptoms vary depending on the cause, but pain is difficult to move, dull pain and discomfort, and stretching the waist will cause long-lasting symptoms of severe pain.

The causes of back pain are very complex and are related to social, psychological, or physical functions. In general, inappropriate mechanical principles, such as heaviness or heavy exercise, account for more than 98%, and the remaining 2% are caused by tumors, infection, spondylitis, endometriosis or nephrolithiasis in the lumbar region.[30]

Structure and Function of Spine

The spine consists of the body's neck to coccyx. It is a pillar of the human body. The spine is divided into 7 cervical vertebra, 12 thoracic vertebra, 5 lumbar vertebra, 5 sacrum and 3~6 coccyx, which are connected with each other and function as a unit. Among these, the lumbar vertebrae are the largest. It is considered to be developed in order to withstand weight and external stress. Behind the vertebral body there is a hole called the vertebral canal. In the middle of it, there is a tube-like tissue called the dura. Among these tubes, the nerve called the cauda equina floats in the fluid. This cauda equina is divided bilaterally between the vertebral body and the vertebral body, passing through the intervertebral disc and out of the spine [Fig. 5.17]. And this is bundled 4~5, become the sciatic nerve and go to the leg. Because of this nervous control principle, back pain is accompanied by numbness in the legs.

As shown in [Fig. 5.17], the seesaw principle of latissimus dorsi (BS) for upper extremity weight (WT) is applied between lumbar vertebrae 3 and 4. Normal adults have a balance of WT and BS, but adults with lordosis or kyphosis are unbalanced in lumbar slope, causing back and leg pain. This principle applies to everyday life as well. For example, in the case of adults who have a sedentary lifestyle, the structure of the lumbar vertebrae is similar to that of lordosis. On the other hand, the examinee who sit on a lower desk have the same structure as kyphosis, causing disability in daily life [Fig. 5.14].

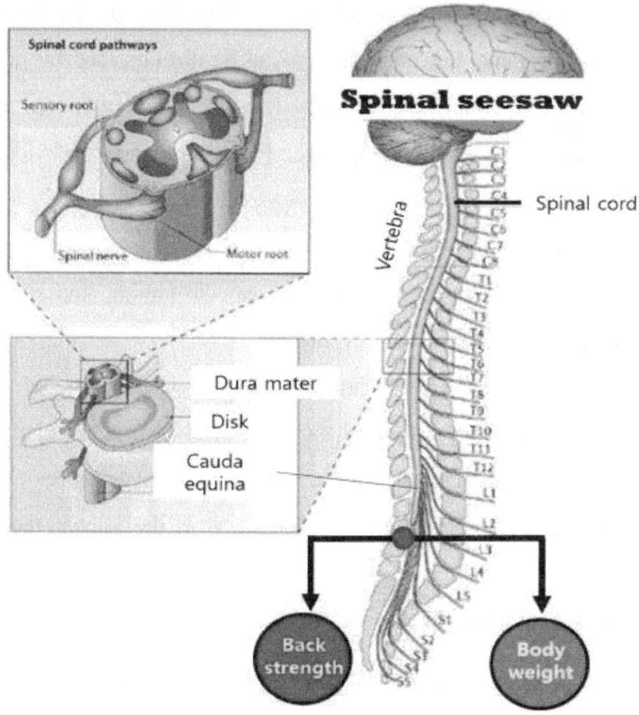

Fig. 5.17 ***Relationship between back strength and body weight***

As shown in [Fig. 5.18], the cartilage of an intervertebral disc is divided into annulus fibrosus and nucleus pulposus. This cartilage contains more than 70% water and overcomes the weight load, provides cushioning action, and responds to the force in all directions to attach the vertebra and vertebra like glue. So, we can think of a soft elephant nose rather than a rigid rod of the spine. The cartilage of the intervertebral disc is the basis for movement and stability of the spinal column. The spinal column, which acts as a pillar of the human body, is not straight like a stick, but curved. The cervical vertebrae and the lumbar vertebrae form an anterior curvature, and the thoracic vertebrae form a curvature in the posterior direction. Overall it is s-shaped. This is a feature only for primates, and there is no curvature for gorillas. There is also no curvature in infants, which is formed when the baby begins to walk.

On the other hand, the third lumbar vertebra is horizontal in standing postures, but the fifth lumbar vertebrae slopes horizontally at 30° and constantly acts as a slipping force, which is very unstable. The disc cartilage and intervertebral joints play an important role in compensating for unstable conditions. In particular, the intervertebral joint located behind the vertebra allows the spinal column to move freely in various directions. However, the lumbar spine can move mainly back and forth due to this joint, and the motion of bending or turning the waist to the side is restricted. The intervertebral joints do not have cushioning like disc cartilage, but are under weight. In the lower lumbar spine, this effect is large, and the load is divided between 3 (intervertebral joints): 7 (disc cartilage). Eventually, the intervertebral joint and intervertebral disc jointly connect the vertebrae to control movement.[89]

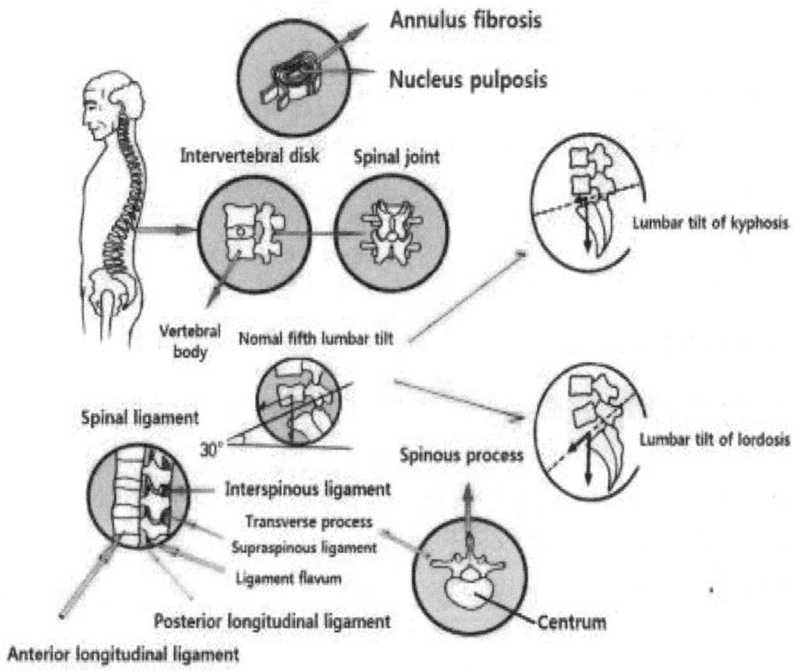

Fig. 5.18 *Spinal Structure and Lumbar Slope*

The spinal ligaments, which are in the shape of a band, are divided into the anterior longitudinal ligament, posterior longitudinal ligament, ligamentum flavum, interspinous ligament, and supraspinous ligament, which are important ligaments connecting the spine and spine. This spinal ligament can be extended up to 1.2 times longer than the circular length, but a stronger breaking action will occur if further extensions occur. Therefore, the ligaments can be said to inspect the range of movement of the spinal column.

As shown in [Fig. 5.19], there are several protuberances in the back of the spine, which are accompanied by small muscles. In the spine, there are several protuberances in the rear, with small muscles attached to it. These muscles are the driving force that moves the spine as desired and stabilize the spinal column by moving the muscles opposite the spinal column simultaneously.

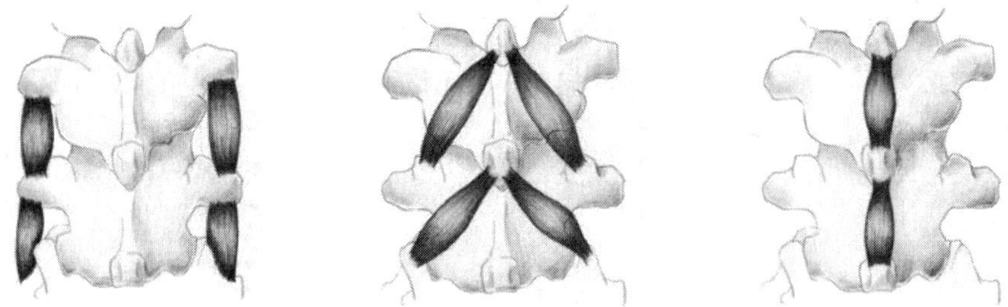

Fig. 5.19 ***Intertransversarii bends the vertebrae outward.***

Transversarii muscle extends the vertebrae laterally. Rotatores rotates the spine to left and right. Interspinales play a role of extending the spine. The origin and insertion of intertransversarii are cervical, lumbar, and thoracic 10th ~ 12th, rotatores muscles stop at the spinous process with all vertebral transversal triggers. Interspinales originate and stop at cervical, lumbar, 1st ~ 2nd thoracic, and 11th ~ 12th thoracic vertebrae.

Spinal Stability

The spinal column removes the muscles and maintains its shape even if the discs, joints, and ligaments are left intact. This is called 'internal stability'. This stability can be tolerated by a weight of about 2 ㎏, but if this load is exceeded, the S-shaped curvature of the spinal column becomes distorted. However, it is possible to stand up even if a much heavier weight is added because the muscles presented above play a role.

Muscles are attached to the spinal column in various directions. This is an important factor in providing 'external stability' that suppresses distortion. The function of the muscles on the spinal column can be considered as an auxiliary rope to build a pole. On the other hand, if weights are applied on the vertebral body connected to the disc cartilage, the disc cartilage will not fracture even if the shape changes temporarily due to the characteristics of the soft tissue, but the vertebral body may be broken. The pressure causing the fracture of the vertebrae is estimated to be about 150 ㎏ for elderly people and about 800 ㎏ for young adults. Therefore, even if external stability is provided by the muscles and the internal stability of the spinal column is maintained, the vertebral body cannot withstand certain loads.

However, the human body acts like a seesaw to maintain balance with whatever weight is placed in front of and behind the body. This is similar to a center line passing a little ahead of the malleolus in the ear canal. At the waist, this center line passes directly in front of the lumbar vertebra. According to one study, the weight load from the waist is said to be 60% of body weight. For example, if a person weighing 70 kg does not stand with the object, it means that 42 kg (70 kg × 60%) of force is always applied to the front of the waist. Therefore, considering the principle of the seesaw, 42 kg of force must be applied to the back of the spine in order to stand straight. The actual measurement of this principle proves that the load on the third lumbar vertebra in the upright state is almost identical to the weight of the person.

On the other hand, if the human body changes posture or takes any action, the load on the lumbar region becomes larger. For example, when the waist is tilted 30° forward, the load on the lumbar vertebrae increases by about three times. In other words, to preserve this posture, it means that the latissimus dorsi needs to use three times as much power. Therefore, when the power of 42 kg (70 kg × 60%) is multiplied by 3, the back lumbar moment of 126 kg is applied to the lumbar spine, and a total load of 168 kg is imposed.

As mentioned above, the spinal column, muscles and ligaments are making endless efforts to maintain stability. However, since the fifth lumbar spine on the sacrum has a slope of about 30° relative to the horizontal, forward sliding force acts on the fifth lumbar spine. For example, when a person weighing 50 kg is standing upright, a sliding force of 25 kg (50 kg × sin 30°) acts on the fifth lumbar vertebra in the vertical direction. Therefore, poor posture increases weight on lumbar lordosis, and the load applied to the intervertebral joint becomes larger, eventually causing back pain.

Posture Correction for Prevention of Lower Back Pain

The importance of proper posture for the human body cannot be overemphasized. In fact, a healthy waist is a state in which you can sit for a long time, be able to stand for a long time, and can bend and stretch your waist freely. A healthy waist can turn into a chronic illness that cannot be rectified due to bad posture. Fortunately, even if you have back pain due to bad posture, correcting it can help prevent and relieve pain significantly.

When Lying Down

Even if you do not have any back pain when you sleep, it is a good idea to change your blanket or bed to a somewhat harder one to minimize the load on your lumbar vertebrae. Also, higher pillows and lean sleep tends to cause back pain due to increased lumbar lordosis. Therefore, you can sleep with your pillow under your knees or with a pillow between your knees, minimizing lumbar lordosis [Fig. 5.20].

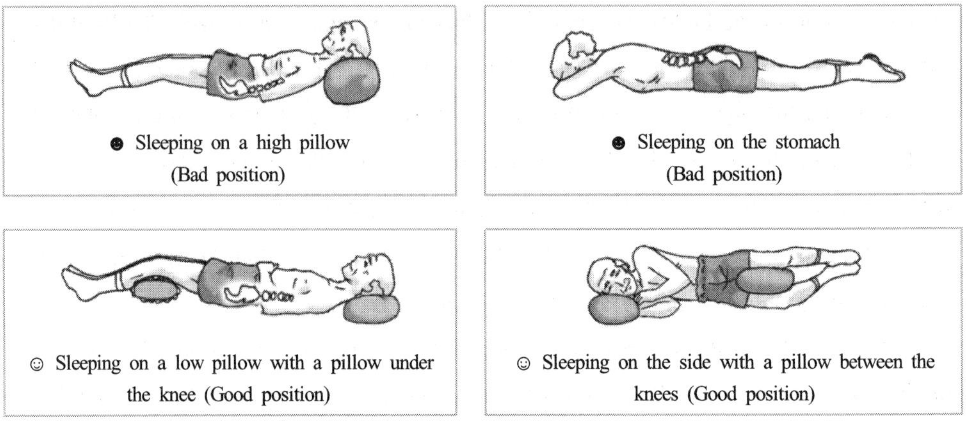

● Sleeping on a high pillow (Bad position)

● Sleeping on the stomach (Bad position)

☺ Sleeping on a low pillow with a pillow under the knee (Good position)

☺ Sleeping on the side with a pillow between the knees (Good position)

Fig. 5.20 ***When Sleeping on the Back***

When Standing

If you stand without your strength, the entire weight of a person weighing about 70 ㎏ will be put on the third lumbar. This can be tolerated by anyone, but when standing for a long time, a sliding force of about 35 ㎏ acts on the fifth lumbar vertebrae, so it is desirable to stand in a good posture as shown in [Fig. 5.20]. Standing bent on the waist increases lumbar lordosis and is bad posture. However, standing with one foot on a 10 ㎝ box or standing wide to increase the base of support leads to relaxation of the iliopsoas muscle that connects the lumbar and leg muscles, reducing the pressure on the lumbar [Fig. 5.21].

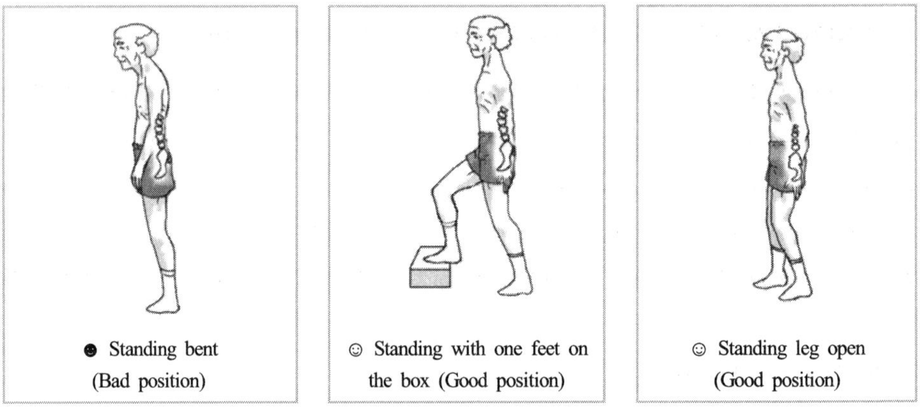

● Standing bent (Bad position)

☺ Standing with one feet on the box (Good position)

☺ Standing leg open (Good position)

Fig. 5.21 ***When Standing***

When Sitting in a Chair

When sitting on a chair without a backrest, about 1.4 times more load is applied to the waist than when standing. This is the same load as the half-bent posture. Therefore, standing rather than sitting on a chair without a back is better for your back. It is also a good idea to sit in a chair with a backrest, sit down with a box under your feet, or alternatively with your legs crossed [Fig. 5.22].

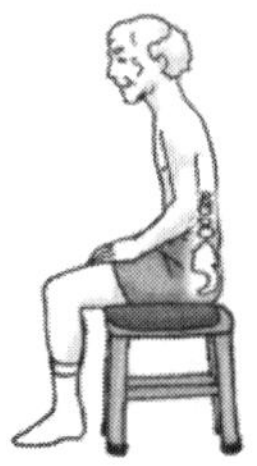

● Sitting on a chair without backrest (Bad position)

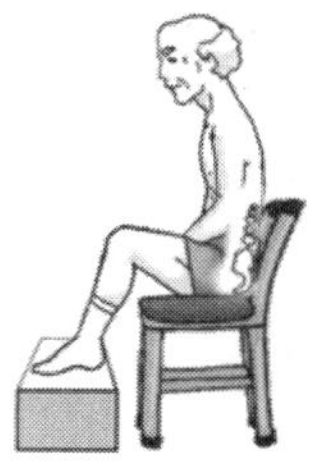

☺ Sitting with the feet on the box (Good position)

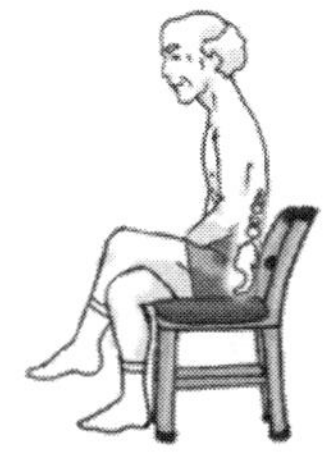

☺ Sitting on a chair with legs crossed alternately (Good position)

Fig. 5.22 *When Sitting on a Chair*

When Sitting on Floor

Sitting crossed-legged on the floor, or with legs straight for a long period of time, increases lumbar lordosis. Therefore, it is better to sit with your back straight or lean against the wall [Fig. 5.23].

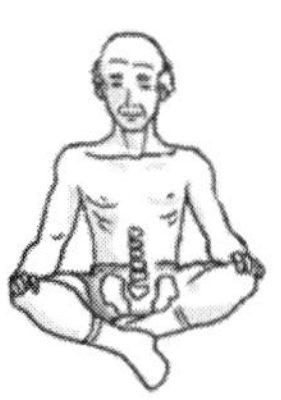

● Sitting crossed-legged (Bad position)

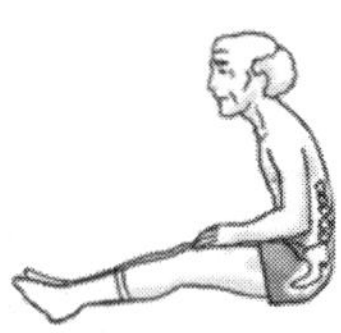

● Sitting with legs straight (Bad position)

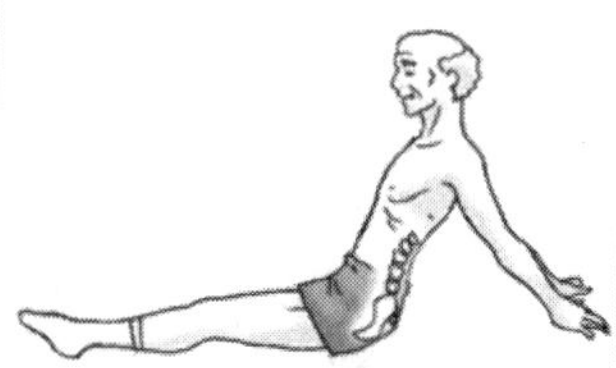

● Sitting back with arms on the floor (Bad position)

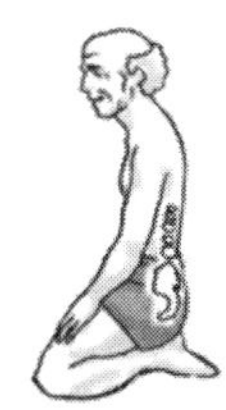

☺ Sitting on knees for a short time (Good position)

Fig. 5.23 *When Sitting on the Floor*

When Carrying Something

If you need to move a bookshelf, pulling the object increases lumbar lordosis and causes back pain. Therefore, as shown in [Fig. 5.24], pushing is less likely to cause back pain because it reduces lumbar lordosis.

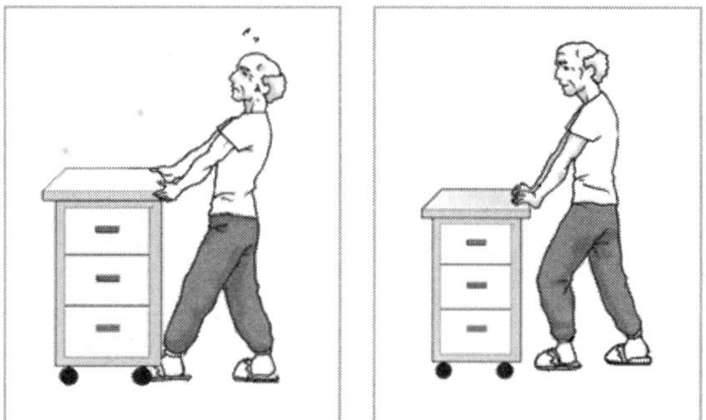

☻ Drawing (Bad position) | ☺ Pushing (Good position)

Fig. 5.24 *When Carrying Something*

When Lifting Something

Even for not-heavy objects, if you lower your arms away from the center of the body, it will increase lumbar lordosis and cause back pain. Therefore, when lifting objects, you should keep it as close to your body as possible to reduce the angle of lumbar lordosis [Fig. 5.25].

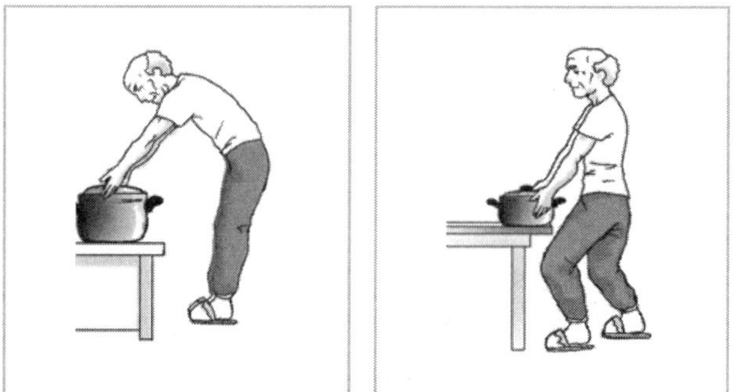

☻ Lifting objects with the back straight (Bad position) | ☺ Lifting objects with the leg bent (Good position)

Fig. 5.25 *When Lifting Something*

When Putting in and Taking out Clothes from a Washing Machine

Washing is an indispensable job in everyday life. Unfortunately, it can cause back pain because you have to bend and stretch your back when putting in or taking out clothes from the washing machine. Therefore, in order to minimize back pain, one leg should be placed in front of the other leg to reduce the load applied to the waist when the waist is bent [Fig. 5.26].

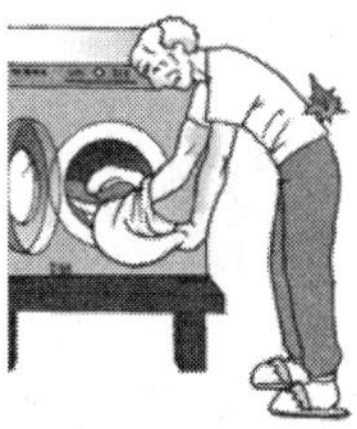

● Taking out laundry with the back muscle (Bad position)

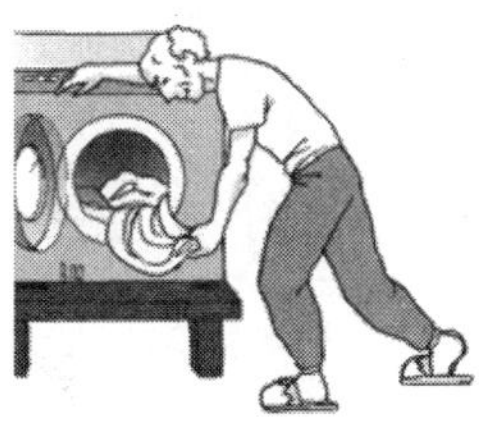

☺ Taking out laundry with the leg muscle (Good position)

Fig. 5.26 *When Putting Clothes in and out of the Washing Machine*

When Putting in and Taking out Something from the Car Trunk

When you put a bag in the trunk of a car or take it out, you have to bend your back, which can cause back pain. Therefore, in order to minimize back pain, placing one's leg on the bumper and taking out the bag will reduce the load on the lumbar [Fig. 5.27].

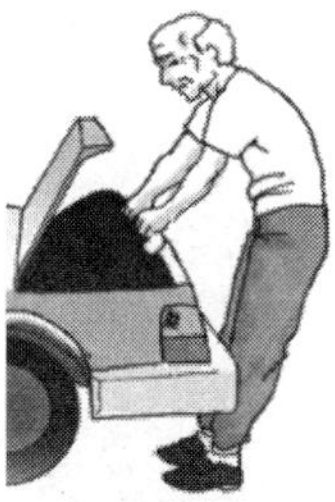

● Taking out a bag with the back straight (Bad position)

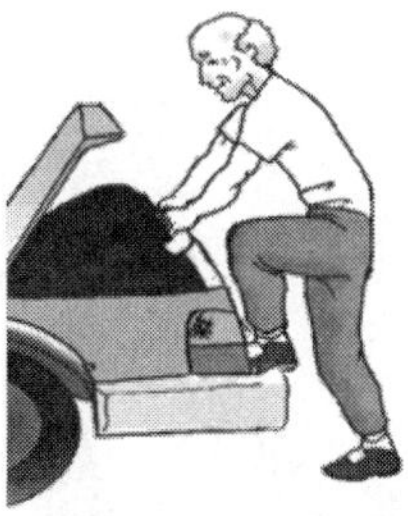

☺ Taking out a bag with bending a leg (Good position)

Fig. 5.27 *When Taking Something out of the Trunk*

When Applying Make Up

When you put on makeup to go out, if you bend your back as you look into the mirror, it is not easy to stand up straight, which can result in back pain. Therefore, do not be in a hurry, straighten your waist, and if the mirror position is low, you can adjust your legs or use a hand mirror [Fig. 5.28].

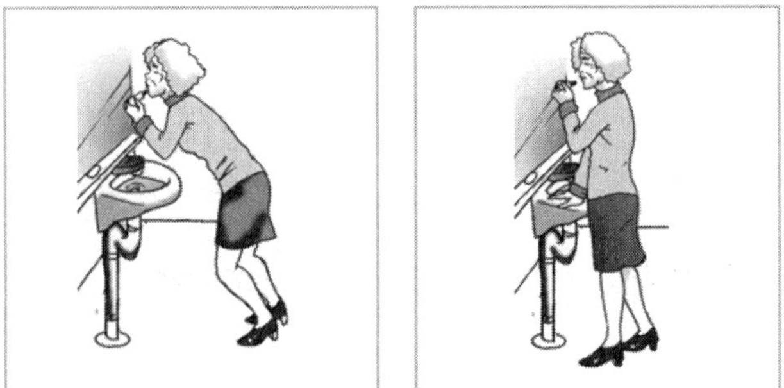

● Bend over and make up (Bad position)

☺ Spread your back and make up (Good position)

Fig. 5.28 ***When Make Up***

Other Bad Posture and Right Posture

Other bad postures that cause back pain are categorized as follows: Sneezing without arm or leg support [Fig. 5.29], changing clothes while standing [Fig. 5.30], sitting on a bed or a chair, stretching your legs and taking off your socks [Fig. 5.31], using excessive force when making bowel movements or holding a bent posture for a long time [Fig. 5.32], showering for a long time with a bent posture [Fig. 5.33], lying in a bath without a base support for the waist [Fig. 5.34].

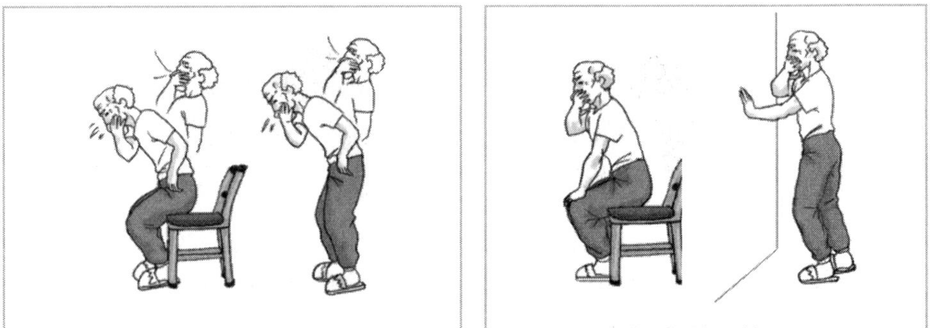

● Bad position

☺ Good position

Fig. 5.29 ***When Sneezing***

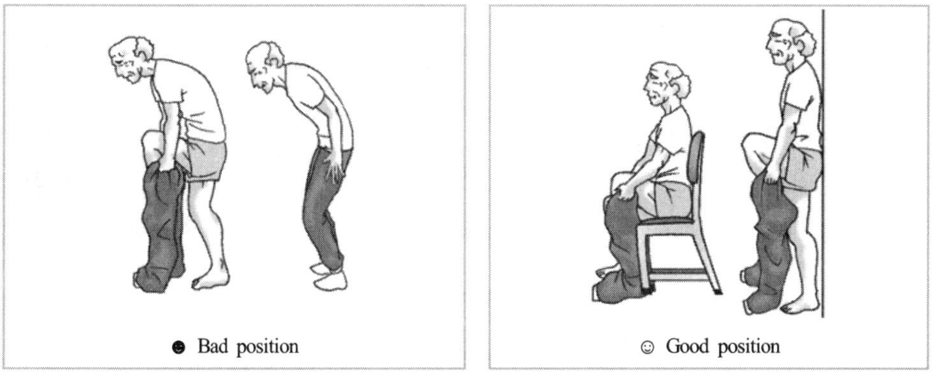

Fig. 5.30 *When Taking off and Putting on Clothes*

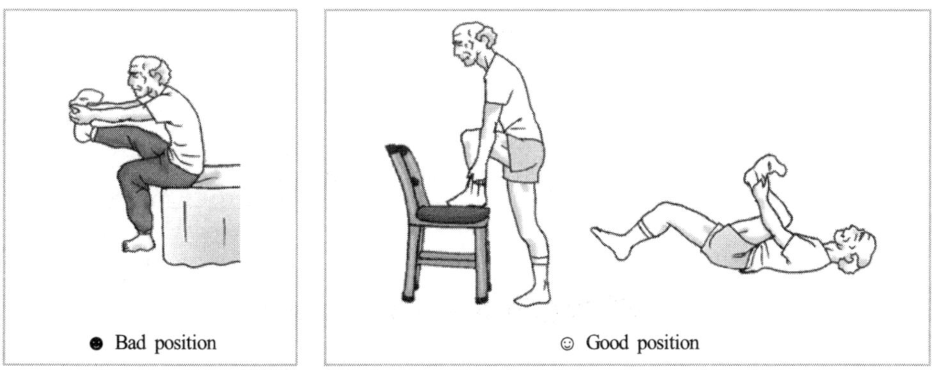

Fig. 5.31 *Putting on and Taking off Socks*

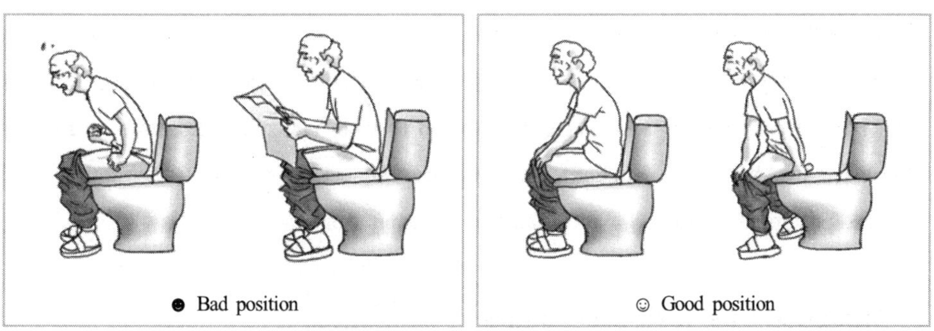

Fig. 5.32 *Sitting on the Toilet*

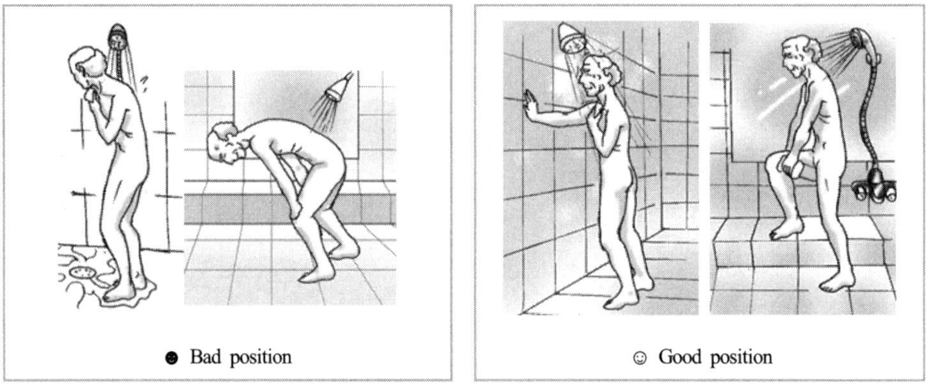

Fig. 5.33 ***When Showering***

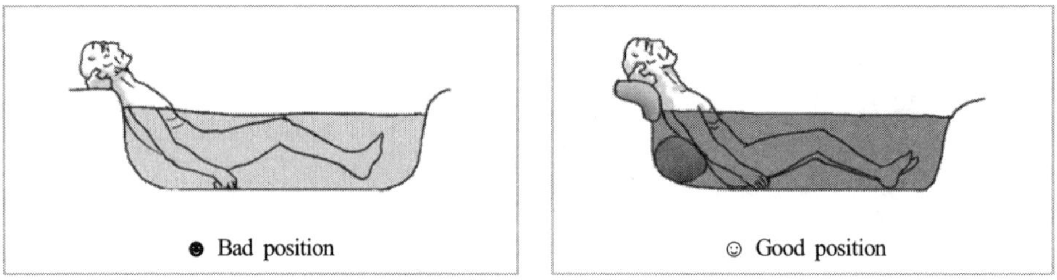

Fig. 5.34 ***When Lying in a Bath***

As described above, our waist appears to be sturdy. However, there is a certain angle between the lumbar spine and the sacrum where the nerves are distributed in several places, so they are very sensitive to small changes and shocks. For anyone who has experienced back pain at least once, it is known that no matter how healthy you may be, the waist can become a handicap since injuries can occur so easily. Therefore, having correct posture is a good way to maintain a strong waist.

Management for Back Pain Patients

Any treatment of back pain can relieve or heal. For example, in the acute phase (within 6 weeks), 80% of patients with back pain can be cured within 8~10 weeks. Patients with neurological symptoms due to the herniation of intervertebral discs can also be cured within about 12 weeks through conservative therapy. However, 1~2% of patients who have not been treated by conservative therapy require surgery.[41] These findings indicate that back pain is likely to recover to normal in a short period of time when treated by appropriate methods.

Guidelines for Rehabilitation Exercise for LBP Patients

The goal of rehabilitation for LBP patients is to reduce the back pain by improving the flexibility of the waist and the tension of the muscles and strengthening the muscles. It is also aimed to calibrate posture, to flex the waist in the correct way, to straighten it, to be able to squat, and to facilitate daily life.

There are two types of exercises for low back pain patients. The first is to relax the muscles passively, such as massaging, and the second is the active way in which the patient stretches or flexes the muscles themselves. Both methods are effective for LBP patients. However, in the case of massages, acute LBP patients have only a short-term effect, and the active method has a long-term effect, although the treatment process is difficult. A massage is basically the application of bare hands to muscles or skin or all tissues between the skin and muscles, and the technique of softly applying pressure and gradually moving in one direction in a rhythmic manner. These techniques may move along the vertebrae, or may be applied in a direction away from the vertebrae, causing the tissue fluid to flow in or out to slowly stretch the tissue. Thus, it is possible to receive a feeling of pain alleviation during the treatment process. Patients who initially start treatment may feel pain due to treatment because the tissue is stimulated by pain. Therefore, massages should be performed smoothly to minimize discomfort and pain. The active method of exercise is the most important method of stretching the muscles and ligaments around the waist of the patients with back pain and properly mixing static muscle strengthening exercises. Also, these exercise methods are safer and more effective when the body temperature is raised. Therefore, during the acute phase of low back pain (1~6 weeks), treatment with cold water for one week reduces the possibility of inflammation. After that, it is advisable to gradually increase the temperature of the waist and then performing light static muscle strengthening exercises. On the other hand, if the patients in the chronic phase (over 12 weeks) can move their legs to some extent, it is better to participate in static muscle strengthening exercises after raising the body temperature using a stationary bicycle.[40] However, increased body temperature due to exercise can increase inflammation in people with back pain, so it is important to minimize inflammation by keeping the area cold before and after exercise. When the muscles of the human body are contracted and relaxed, new blood is supplied smoothly to the tissues and plays a major role in eliminating inflammation. In addition, muscle contraction and relaxation are necessary to move body fluids into inflamed tissues. Ultimately, pain after treatment is relieved and muscles are fully stretched to improve the ROM in the waist.

Types of LBP Exercise Therapy

The waist should be flexible and sturdy enough to bend, stretch, twist, and move smoothly. Therefore, exercise methods that can meet this purpose have been made by many clinicians in the past. McKenzie movement and Williams movement are recognized forms of exercise.

❶ Lying Prone

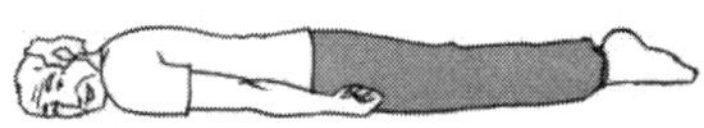

▪ Put your left face on the floor and lay down for five minutes. Face the other side and do the same 6 to 8 times.

❷ Progress to Elbows

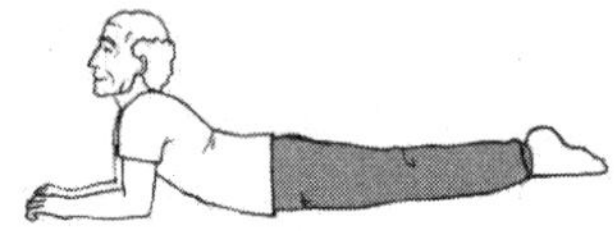

▪ Perform 2~3 minutes (to orient the nucleus pulposus in the disc toward the abdomen).

❸ Full Press Up

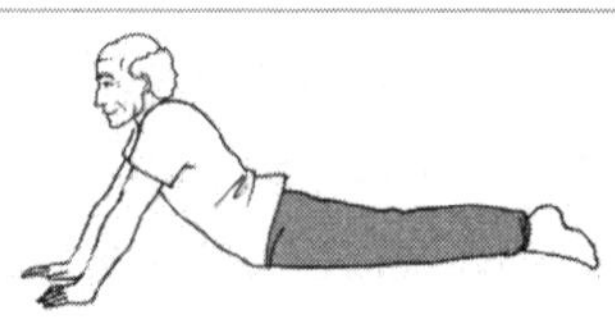

▪ If you feel that you are maximally stretched, stop and fix for 2 to 5 seconds. Repeat twice.

❹ Knees to Chest Lying Supine

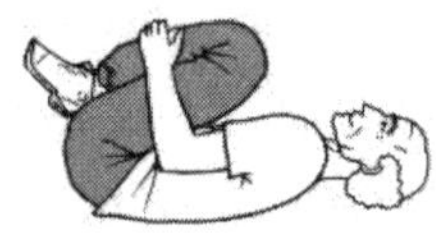

▪ Put knees on the chest and stop for 3 seconds. Repeat four times.

❺ Flex with Hands Beneath Seat

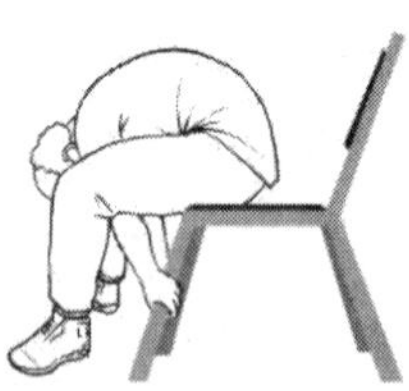

▪ Breathing in a relaxed posture, hold the chair leg and stop for 3 seconds. Repeated twice.

❻ Spread the Back and Lift Leg

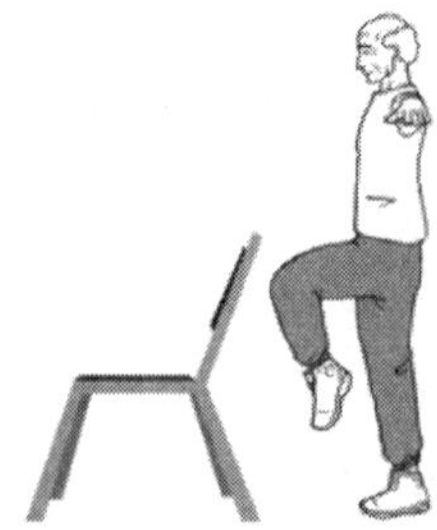

▪ (Application of McKenzie exercises) Stand up from a chair, spread the back and stop for 3 seconds. Then hold a leg for 2 seconds to stop.

Fig. 5.35 McKenzie Lumbar Extension Exercises

McKenzie Extension Exercise

As shown in [Fig. 5.35], the McKenzie exercise can strengthen back muscles, stretch soft tissues, and restore lumbar lordosis. It is effective for patients with disc herniation, but it is preferable to avoid patients with spinal stenosis, spondylolysis, and spondylolisthesis. In the case of acute abdominal pain, only ①, ②③, ② should be performed. If the pain has decreased to some extent after several days, perform ① to ⑥.

In order to prevent recurrence after disc surgery, figures ③ and ⑤ should be regularly performed every day, and ⑥ can develop balance and lower limb muscles by applying motion with the goal of 10 reps a day for 10 seconds each.

Williams Flexion Exercise

As shown in [Fig. 5.36], Williams' lumbar flexion exercises are effective for patients with spinal stenosis, spondylolysis, and spondylolisthesis because they strengthen abdominal muscles, stretch lumbar muscles and soft tissues, and widen the intervertebral foramen and articular process.

❶ Abdominal Strengthening Exercise

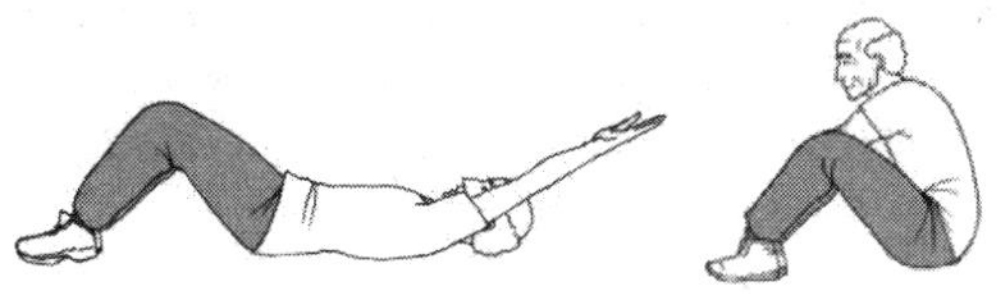

▪ Try to reach the knees and ankles with both hands. Repeat 3 sets of 15 reps.

❷ Gluteus Maximus Strengthening Exercise

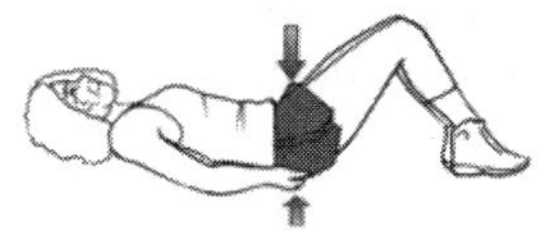

▪ Press the floor with hips. Stop for 10 sec. Repeat 3 times.

❸ Waist Strengthening Exercise

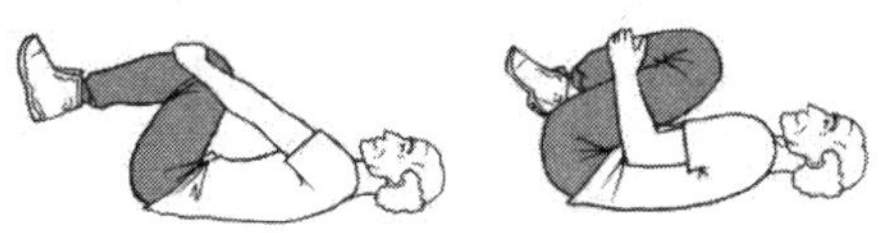

▪ Attach both knees to the chest while breathing. Repeat 3 sets of 15 reps.

❹ Waist and Hamstring Stretch

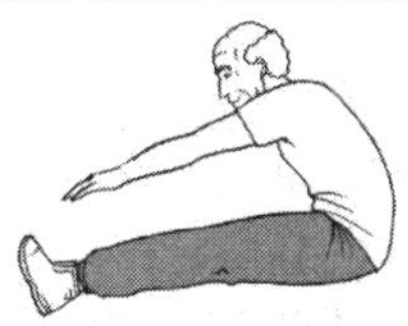

▪ Try to reach the feet with both hands. Repeat 3 sets of holding 10 sec.

❺ Hip Joint/Lower Limb Stretch

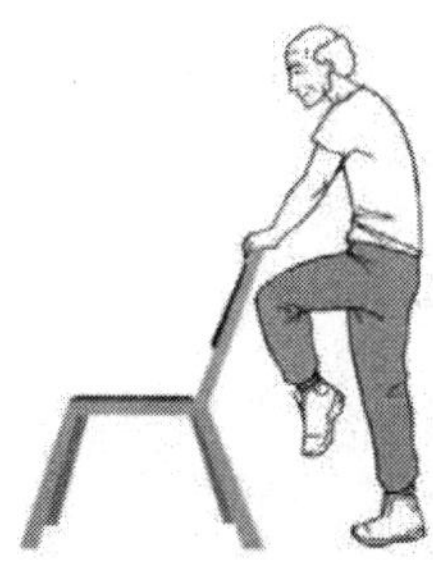

▪ Hold the chair and attach one leg to the chest. Repeat 3 sets of 5 reps.

❻ Waist/Lower Limb Exercise

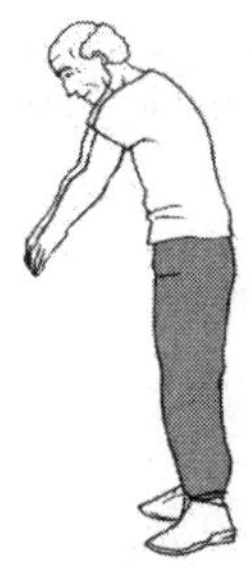

▪ Stand up and sit down in a bent posture. Repeat 3 sets of 5 reps (application of Williams exercises for stability problem).

Fig. 5.36* *Williams Lumbar Flexion Exercises

❶ Stretching

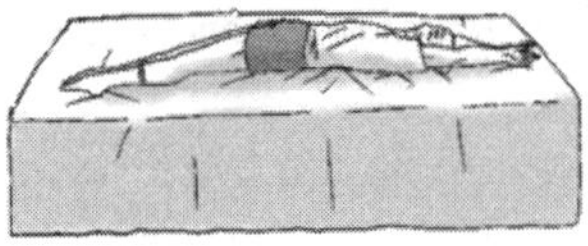

- Keep stretching in relaxed position and holding for 10 seconds. Repeat 2 times.

❷ Attaching One Leg to the Chest

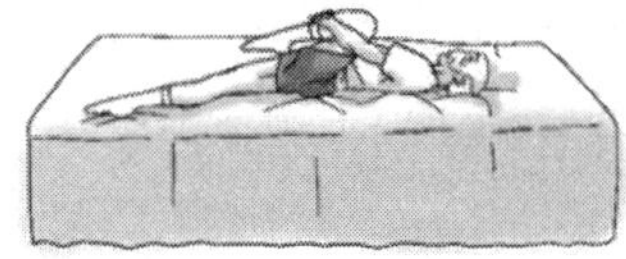

- The right leg is stretched, and the left leg is attached to the chest and held for 10 seconds. Change the legs and repeat each 2 times.

❸ Attaching to Both Legs

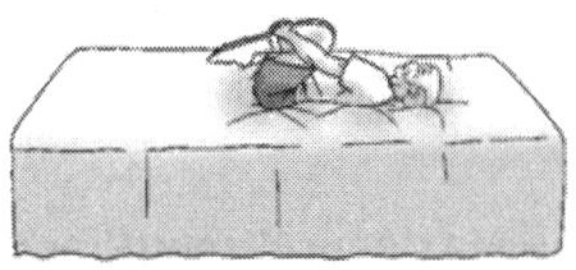

- Hold both legs to chest for 10 seconds. Breathing is natural and repeats twice. Try to attach the nose to the knees when want to improve more.

❹ Cross Legs to Chest

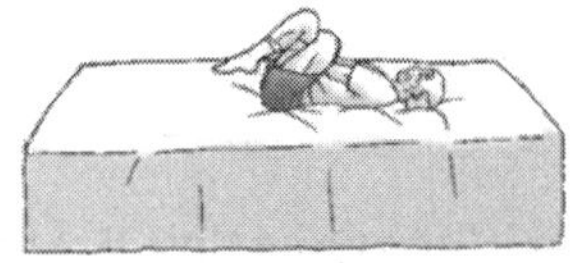

- The left leg is overlaid on the right leg, and both hands are put in and out of the thigh, holding the pod and holding the knee. Put your right leg on your chest with both hands. Repeat 2 times every 10 seconds.

❺ Static Abdominal Exercise

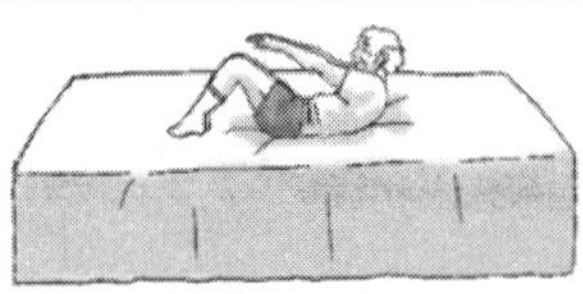

- Try to put the hands on the knees and give strength to the belly. Keep for 15 seconds and repeat 2 times.

❻ Waist Up

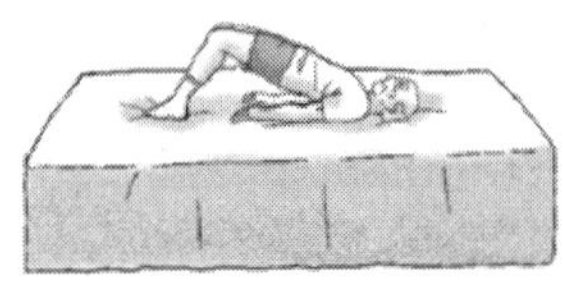

- Hold the waist toward the ceiling and stop for 15 seconds. At this time, respiration maintains exhalation state. Repeat 2 times.

❼ Relax the Pelvis on the Corner

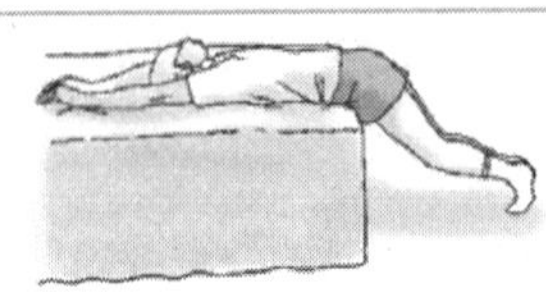

- Spread the pelvis on the edge of the bed and rest for 5 to 10 minutes. At this time, the two legs are completely relaxed.

❽ Lift One Leg

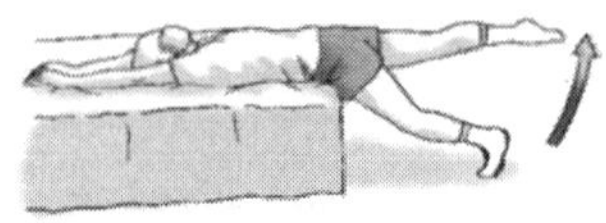

- Lift one leg and stop for 10 seconds. The opposite leg is carried out in the same manner and repeated twice.

❾ Lift Both Legs

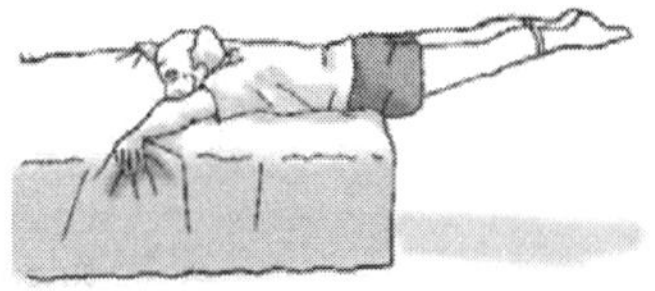

- Grab the corner of the bed with both hands, lift both legs, hold for 5 to 10 seconds, and repeat twice.

❿ Ice Pack Lumbar

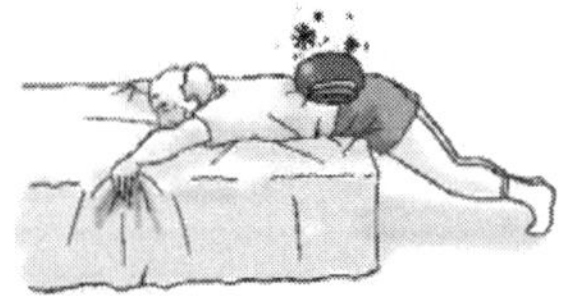

- After all the work is done, put the ice bag on a thin towel and put it on the waist for 10 minutes.

Fig. 5.37 *Home exercise for LBP*

In [Fig. 5.36], ⑤ operation can be done sitting on the floor, but it is safe to stand in order to reduce the burden. The six movements of Williams' flexion movements are repeated two or three times a day, and it is good to put a pad with a cushion on the floor. It is recommended that the number of actions be repeated 5 times for each item. However, patients with severe back pain should first consult an expert. After performing the two waist exercises mentioned above, aggressive exercise using a specific Lumbar Extension machine should be applied to strengthen the muscles and ligaments around the waist so that it can be effective in preventing recurrence later.

Home Exercise for LBP

This method of exercise is called Bed Exercise. Stretching exercises and muscular strengthening exercises to improve the flexibility of the lumbar and abdominal muscles are the main focus of this program. The low back exercises shown in [Fig. 5.37] can easily be carried out on a bed or a desk, and have been proven to be suitable for the elderly and the weak. Ultimately, the prescribing practitioner needs to know the test methods of LBP patients presented in [Table 5.68], the medicine to be administered, and the special considerations before giving the details of the method to the patient. The specific management program is shown in [Table 5.69].[3,5,22,25,88,89]

Table 5.68 ***Exercise test, drug, and specific considerations for LBP Patients***

Test Item	Measurement items	Recommended Stopping Point	Remarks
Aerobic Power Ability			▪ Only when there are signs and risks of CAD.
Myofunction	▪ Isokinetic lumbar test	▪ Myofunction curve ▪ Ratio of extension / flexion	▪ Review of lumbar motion and peak torque. ▪ Sudden motion causes pain.
Flexibility	▪ Sit-and-reach ▪ Stretching the bridge		
Considerations	▪ During the first four weeks of symptoms of back pain, the test is not helpful. ▪ Exercises that impact such as running should be avoided.		

Table 5.69 ***Management program for LBP Patients***

	Type	Goal	Intensity/Frequency/Time	Period
Strength Exercise	■ Sit-up ■ Back muscle extension	■ Strength development of body including lumbar	■ Less than 50 years old: 10 to 15 reps / days ■ 50 years or older: 8 to 12 reps / more than 2 days per week	■ 2~4 week
Flexibility Exercise	■ Standardized flexibility exercises without causing LBP	■ ROM increase in body and hip flexor and extensor muscles	■ Two minutes per muscle ■ Maintain one motion for 3 reps (10 seconds stretch)	
Function Exercise	■ 5 min walking ■ Sit in a chair for one min Stand up	■ Increase the flexibility of the body	■ Brisk walk 3~5 days / week ■ Sit at the chair, stand up, 2~3 days / week	
Considerations	■ The high-impact movement is skipped. ■ It is advisable to start low-load aerobic activity safely for the first two weeks after back pain and to initiate fuselage at least two weeks later.			

Cancer

Overweight and obesity are increasing worldwide. The increase in such patients was easily found in advanced countries, but has recently been increasing in Asian and developing countries, including Korea. It is a common opinion among scholars that the cause of the increase in these patients is derived from an unhealthy lifestyle and a high-calorie diet. Moreover, some scholars argue that being overweight and the lack of exercise cause Type 2 diabetes, hypertension, hyperlipidemia, stroke, and cancer, including heart disease.

The World Health Organization's International Agency for Cancer on Research reports that obesity and lack of exercise increase colon cancer, breast cancer, uterine cancer, kidney cancer, and esophageal cancer in women after menopause. When the BMI is between 23 and 30 ㎏/㎡, the risk of colon cancer is higher in women by about 1.25 times and in men by about 1.5 times. When the BMI was over 24 ㎏/㎡, women who did not receive hormone treatment had a significantly increased incidence of breast cancer. However, the relationship between BMI and rectal cancer and prostate cancer has not yet been established.

Table 5.70 BMI Evaluation (㎏/㎡)

Category	Male	Female
Normal	24~27	23~26
Overweight	28~31	27~32
Obesity	More than 32	More than 33

On the other hand, uterine cancer is highly prevalent in all women before and after menopause with a BMI of 25 ㎏/㎡ or more. Renal cancer is two to three times as high in both men and women with a BMI greater than 30 ㎏/㎡. However, the relationship between weight and cancers such as the thyroid gland, ovaries, testis, liver, pancreas, gallbladder, and lungs has not yet been concluded.

Relationship among Cancer, Physical Activity, and Being Overweight

Recently, many researchers have reported that regular exercise reduces the risk of colon cancer by about 40% through epidemiological surveys. It is reported that the effect is increased by raising exercise intensity, exercise frequency, or exercise time. In other words, exercising more than 30~60 minutes per day produces a more positive effect. Particularly, the risk factors for breast cancer are reduced 20~40% when participating in physical activity regardless of menopausal state, exercise form, and exercise intensity.

So, for what reasons do regular exercise have a positive effect on many cancer risk factors? This may be related to the mechanism by which physical activity affects the colon, breasts, and uterine. Prostate cancers prevent weight gain and reduce overweight and obesity that can occur after menopause. The International Agency for Cancer on Research has measured the effects of being overweight and physical inactivity to demonstrate common cancer induction processes. Results have shown that 11% of colon cancer was due to high BMI and 13~14% was due to low physical activity. In particular, after menopause, about 10% of breast cancers were caused by being overweight, while the other 10% were caused by physical inactivity. However, uterine cancer, renal cancer, and esophageal cancer were not associated with the lack of exercise. Only BMI was accountable for 39% (uterine cancer), 25% (kidney cancer), and 37% (esophageal cancer), respectively. Ultimately, obesity and lack of exercise can be said to be related to various types of cancer, as shown in [Fig. 5.38].

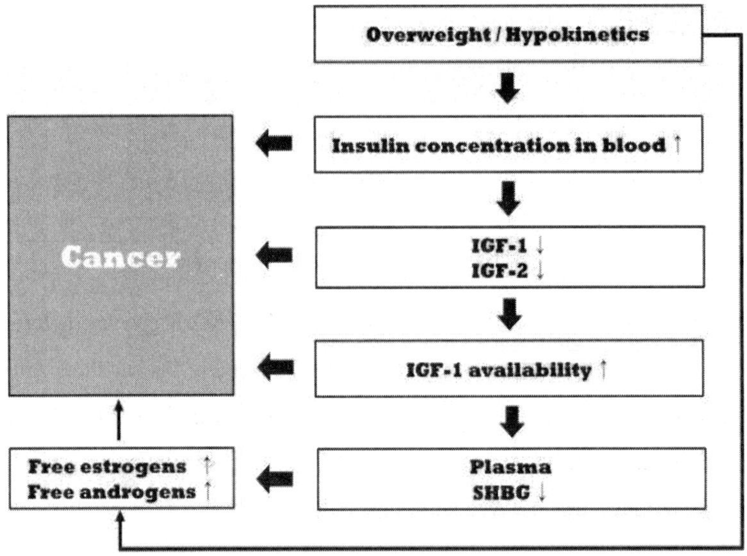

Fig. 5.38 *Mechanism of Pathogenesis of Cancer*

As shown in [Fig. 5.38], overweight or obesity and lack of exercise cause insulin resistance and chronic hyperinsulinemia. This can lead to cancer, and if it persists, it can also cause cancer by decreasing IGF-1 (insulin like growth factor) and IGF-2. Decreases in IGF-1 and IGF-2 can lead to cancer by increasing IGF-1 in the blood and decreasing sex hormone binding globulin (SHBP), thereby increasing estrogen and androgen. Increased blood estrogen levels are associated with breast and uterine cancer in postmenopausal women. Increased blood androgen is thought to be associated with a lack of intrauterine progesterone in premenopausal women.[30]

Recommendations to Reduce Cancer Risk

In recent years, efforts to reduce the risk of cancer have been increasing epidemiologically and experimentally, and these studies report that weight control and physical activity have a very beneficial effect. As mentioned above, regular exercise can reduce insulin levels, sex hormones, and the activity of IGF-1.[30] In this regard, the International Agency for Cancer on Research recommends that it is desirable to maintain a healthy life at a young age. Furthermore, it is recommended that the BMI be maintained in the range of 18.5~25 kg/m^2 and that the weight of for adults should not be increased by more than 5 kg. Particularly, in the case of overweight or obese patients, it is desirable to avoid additional weight gain first and then to reduce weight by 5~10%. Ultimately, this can easily be achieved by walking or quick pacing an hour or so a day.

Exercise and Cautions for Cancer Patients

There are many types of exercises that can be very beneficial for cancer patients. Many cancer patients who could benefit from physical activity or exercise were told by some experts that they should be "stable" or "relaxed." Proper exercise can develop or maintain the functional capacity of the human body, while inactivity can result in fatigue and frailty. Of course, it is not easy for cancer patients to exercise. However, like normal people, cancer patients are at risk of complications such as heart disease, diabetes, hypertension, and back pain. As a result, psychological depression or poor quality of life are added to the bad conditions. Therefore, cancer patients must exercise, and after exercising regularly, there should be positive physical and mental changes. The cancer patient must exercise and believe that he or she can change mentally or physically.

Considerations before Exercise

Regular exercise can improve functional capacity and improve the quality of life for cancer patients, but most importantly, it is "stability assurance". This stability is achieved by examining the medical and functional status of each patient, including the type and management of cancer. Also, patients receiving medication or chemotherapy should observe the response of the treatment and progress of the disease during the period of participating in the exercise program. [Table 5.71] shows the details of pre-exercise considerations.

Table 5.71 ***Pre-exercise considerations for cancer patients***

- Daily activity or exercise performance status
- Presence for other diseases other than tumor (i.e., cardiovascular disease, pulmonary disease and diabetes)
- Cancer status (type, degree, location, metastasis position, and degree of malignancy
- Complications from tumors or metastatic sites
- Actual or potential complications from treatment type and treatment

Table 5.72 ***Zubrod and Karnofsky scale: exercise performance classification***

Activities and Symptoms	Zubrod	Karnofsky
■ Normal activity possible and no limitations	0	90~100%
■ Have symptoms but can walk, can participate in self-care	1	70~80%
■ You can walk more than 50% and need help from an occupational therapist	2	50~60%
■ Walking less than 50%, requiring nursing care	3	30~40%
■ Admission is required for stable bed	4	10~20%

The ability of cancer patients to participate in exercise programs should be assessed in detail. These assessments should primarily be designed to assess exercise performance based on functional abilities. Among the many evaluation forms, scale maps developed by Zubrod and Karnofsky are mainly used [Table 5.72].

Exercise Intensity and Time

Standardized aerobic exercise is recommended only for patients with a Zubrod scale of 0~1 or a Karnofsky scale of 70~100%. In other words, patients who have full functional ability, or who have had a very active lifestyle prior to diagnosis, need to be encouraged to maintain their form of exercise that they are enjoying. On the other hand, an exercise program that can start in a short time is effective for patients with some functional impairment whose Zubrod scale is 2 (50~60% of Karnofsky scale). For example, repeating 5 minutes / 10 minutes of rest two or three times a day is a way to reinforce their physical strength. At this point, the goal of exercise is to increase the exercise time so that the patient can walk for 30 minutes without dyspnea. This limited exercise program is particularly good at preventing adverse effects due to rest and preventing exercise performance from falling. Furthermore, even in patients with two levels of a Zubrod scale, in the presence of supervision and observation of clinical exercise prescribers, they can also participate in high-stakes programs, which are 60~75% of their maximum heart rate.[30] However, exercise prescribers must make sure that these patients are provided with detailed information on the patient's tumor course, special cautions, and therapeutic effects, before engaging in training.

Type of Exercise

The most important thing in prescribing the type of exercise is to first determine the stability before selecting the items that the patient likes and is comfortable with. The presence or absence of stability needs to be verified in detail through the regular blood test (CBC75)) in [Table 5.73]. For patients with low platelet counts or bone metastases, it is desirable to avoid exercise items such as rope skipping, jogging, or running because they can lead to hemorrhagic arthropathy or stress fractures (see Table 5.73). Physical injuries such as fatigue fractures and shin splints76) may be positive on radiologic examination, and metastatic bone tumor may also be mistaken for injuries.[30] Therefore,

75) CBC: complete blood count.

76) Shin splint: Stiffness in the front of the shins when running on a hard surface or running suddenly.

active patients who are at risk for metastatic bone tumor or fatigue fractures should choose low intensity activities such as a cycle ergometer or arm ergometer to reduce the likelihood of fatigue fractures.

Table 5.73 ***Limitations of exercise based on CBC***

- White blood cell : 3,000 cells/㎣ or less
- Absolute granulocyte count: 2,500 cells/㎣ or less
  - Pay attention to infection. Avoid places with a lot of people in particular.
  - The risk of infection should be minimized by avoiding swimming pools, etc.
- Platelets: 50,000 cells/㎣ or less
  - Limit activity due to the risk of bleeding.
- Hemoglobin: less than 10 g/dl.
  - Avoid severe activities.

Exercise Prescription for Cancer Patients

The walking is the most convenient and effective means of maintaining their daily lives for the cancer patients not included in exercise contraindication. It is recommended for patients who have never had any exercise experience. The cycle ergometer is also one of the preferred training methods. The feature of bicycle riding is that it can be carried out in a small space, affordable, convenient, and has the advantage of being able to control the intensity of exercise accurately.

Exercise intensity is a very important factor for cancer patients. The setting of this exercise intensity should be prescribed between the "effective limit" to get an effect on the stimulus of exercise and the "safety limit" to prevent injury. Generally, the limit of exercise intensity for cancer patients is differentiated according to physical fitness levels, age, sex, and mobility, but it is usually desirable to set it between 40~70% of the maximum limit (maximal heart rate or $\dot{V}O_2max$). In other words, 40% of exercise intensity refers to the effective limit and 70% refers to the safety limit. This represents the target heart rate zone. These "limit" points are routinely based on heart rate, but heart rate during exercise, calculated from actual or predicted maximal heart rate, can be affected by the two causes listed below.

First, the resting heart rate of cancer patients tends to be higher than that of normal people.
Second, the ability of the cancer patients to metabolize aerobic is generally low.

The above two points can be expressed by changing the maximum metabolic equivalent (METmax) to 3~5 METs in patients with cancer of the foot, which refers to the amount of activity that patients can walk on level ground or walk more quickly. The heart rate formula for determining exercise intensity is calculated as {(220 - age) - rest heart rate} × exercise intensity (40~70%) + rest heart rate. For example, in a 50-year-old cancer patient with a rest heart rate of 90 bpm and a maximum heart rate of 170 bpm (220 - age), the target heart rate range is (170 to 90) × (0.4 to 0.7) + 90 = 122~146 bpm.

Table 5.74 ***Contraindications during exercise for cancer patients***

- If you have skeletal system or back pain before exercise
- Sudden breathing difficulty
- If you received intravenous chemotherapy before 24 hours
- If you have an irrigation drug before exercise
- If you have nausea during exercise
- If you have nausea or vomiting before 24~36 hours
- If you experience fatigue that you have not experienced
- If you have inflammatory disease
- If you have cachexia

Patients without metabolic abnormalities or those without cardiopulmonary disease can lead to functional improvement by prescribing their heart rate at 60~85% of their maximum heart rate. At this time, it is good to use the intermittent method of motion form. In other words, high and low rates of exercise intensity are favored by patients who are functionally restricted or easily fatigued. After that, patients whose functional abilities are 1~2 on the Zubrod scale can walk without rest for 20 minutes during the first exercise period and not show fatigue, stiffness, or pain after exercise. However, it is advisable to stop the exercise if symptoms such as those listed in [Table 5.74] appear during exercise.

Patients who have lost physical strength after surgery or who have been receiving long-term hard-wired therapy (1~2 of Zubrod scale) can help improve their aerobic capacity by cycling or walking. However, these patients should not exercise more than 60% of the exercise intensity using heart rate, and it is beneficial to repeat the method of walking and resting for a short period. If the exercise intensity is low or the exercise time is too short, it is effective to prescribe the exercise amount again. Patients with a 2~3 of Zubrod scale are recommended to walk several times a day for 5~10 minutes, but if exercise endurance is improved, exercise time should be increased to 30~60 minutes.

Many people with fragile cancer know that tiredness and frailty can be triggered without warning in advance. For patients with a 2~3 of Zubrod scale, try to assess how far they can walk without getting tired to find the point of triggering fatigue or weakness. Then have them sit on the chair and rest until fatigue is restored, and then have them walk again as soon as they recover. The purpose of these activities is to ensure that the walking is completed smoothly without reaching the exhaustion point. This can be done several times a day to prevent or alleviate various complications resulting from long-term bed rest. If the disease process is gradual, the goal of exercise is to ensure that the patient's endurance does not decline.

Table 5.75 ***Exercise test, drug, and specific considerations for cancer patients***

	Test Item	Measurement	Recommended Stopping Point	Remarks
Aerobic Power Ability	■ Walking on a treadmill (1~2 Mets / step) ■ Bicycles ① Ramp Protocol 17W / min ② 25~50W / 3 min ■ Walk for 6 minutes	■ 12 lead ECG ■ HR	■ Maximum oxygen uptake / uniformity ■ Severe arrhythmia ■ > 2 ㎜ ST segment fall / rise ■ Ischemic threshold ■ T-wave inversion with ST change	■ Most cancer patients have decreased aerobic capacity.
		■ BP	■ SBP/DBP >250/115 ㎜Hg ■ When hypertension or hypotensive response time	
		■ RPE	■ Time to stop voluntarily	
Myofunction	■ Isotonic ■ Isokinetic	■ 1RM or 3RM ■ Peak torque		■ Atrophy and weakness.
Flexibility	■ Goniometer ■ Sit-and-reach		■ Flexion / Extension angle ■ Distance	■ Measurement of upper limb ROM in patients with mastectomy.
Functional Ability	■ Activities of daily living (ADL) ■ Sit up Stand up ■ Stair climbing	■ Speed ■ Time ■ Number of repetitions		■ Observation of nerve abnormalities after chemotherapy (including radiation).
Pharmacotherapy	■ Radiation : Causes cardiomyopathy and may promote atherosclerosis. ■ Bleomycin : May cause lung fibrosis. ■ Vincristine : May cause limb neuropathy. ■ Daunorubicin : May cause cardiomyopathy.			
Considerations	■ Peripheral and limb amputation require special orthopedic devices and may lead to bone disease in the remaining bone. ■ If cancer patients have CAD-related complications, see How to Manage Myocardial Infarction and CAD.			

Table 5.76 ***Management program for cancer patients***

	Type	Goal	Intensity/Frequency/Time	Period
Aerobic Exercise	▪ Biking ▪ Walking ▪ Swimming	▪ Increase and maintain maximum oxygen uptake / power / endurance ▪ Decrease in Zubrod scales ▪ Increase of Karnofsky scale	▪ 40~60% of HRR ▪ 3 to 5 days a week ▪ 20 to 60 minutes / once exercise (intermittently deformed when fatigue soaring)	▪ 12 month+
Strength Exercise	▪ Circuit training ▪ Gym exercises	▪ Increased strength and muscle endurance	▪ 1RM 40~60% ▪ 20 to 30 min a week 2~3 days ▪ Repeat 3 to 5 reps / 1 to 3 sets (aiming at 8 to 15 reps) ▪ RPE 11~13	▪ 12 month+
Flexibility Exercise	▪ Stretching ▪ Chair Gymnastics	▪ Increase and Maintain ROM	▪ 20 to 30 seconds stretching ▪ Repeat 2 to 4 reps per stretch ▪ 5 to 7 days a week	▪ 6~12 weeks
Neuromuscular Exercise	▪ Walking ▪ Balance movement	▪ Improvement of walking, balance, coordination ability		
Functional Exercise	▪ Increase of activities of daily living (ADL)	▪ Increase ADL ▪ Return to work ▪ Improving the QoL	▪ Daily	
Pharmacotherapy	▪ See Pharmacotherapy during testing			
Considerations	▪ Setting Intensity, Time, and Frequency is not easy. The reason for this is that the prior information is insufficient, and the type of cancer and the condition of each patient are extremely changed, making it difficult to provide such a form. However, some cancer patients (colon cancer, prostate cancer, breast cancer, etc.) have experienced the benefits of postoperative recovery. Although there are not many, there are some proven results in some previous studies, so it is desirable to actively participate in exercise programs with hope.			

Occasionally, the therapeutic range makes patients unable to tolerate several days, but they recover quickly after the treatment process is over. These patients also undergo positive changes, starting at 3 and falling from 2 to 1, on the Zubrod scale. The goal of this period of exercise is to prevent the decline in physical and mental fitness through chemotherapy and active rehabilitation therapy. The speed of the walking program for patients with a 0~2 of Zubrod scale can be increased until the heart rate reaches approximately 80% of the maximum heart rate during exercise. Younger cancer patients not included in exercise contraindication may progress to a walking-jogging program at this point. For intermittent bicycle programs, workload can be increased by 12.5 watts. A program that keeps the lower speed and the pedaling speed faster, increases the time spent on exercise, making the legs feel less tired. However, this condition only allows patients with a 0~1 of Zubrod scale to increase the pedaling speed or increase the load only if the exercise intensity does not reach 75~85%. However, increasing the pedaling speed and exercise load at the same time should not be allowed.[30]

It is desirable to reduce the exercise program somewhat after difficult treatment or infection treatment. To avoid excessive exercise during recovery, the statement 'Too much is as bad as too little' should be recalled. If the patient participates in the original exercise program again, keep the exercise less than 1 week before stopping exercise, and monitor their heart rate more closely. If the heart rate exceeds 75% of their maximum heart rate, lower their effort level. If their heart rate is between 60 and 75%, they should maintain at least twice that amount before increase the workout.

Ultimately, as shown in [Table 5.75], exercise prescribers should be familiar with the exercise test methods for cancer patients, medications being prescribed, and special considerations. It is necessary to give this information to the patient in detail. The specific management program is shown in [Table 5.76].[3,5,22,83,88,92]

Stroke and Brain Injury

Pathophysiology of Stroke and Brain Injury

Stroke refers to local neurological deficits caused by abnormalities in the cerebral blood flow. It occurs when the blood flow in a specific brain area is blocked, causing the function of the brain to decrease rapidly for 24 hours or until just before death. Stroke, on the other hand, is a term for symptoms. It is sometimes referred to as a cerebrovascular accident (CVA) or cerebrovascular stoke (CVS) when it is referred to as a medical illness. Though often called paralysis, the term paralysis is a broad expression.

Eighty-seven percent of strokes are caused by ischemia due to thrombosis or embolism. 10% is caused by a cerebral hemorrhage in which blood vessels in the brain rupture and leak blood to the brain tissue or cerebrospinal fluid. In the United States, stroke is the third leading cause of disability and is the third leading cause of death. Approximately 20% of stroke patients require more than 3 months of long-term inpatient treatment, and 15~30% have a permanent disability. The Korean Stroke Society reported that 98% of patients in the stroke patients visited the hospital because of hemiplegia, speech disorder, visual disturbance, dizziness, and severe headache. Patients should go to a hospital within 3 hours to prevent the occluded blood vessels from penetrating or progressing to a cerebral infarction. In recent years, the mortality rate for strokes have been steadily declining as treatment techniques improve.[1]

The brain weighs about 2% of the body. However, cerebral blood flow accounts for 15% of cardiac output, and 20% of $\dot{V}O_2max$. In addition, since the brain uses only glucose as an energy source, it is easy for necrosis to occur even if the energy supply is temporarily stopped. Therefore, it is not an exaggeration to say that the abnormality of cerebral blood flow is closely related to brain damage.

On the other hand, elderly people over 60 years old are likely to have a new stroke or are likely to recur an already existing stroke. In particular, the elderly who are 74 years old have a 1.25~1.5 times higher risk of stroke than younger men. The risk factors for stroke are: hypertension (the most important risk factor in stroke), hyperlipidemia, smoking (causing a double increase in stroke), diabetes, heart or arterial disease, atrial fibrillation, metabolic syndrome, and unhealthy dietary habits.[70,71]

One of the strongest predictors of stroke is transient ischemic attacks (TIAs), also known as a 'mini-stroke'. This appears to be a stroke-like symptom but does not cause sustained brain damage. Patients who had one or more TIAs were 10 times more likely to progress to a stroke than those who did not. 23% of stroke patients are those who had a stroke in the past, and the 30-day survival rate is only 88% for ischemic versus 62% for hemorrhagic causes. The 25% of stroke patients die from complications from the disease. Nearly 50% have serious health problems or develop into mid- to long-term disabilities. Only the remaining 25% of patients are able to recover before the stroke.

As mentioned earlier, during the stroke, brain blood flow shortage causes primary necrosis of the nerve cell and secondary lesion. Neurologic lesions differ according to their size, location and extent of involvement. Blood flow in the medial side occurs, slowly forming lesions and leaving only minor damage. After the stroke, patients may experience the following problems: First, there is a problem in controlling the motion of the human body, such as paralysis. Paralysis is one of the most common disorders caused by stroke. Paralysis affects the face, one arm, one leg or the entire arm and leg, with symptoms on the opposite side of the brain damaged by the stroke. When the cerebellum is damaged, it causes physical disability called ataxtia, making it difficult to maintain posture, walk and balance. Second, the sensory disorder in the affected part leads to loss of ability to tactile, pain, temperature, and location. Third, about 25% of patients with stroke have aphasia, and their ability to speak and write is lost. Fourth, problems can arise in thinking and remembering, and attentiveness is greatly reduced. Fifth, emotional disturbance causes fear, anxiety, frustration, and negative emotions about their physical and mental loss of ability.[70,71]

On the other hand, traumatic brain injury (TBI), which occurs in the developing world, is caused by striking, impacting or penetrating the head [Fig. 5.39].[75] TBI permanently damages the brain, resulting in functional or partial brain malfunctions or psychosocial disorder. After TBI, problems arise in one or more cognitive functions such as memory, attention, abstract thinking, judgment, problem solving ability, sensory ability, psychosocial behavior, physical function, information processing, and language function.

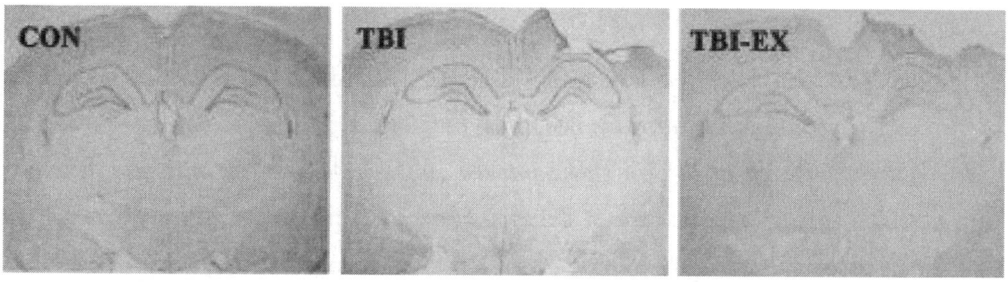

Fig. 5.39 ***Brain Tissue Recovery from TBI after Rehabilitation Exercise***

In general, TBI is most likely to occur between 0 and 4 years of age, between 15 and 19 years of age, or after 75 years of age. Once TBI occurs, it bruises the area under the head, where the main damage occurs at the bottom of the directly hit area. The damage also occurs at the opposite side of the original impact. The gelatin-like brain inside the rigid skull collides with the sharp, irregular bone structure and the dural end of the cranium from sudden deceleration and acceleration. This causes torn nervous tissue and the axons in the myelin stretch or burst. Secondary impairment may be accompanied by TBI and stroke, and may result in permanent damage to the more extensive parts of the brain. Edema caused by secondary neurological impairment destroys the metabolic process by reducing the oxidized blood supply to the affected tissue by compressing the surrounding tissue of the affected side.

Damage by TBI is more sporadic than general damage by stroke. Physical disability that occurs after moderate TBI affects the movement of the body and permanently disrupts limb, neck, and trunk control. Damage to upper motor neurons causes spasticity, clonus, and athetoid. Brainstem and cranial nerves can be invaded, which in turn affects the functions needed to maintain life. When lesions are present in the cerebellum, it is difficult to control the degree and timing of body movement, loss of balance, and loss of coordination (ability to communicate between the nerves and the muscles). Finally, the factors that limit independent function after mild brain damage are behavioral and cognitive disabilities.[4,5] Examples include excitement, confusion, impulsivity, attention deficit, memory impairment, anesthesia, poor judgment, and lack of learning.

Response to Exercise in Stroke Patients

The overall functional capacity of stroke or TBI patients is significantly reduced compared to the general population. When a stroke occurs, the oxygen uptake capacity at the submaximal level increases, but the $\dot{V}O_2peak$ decreases. This $\dot{V}O_2peak$ is only about 50% in healthy people of the same age group. After TBI, aerobic capacity is 67~74% of the prediction based on height and age. The lowered cardiac response and exercise performance of these patients is due to the partial damage of motor function due to brain trauma. Only 20 to 34% of stroke patients can reach 85% of the maximum heart rate (220 - age) by age. Because of the associated body injuries, TBI patients have a much higher heart rate than the average person when performing on a bicycle ergometer. Even with little or no physical deficits, response variables (submaximal $\dot{V}E/\dot{V}O_2$, oxygen pulse, maximal heart rate, $\dot{V}E$, $\dot{V}O_2$) to exercise appear less efficient.

The degree of functional impairment in patients with stroke or TBI makes breathing difficult. Fatigue sets in 2.5 times faster, and mobility and activities of daily living deteriorate. This increase in fatigue and decrease in endurance reduces productivity in the workplace.

Effects of Exercise Training on Stroke Patients

Recurrent stroke and CAD are the main causes of death after stroke. However, recent studies have reported that even if exercise alone is performed, the mortality rate can be reduced by 20% or more. Stroke patients can increase the $\dot{V}O_2peak$ by 60% when exercising. Treadmill exercise can improve $\dot{V}O_2peak$, load response, blood pressure, resting heart rate, and cholesterol levels. Additionally, exercise after stroke can increase walking speed, reduce walking aids, and improve functional mobility.

The benefits of certain exercise programs are somewhat limited. For example, aerobic training improves physical fitness and gait, but it does not improve activity in everyday life. Therefore, the American Heart Association recommends stretching, flexibility training, balance training, and coordination training to be conducted two to three days a week. It also recommends that you use an additional 2~3 days per week of weight training with light weights due to muscle weakness after a stroke. Strength training after a stroke is very beneficial in improving the activities of daily living, and in increasing speed and endurance. On the other hand, in institutions that provide exercise training to brain injured patients, it has been reported that excessive exercise of gait training or strength training may cause potential damage.

Patients with TBI are mostly young, but their physical abilities and endurance can be severely limited by the trauma sustained. However, exercise significantly improves $\dot{V}O_2$peak, endurance, and muscle strength, allowing greater independence, more efficient walking ability, and better vocational competency. Furthermore, patients with TBI after exercise have low rates of depression and good cognitive function.

Management and Medicine of Stroke Patients

Medical treatment for stroke patients should include the following: [Table 5.77].

Table 5.77 ***Medical Treatment of Stroke Patients***

- Use of anticoagulants in a short period of time and use of platelet inhibitors (heparin, coumadin, aspirin) for long periods of time.
- If vasospasm of the cerebral artery is suspected, use vasodilators (hydralazine, clonidine, Isordil).
- An antihypertensive agent (ACE inhibitors, beta blockers, calcium channel blockers, diuretics, sympathetic nerve inhibitors) is used for hemorrhagic stroke patients who need strict blood pressure control.

Some patients with brain damage require intensive postacute medical care. Seizures and convulsions may require long-term anticoagulants and anticonvulsants. Side effects of these medicines are reported to be slow cognitive function. Taking medicine that helps seizures can be stopped only if seizures did not occur for one year or longer. The medicines that prevent seizures are listed below [Table 5.78].

TBI may also cause dizziness, hypotension, and altered arousal states, which may lead to depression and anxiety, thus also requiring medical treatment [Table 5.78]. On the other hand, after stroke or TBI, hypertonia of the muscles occurs, which makes the muscles unusually tense. Medicines can reduce hypertonia, but may also be accompanied by a decrease in alertness and cognitive function. Medicines commonly used for hypertonia or other behavior-related problems are listed in [Table 5.78]. Finally, medicines that can reduce cognitive deficits in patients with TBI or stroke are also shown in [Table 5.78].

Table 5.78 Drugs required for Stroke and TBI Patients

Seizure prevention	Antidepressants/Anxiolytics	Tension reduction	Anticognitive defects
▪ Phenobarbital	▪ Venlafaxine	▪ Dantrolene	▪ Tacrine
▪ Clonazepam	▪ Amitriptyline	▪ Diazepam	▪ Sinemet
▪ Gabapentin	▪ Desipramine	▪ Baclofen	▪ Aricept
▪ Carbamzepine	▪ Nortriptyline		▪ Ritalin
	▪ Fluoxetine		▪ Dexedrine
	▪ Sertraline		▪ Cylert
	▪ Lorazepam		
	▪ Diazepam		
	▪ Alprazolam		

On the other hand, some medications also affect short-term physiological responses during exercise testing. In particular, the vasodilator needed to prevent hypotension may prolong the time for clean-up. Medications that limit cardiac output by reducing heart rate can reduce peak heart rate. Diuretics may also cause arrhythmia by decreasing plasma volume and altering electrolyte balance.

Recommendations for Exercise Testing

Patients who had a stroke or at risk of stroke should undergo ECG monitoring under the supervision of a physician. The pauses in exercise testing of these patients are similar to those of other high-risk patients or patients with CAD. In the presence of neurological deficits, exercise testing may involve more than a human body part that is not available. On the other hand, the type of exercise test can be evaluated variously according to the degree of physical impairment of stroke patients [Table 5.79].[3-5,22,88,92]

Leg Cycle Ergometer Test

A standard leg bike ergometer is used when a stroke or TBI patient is sitting in balance on the seat. The ramp protocol can be increased by 5~10 watts per minute, or by increasing the load by 20 watts per step so that the patient's maximum aerobic capacity can be determined. If the patient is unbalanced, a semi recumbent cycle or a recumbent cycle may be used. It is better to personalize the test protocol based on the patient's strength status. A recommended protocol is to maintain a pedal speed of 50 rpm and a protocol that starts at 20 watts and increases by 20 watts per step.

Table 5.79 ***Exercise test, drug, and specific considerations for brain injured patients***

	Test Item	Measurement	Recommended Stopping Point	Remarks
Aerobic Power Ability	■ Bicycle (5~10 watts / ramp protocol) ■ Treadmill (0.5~2 METs / step) ■ Combined ergometer ■ Seated stepper ■ Arm ergometer	■ 12 lead ECG	■ Severe arrhythmia ■ > 2 mm ST segment descending / rising ■ Ischemic threshold ■ T wave inversion with ST change	■ CAD is a major risk factor for CVA.
		■ Heart rate(HR) ■ Awareness	■ Sudden increase ■ Sudden fatigue increase	■ Useful for prescribing Intensity.
		■ SBP／DBP	■ More than 250/115 mmHg ■ If there is no change in SBP despite increasing Intensity	■ Hypertension is a major risk factor for CVA.
		■ $\dot{V}O_2$peak	■ Only necessary for the purpose of conducting research.	
Endurance	■ 6 minutes / 12 minutes walking ■ Leg ergometer ■ Combine ergometer	■ Distance the patient walked ■ Peak power 60% exercise time	■ Time, Distance ■ Symptoms of Stability	■ Applied to patients who need help with gait.
Muscular Strength	■ Manual muscle test ■ Computerized machines	■ Power output ■ Peak torque per weight ■ Maximal work per weight	■ Pounds, kilograms, repetitions ■ Maximum torque	■ Use when the patient is able to perform an operation.
Flexibility	■ Goniometer	■ ROM measurement of damaged limb ■ Distance	■ Overall flexion / extension angle ■ Total arc	
Neuromuscular	■ Gait analysis ■ Berg Balance ■ Functional reach ■ Tinetti	■ Walking speed ■ Symmetrical balance of motion		■ Useful for stability and efficiency of operation.
Functional Ability	■ Duke mobility ■ Functional independence measure ■ Inspection by individual criteria			■ It is useful for observing the recovery ability of ADLs.

Treadmill Inspection

If minimal motor nerve damage occurs, the Balke protocol is appropriate. The patient should be balanced when standing, or able to walk independently without assistance. The treadmill must choose to have a "zero start" as it should not cause a sudden speed change and fall. Because patients prefer a slower rate, the rate of treadmill testing should be slowed down to match the rate. Energy expenditure at a specific exercise rate is only 55~64 percent less than people without a stroke, so they do not require more tests. For patients with stroke or TBI, the appropriate protocol is Norton-Balke or a modified Balke protocol. This is generally considered to be safe because it requires 0.5~2 METs of energy consumption every three minutes.

Combination Arm-Leg Ergometer Test

When the test is performed on the unaffected side because the patient cannot pedal on the affected side due to convulsions or muscle weakness, the heart may be inflicted with other problems. At this time, it is preferable to use a combination arm-leg ergometer. This device has been evaluated to be very safe because it can only be performed using the limb of the unaffected side or performing the test with the help of the affected side.

Muscle Strength Test

The muscle strength test is preferably performed by a computer controlled power device. Isokinetic machine is popularized in Korea. The device measures the extent to which the patient maintains a constant resistance at the inspection position or withstands the amount of applied resistance. The reliability of a muscle strength test is affected when the patient's joint motion cannot be fixed.

Exercise Program for Brain Injury Patients

Stroke patients are recommended to take 3 weeks of stability without exercise to regain the tissue and blood vessels of the damaged brain and to control blood pressure. After 3 weeks, it is good to start active and passive joint exercises immediately for stroke patients. In patients with cerebral hemorrhage, passive joint exercises should first be performed on the limb. Patients should be instructed to move or massage the paralyzed side with a movable arm. If this is not possible, the caregiver should passively perform full motion of the joint at least twice a day to prevent joint stiffness. Most importantly, it gives patients confidence. Allow the patients to move steadily, and if they are able to stand, practice the position in multiple directions.

Patients with brain damage should be instructed to perform aerobic exercise such as the treadmill and the stepper, gradually starting from the bicycle which does not impact the head. The intensity of aerobic exercise should start at 40% of $\dot{V}O_2$peak and can be increased gradually to 70%. Exercise time should be 20~60 minutes, 3~5 days per week, but 3 days a week (every other day) is better [Table 5.80].

In the case of strength exercise, isometrics, such as weight machines and free weights, can be used to increase daily activity and living ability. Neuromuscular movements should be included when performing muscle strength exercises. Before and after exercise, flexibility exercises including stretching are applied to prevent not only increase of ROM, but also contracture [Table 5.80].[3-5,22,88,92]

Table 5.80 Management program for brain injured patients

	Type	Goal	Intensity/Frequency/Time	Period
Aerobic Exercise	■ Upper and lower ergometer ■ Lower ergometer ■ Treadmill ■ Seated steppe	■ Increase in activities of daily living skills ■ Increased walking speed ■ Reduction of cardiovascular disease	■ 40 to 70% of $\dot{V}O_2$peak ■ 3 to 5 days a week ■ 20 to 60 min (10 min for intermittent exercise)	■ 2~4 month
Strength Exercise	■ Isometric exercise ■ Weight Machine ■ Free weight	■ Increase in activities of daily living skills	■ 8~12 reps × 3 sets ■ 1~2 sets ■ 2 days per week	■ 2~4 month
Flexibility Exercise	■ Stretching	■ Increase of ROM ■ Prevention of muscle contracture	■ 2 days per week - Conducted before or after aerobic or strength training	■ 2~4 month
Neuromuscular Exercise	■ Coordination / balance sense exercise	■ Increased stability in daily activities	■ 2 days per week - Conducted on the day that includes strength training	■ 2~4 month

Because of the high risk of stroke recurrence, it is advisable to regularly consult with a specialist to continue exercise therapy according to his or her abilities after regular treatment.

❖ Study Questions

1. Obesity is defined as the percentage of body fat (*25*)% for men and (*30*)% for women.

2. The distribution of fat varies between males and females because of differences in hormones that regulate (*lipoprotein*) enzymes.

3. The type of obesity in men is called (*apple type*) obesity, and the type of obesity in women is called (*pear type*) obesity.

4. In the genetic characteristics of obesity, more than 200 factors have been proposed, mainly genes and chromosomal abnormalities affecting energy consumption, dietary intake, and fat metabolism. The major genes for such variation are (*leptin*), (*leptin receptors*), beta-3 adrenergic receptors, Neuropeptide Y, Uncoupling protein, Pro-opiomelanocortin, Tubby-like protein and Peroxisome proliferator-activated receptor.

5. When measuring obesity for the elderly, most of the indicators should be corrected. The reason is that when the elderly people lose height, the reliability of the (*body mass index*) using height and weight is lowered, and the skinfold method is inaccurate because of (*skin slackening*) caused by skin aging.

6. Exercise intensity for obese patients is (*40~60*)% of peak oxygen uptake, the frequency is 5 days or more per week, and exercise time is (*30~60*) minutes.

7. It is suggested that the cause of type 1 diabetes may be (*Coxsackie*) or (*Mumps*) virus.

8. Three common symptoms of the diabetic patients are (*polyuria, polyphagia, and polydipsia*). In addition, weight loss and increased fatigue are characteristic of diabetes.

9. Diabetes mellitus is defined as fasting plasma glucose above (*126*) mg/dℓ, and two-hour plasma glucose above (*200*) mg/dℓ.

10. Fasting plasma glucose levels of between 111 mg/dℓ and 125 mg/dℓ are called (*impaired glucose tolerance*).

11. Diabetes mellitus may be accompanied by various complications, but it may be accompanied by neurological disorders. (*peripheral neuropathy*) is common in the hands and feet and causes symptoms of tingling and burning. On the other hand, (*autonomic neuropathy*) may cause a transient incapacity state during exercise and may not increase heart rate.

12. Appropriate blood glucose level before exercise is (*150~249*) mg/dℓ.

13. Exercise intensity for diabetic patients is (*50~80*)% of peak oxygen uptake, the frequency of 4 to 7 days per week and the time of (*20~60*) minutes.

14. Total cholesterol level is the overall amount of cholesterol found in the blood, in which (*HDL-C*) accounts for about 17%, (*LDL-C*) 70%, and (*VLDL-C*) 13%.

15. Hyperlipidemia is defined as a condition in which total cholesterol is (*200*) mg/dℓ or more, LDL-C is (*130*) mg/dℓ or more, HDL-C is (*35*) mg/dℓ or less, and triglyceride is (*250*) mg/dℓ or more.

16. Exercise for atherosclerosis should be (*40~70*)% of the maximum oxygen uptake, (*40*) minutes per day, 5 ~ 7 days per week.

17. Fatty liver patients should begin exercise after the GPT level drops to (*100*) IU.

18. Hypertension is defined as the period when SBP is greater than (*140*) mmHg and DBP is greater than (*90*) mmHg as a result of regular blood pressure measurements.

19. (*Essential*) hypertension accounts for 95% of all patients and (*secondary*) hypertension accounts for 5%.

20. Ideal hypertension management does not use many medicines but lowers blood pressure without (*side effects*) considering the (*economy*).

21. The 'antihypertensive program' emphasizes weight loss, (*regular exercise*), ingestion of high content of (*potassium*) and magnesium, inhibition of alcohol and salty foods, and smoking cessation.

22. Exercise for hypertension patients should be (*40~80*)% of maximum heart rate, 4~7 days a week, and exercise time (*30~60*) minutes. It should consume between (*700~2,000*) kcal per week.

23. Among the drugs for CAD, (*verapamil*) and diltiazem reduce heart rate by slowing the conduction of SA-node and AV-node.

24. CAD patients are safe to exercise.
   ① There is no ischemia at the exercise intensity of (*6*) METs or less.
   ② No exercise-induced (*ventricular tachycardia*), exercise-induced (*hypotension*), or exercise-induced (*cardiac arrhythmia*).
   ③ More than 50% of (*ejection fraction*).
   ④ myocardial infarction, (*coronary artery bypass graft surgery*), angioplasty and resection without complications.

25. Patients who are not suitable for weight loading exercise
① Patients with uncontrolled (*hypertension*)
② Patients with congestive (*heart failure*)
③ Patients with uncontrolled arrhythmia
④ Patients with severe (*valve disease*)
⑤ Patients with aerobic capacity below 5 METs

26. Exercise intensity for patients with myocardial infarction is (*40~80*)% of maximum oxygen intake, the frequency is 3 days or more per week and exercise time is (*20~60*) minutes.

27. General treatment includes treatment of causes of weakening (*left ventricular*) function and weight loss, (*anemia*) treatment, low sodium diet, and diuretic use.

28. The drug that helps only patients with atrial fibrillation is (*digitalis*).

29. It is extremely dangerous if the systolic pressure difference is greater than 50 ㎜Hg or if the valve opening area is less than (*0.4*) cm^2/m^2.

30. Exercise intensity for valve patients is (*40~80*)% of THR, 4~7 days per week, and exercise time is (*20~60*) minutes.

31. In patients with hypertrophic cardiomyopathy, contraindications to exercise are the family history of (*sudden death*), severe (*ventricular*) hypertrophy, cardiac output less than (*40*) ㎜Hg at rest, and young patients with exercise-induced syncope.

32. Diseases that can cause sudden death are severe hypertrophic cardiomyopathy, severe (*aortic*) stenosis, severe (*left ventricular systolic*) dysfunction, exercise-induced complex ventricular arrhythmia, exercise-induced (*hypotension*), exercise-induced (*angina*), past history of ventricular fibrillation, patients with angina who experience ventricular arrhythmia, patients with delayed QT intervals and a history of syncope.

33. Treatment of chronic lung disease is aimed at reducing (*functional impairment*), not improving disease.

34. When CLD patients exercise, endurance improves and (*dyspnea*) decreases.

35. The vital capacity and FEV_1 of patients with CLD are less than (*70*)% of those of normal subjects, so excessive rehabilitation should be avoided.

36. According to the general management guidelines for lung disease patients, the vaccine against pneumococcus should be inoculated once every (*6*) years.

37. (*Oxygen*) therapy is inevitable for patients with hypoxia.
38. Breathing exercises should include (*diaphragmatic*) breathing and (*mouth*)

exercises and should be performed regularly.

39. (*Intermittent*) exercise should be performed when patients with pulmonary disease are unable to perform the continuous exercise.

40. Patients with pulmonary disease are difficult to measure oxygen uptake, so it is advisable to repeat 1 to 2 repetitions per day in the range of (*11~13*) of RPE.

41. (*Ipratropium bromide*) is the most effective treatment for CLD.

42. CF is characterized by many causes, but it is known as (*genetic*) disease.

43. CF patients do not have (*immunological*) competence for microorganisms.

44. Patients with CF can be treated with antibiotics, (*bronchodilators*), airway remedies, and dietary therapy.

45. In CF patients, furosemide is good for hyponatremia and (*diuretic*) is effective for patients with severe edema.

46. Patients with the pulmonary disease show a significant improvement even after only (*3~4*) weeks of exercise.

47. One of the effects of exercise therapy in patients with lung disease, (*dyspnea*) level is reduced by 30%.

48. Patients with CLD should undergo a (*symptom-limited*) GXR before participating in an exercise program.

49. GXR in patients with CLD has the advantage of detecting (*40~50*)% blood disease and exercise-induced (*bronchial*) spasm.

50. Patients with severe pulmonary disease set their exercise intensity at a heart rate equal to (*80*)% of the maximal work.

51. If a mild pulmonary disease patient cannot perform an exercise test, use a (*dyspnea scale*) or awareness.

52. Patients with the pulmonary disease should perform (*big muscle*) movements to control breathing sensation.

53. Patients with asthma may experience (*dyspnea*), (*wheezing*), and chest pain periodically, accompanied by coughing.

54. The most important goal of treatment for asthma patients is to maintain normal (*pulmonary function*).

55. Peak flow is reduced by (*12.5*)% during or after exercise is mobility asthma.

56. Athletic items that do not cause bronchospasm have (*advantages*) in a warm and humid environment.

57. Patients with asthma are less likely to experience symptoms of less than (*2*) on the dyspnea scale.

58 Patients with pulmonary disease are prevented from exercising if they have congestive (*heart failure*), uncontrolled (*arrhythmia*), or severe (*valve disease*).

59. When a patient with pulmonary disease intends to undergo weight-bearing exercise, an initial load of (*30~50%*) of 1RM is recommended.

60. When patients with pulmonary disease are trying to undergo weight bearing exercise, the degree of breathing difficulty should not exceed (*3~6*).

61. Arthritis arising from abnormalities of an autoimmune body is a (*rheumatoid arthritis*).

62. Drugs in patients with (*rheumatoid arthritis*) include analgesics, glucocorticoids and (*nonsteroidal anti-inflammatory*) drugs.

63. When arthritis patients are to undergo weight-bearing exercise, a load of (*11~16*) is recommended for self-awareness.

64. Patients with rheumatoid arthritis are divided into four categories: patients who are uncomfortable but who are capable of normal life are classified as type (*2*).

65. Patients with rheumatoid arthritis who are suitable for walking and stationary bicycle riding are (*1~3*) type.

66. Osteoporosis results in the release of calcium into the blood by (*osteoclasts*).

67. The osteoporosis is judged to be (*-2.5*) or more in the bone mineral density test.

68. Elderly women with osteoporosis over 65 years of age should be given (*1,500*) mg calcium.

69. The drug that promotes bone growth without causing cancer in patients with osteoporosis is (*alendronate*).

70. Calcium and (*vitamin D*) supplements are effective for osteoporosis and cardiovascular disease when combined with exercise.

71. The most effective exercises for osteoporosis are walking, (*brisk walking*), swimming, underwater walking and resistance exercise.

72. Patients with osteoporosis should be given 3 to 5 days per week and (*30~60*) minutes per day for (*40~70*)% of the maximum heart rate for aerobic exercise. Resistance exercise is effective at (*75*)% of 1RM, (*8~12*) times, 2~3 days per week and exercise time of (*20~40*) minutes.

73. Low back pain is a pain syndrome caused by the spinal nerve ending from the second lumbar vertebra to the cephalic bones (*sacroiliac joint*) range.

74. (*McKenzie extension exercise*) is effective for patients with disc herniation.

75. (*Williams flexion exercise*) are effective for patients with spinal stenosis or spondylolysis.

76. Regular exercise reduces the risk of (*colon cancer*) by about 40%.

77. The scale that distinguishes the activities and symptoms of cancer patients is Zubrod scale and (*Karnofsky*) scale.

78. If cancer patients receive intravenous chemotherapy, exercise should be performed after (*24*) hours.

79. Choose the wrong thing to consider before exercising for cancer patients. (*A*)

A. The usual state of sleep or exercise

B. Presence of other diseases other than tumor

C. Complications from tumors or metastatic sites

D. Potential complications that may result from treatment type

80. When prescribing exercise for a cancer patient, choose something that does not fit when checking with a complete blood count. (*C*)

A. If the white blood cell count is less than 3,000 cells / mm^3

B. When granulocytes are less than 2,500 / mm^3

C. If the platelet count less than 5,000 / mm^3

D. If the hemoglobin level is 10 g / mm^3 less

Suggested Readings

Chapter 1. Exercise and Health

[1] Brooks G, Mercier J. Balance of carbohydrate and lipid utilization during exercise: The "crossover" concept. J Appl Physiol (1985) 1994;76:2253-2261.

[2] Chwalbinska-Moneta J, Robergs RA, Costill DL, Fink WJ. Threshold for muscle lactate accumulation during progressive exercise. *J Appl Physiol* 1989;*66*:2710-2716.

[3] Smith JC, Hill DW. Contribution of energy systems during a Wingate power test. Br J Sports Med 1991;25:196-199.

[4] Crabtree B, Higgins SJ, Newsholme EA. The activities of pyruvate carboxylase, phosphoenolpyruvate carboxylase and fructose diphosphatase in muscles from vertebrates and invertebrates. *Biochem J 1972;*130:391-396.

[5] Gollnick PD, Bayly W, Hodgson D. Exercise intensity, training, diet, and lactate concentration in muscle and blood. *Med Sci Sports Exerc 1986;*18:334-340.

[6] Gollnick PD, Saltin B. *Fuel for muscular exercise: Role of fat. In:* Horton ES, Terjung RL, editors. *Exercise,* nutrition, and energy metabolism. NY: Macmillan; 1988. p. 72-88.

[7] Gollnick PD. Metabolism of substrates: Energy substrate metabolism during exercise and as modified by training. *Fed Proc 1985;*44:353-356.

[8] Henrikson EJ, Bourey RE, Rodnick KJ, Koranyi L, Permutt MA, Holloszy JO. Glucose transporter protein content and glucose transport capacity in rat skeletal muscle. *Am J Physiol 1990;259*:E593-598.

[9] Holloszy JO. *Utilization of fatty acids during exercise.* In: Taylor AW, editor. Biochemistry of Exercise, 7th ed. Champaign, IL: Human Kinetics; 1990. p. 319-328.

[10] Ko IG, Jeong JW, Kim YH, Jee YS, Kim SE, Kim SH, Jin JJ, Kim CJ, Chung KJ. Aerobic exercise affects myostatin expression in aged rat skeletal muscles: a possibility of antiaging effects of aerobic exercise related with pelvic floor muscle and urethral rhabdosphincter. Int Neurourol J 2014;18:77-85.

[11] Newsholme E, Leech A. *Biochemistry for the medical sciences.* Chichester: Wiley; 1984. p. 25-36.

[12] Powers SK, Howley ET. *Exercise physiology.* 3rd ed. WCB McGrow-Hill; 1997. p. 21-61.

[13] Robers RA, Roberts SO. *Exercise physiology.* WCB McGrow-Hill; 2000. p. 26-54.

[14] Saltin B, Gollnick PD. *Fuel for muscular exercise: Role of carbohydrate.* In: Horton ES, Terjung RL, editors. Exercise, nutrition, and energy metabolism. NY: Macmillan; 1988. p. 45-71.

[15] Wilson RW, Jacobsen PB, Fields KK. Pilot study of a home-based aerobic exercise program for sedentary cancer survivors treated with hematopoietic stem cell transplantation. *Bone Marrow Transplantation 2005;*35:721-727.

[16] Boughton B. Exercise could improve colorectal-cancer survival. Lancet Oncol 2006;7:713.

Chapter 2. Exercise and Nutrition

[1] Coaching and Sports Science Division. *Body composition.* United States Olympic Committee. 2001.

[2] Costill DL. *Nutritional requirements for endurance athletes.* In: Burke EJ, editor. Toward an understanding of human performance. Movement publication; 1980.

[3] Coyle EF, Coggan AR, Hemmert MK, Ivy JL. Muscle glycogen utilization during prolonged strenuous exercise when fed carbohydrate. J Appl Physiol (1985) 1986;61:165-172.

[4] Jee YS, Kim MH, Han JW, Ahn HJ, Lee CH, Kim JH. The influence of all-out exercise on antioxidant enzymes activity and MDA level in judo athletes. Korean Journal of Physical Education 1999;38:617-626.

[5] Jee YS. Athletes and nutrition. Journal of Coaching Development 2000;2:26-38.

[6] Ji LL. Exercise, Oxidative Stress, and Antioxidants. *Am J Sports Med 1996;*24:S20-24.

[7] Katch FI, McArdle WD. *Nutrition, weight control, and exercise.* Philadelphia: Lea & Febiger; 1988.

[8] Lin DJ. Free Radicals and Disease Prevention. Keats Publishing Inc; 1993. p. 74-77.

[9] Robergs RA, Roberts SO. *Fundamental principles of exercise physiology for fitness, performance, and health.* McGraw-Hill College; 2000.

[10] Roberts KM, Noble EG, Hayden DB, Taylor AW. Simple and complex carbohydrate-rich diets and muscle glycogen content of marathon runners. Eur J Appl Physiol Occup Physiol 1988;57:70-74.

[11] Rudman D, Williams PJ. Mega-dose vitamins: Use and misuse. N Engl J Med 1983;309:488-490.

[12] Tarnopolsky MA, MacDougall JD, Atkinson SA. Influence of protein intake and training status on nitrogen balance and lean body mass. J Appl Physiol (1985) 1988;64:187-193.

Chapter 3. Clinical Exercise Prescription

[1] Alderink GJ, Kuck DJ. Isokinetic shoulder strength of high school and college-aged pitchers. *J Orthop Sports Phys Ther 1986;7*:163-172.

[2] American College of Sports Medicine. *ACSM's guidelines for exercise testing and prescription.* 9th ed. Philadelphia: Lippincott Williams & Wilkins; 2013.

[3] Appen L, Duncan PW. Strength relationship of knee musculature: effects of gravity and sport. *J Orthop Sport Phys Trer* 1986;7:232-5.

[4] Jee YS. Exercise rehabilitation, work to revive the human becoming the driving force of the country. J Exerc Rehabil 2013;9:395-396.

[5] Jee YS. Usefulness of measuring isokinetic torque and balance ability for exercise rehabilitation. J Exerc Rehabil 2015;11:65-66.

[6] Barton TM, Torg JS. Natural history of the posterior cruciate ligament deficient knee. *Am J Sports Med 1986;*13:439.

[7] Bassey EJ et al. Health professional view on exercises: A study. *J R Soc Health 1984;*104:225-228.

[8] Blumenthal JA, Emery CF, Madden DJ, Schniebolk S, Walsh-Riddle M, George LK, McKee DC, Higginbotham MB, Cobb FR, Coleman RE. Long-term effects of exercise on psychological functioning in older men and women. J Gerontol 1991;46:P352-361.

[9] Borg G. Psychophysical bases of perceived exertion. *Med Sci Sports Exerc* 1982;14:377-381.

[10] Cain TE, Schwab GH. Performance of an athlete with straight posterior knee instability. *Am J Sports Med 1981;*9:203-208.

[11] Chan KM, Maffulli N, Korkia P, Li RCT. *Principles and practice of isokinetics in sports medicine and rehabilitation. Hong Kong:* Williams & Wilkins; 1996.

[12] Chisholm DM, Collis ML, Kulak LL, Davenport W, Gruber N. Physical activity readiness. *Br Columbia Med J 1975;*17:375-378.

[13] Costill DL, Coyle EF, Fink WF, Lesmes GR, Witzmann FA. Adaptations in skeletal muscle following strength training. J Appl Physiol Respir Environ Exerc Physiol *1979;*46:96-99.

[14] Computer Sports Medicine Inc. (CSMI). HUMAC /NORM™ Testing & Rehabilitation System User's Guide. Stoughton, MA, 2006;5:63–67.

[15] Davies GJ. *A compendium of isokinetics in clinical usage:* Workshop and clinical notes. LaCrosse, WI: S&S Publishers; 1985.

[16] Farmer ME, Locke BZ, Mościcki EK, Dannenberg AL, Larson DB, Radloff LS. Physical activity and depressive symptoms: the NHANES I Epidemiologic Follow-up Study. Am J Epidemiol 1988;128:1340-1351.

[17] Figoni SF, Morris AF. Effects of knowledge of results on reciprocal, isokinetic strength and fatigue. *J Orthop Sports Phys Ther* 1984;6:190-197.

[18] Gettman LR. Fitness testing. In: Blair S, Painter P, Pate R, Smith L, Taylor C, editors. *Resource manual for guidelines for exercise testing and prescription.* Philadelphia: Lea & Febiger; 1988. p. 161-170.

[19] Glick JM. Muscle strain: Prevention and treatment. Phys Sportsmed. 1980;8:73-77.

[20] Grace TG, Sweetser ER, Nelson MA, Ydens LR, Skipper BJ. Isokinetic muscle imbalance and knee-joint injuries. A prospective blind study. J Bone Joint Surg Am 1984;66:734-740.

[21] Green HJ. Muscle power: Fiber type recruitment, metabolism and fatigue. In: Jones NL, McCartney N, McComas AJ, editors. *Human muscle power.* Champaign, IL: Human Kinetics; 1986. p. 65-79.

[22] Hage P. Primary care physicians : First stop for exercise advice? *Phys Sportsmed* 1983;11:149-152.

[23] Hald RD, Bottjen EJ. Effect of visual feedback on maximal and submaximal isokinetic test

measurements of normal quadriceps and hamstrings. *J Orthop Sports Phys Ther 1987;*9:86-93.

[24] Heyward VH. *Advanced Fitness Assessment & Exercise Prescription.* Champaign, IL: Human Kinetics; 1991.

[25] Hinson MM. *Kinesiology.* Dubuque, Iowa: Wm. C. Brown; 1977.

[26] Jackson AW, Morrow JR Jr, Brill PA, Kohl HW 3rd, Gordon NF, Blair SN. Relations of sit-up and sit-and-reach tests to low back pain in adults. J Orthop Sports Phys Ther 1998;27:22-26.

[27] Jee YS, Han JW. The changes of subjective pain degree and isokinetic abductor/adductor in baseball pitchers with shoulder joint injury after rehabilitative exercise therapy. Journal of Sport and Leisure Studies 2002;18:1405-1420.

[28] Jee YS. The changes of pain degree, ROM, and musculo-articulation functions in athletes with isolated posterior cruciate ligament injury. Korean Journal of Physical Education 2002;41:501-515.

[29] Park JS, Oh HY, Park EK, Ko IG, Kim SE, Kim JD, Jin JJ, Jee YS. Effects of rehabilitation program on functional scores and isokinetic torques of knee medial plica-operated patients. Isokinetics and Exercise Science 2013;21:19–28.

[30] Kannus P, Alosa D, Cook L, Johnson RJ, Renström P, Pope M, Beynnon B, Yasuda K, Nichols C, Kaplan M. Effect of one-legged exercise on the strength, power, and endurance of the contralateral leg. A randomized, controlled study using isometric and concentric isokinetic training. Eur J Appl Physiol Occup Physiol *1992;*64:117-126.

[31] Kannus P, Cook L, Alosa D. Absolute and relative endurance parameters in isokinetic tests of muscular performance. J Sport Rehabil *1992;*1:2-12.

[32] Kannus P, Järvinen M. Prediction of torque acceleration energy and power of thigh muscles from peak torque. Med Sci Sports Exerc 1989;21:304-347.

[33] Kannus P. Isokinetic evaluation of muscular performance: Implication for muscle testing and rehabilitation. *Int J Sports Med 1994;*15:S11-18.

[34] Kannus VP. Isokinetic peak torque and work relationship in the laterally unstable knee. Can J Sport Sci 1989;14:17-20.

[35] Kannus P. Peak torque and total work relationship in the thigh muscles after anterior cruciate ligament injury. *J Orthop Sports Phys Ther 1988;*10:97-101.

[36] Kannus P. Relationship between peak torque and total work in an isokinetic contraction of the medial collateral ligament insufficient knee. *Int J Sports Med 1988;*9:294-296.

[37] Karvonen MJ, Kentala E, Mustala O. The effect of training on heart rate: a longitudinal study. *Am Med Exp Biol Fenn 1957;*35:307-315.

[38] Kim JJ, Wang MJ, Lee YJ, Jeon SJ. Electrocardiography. Seoul: Hyunmoonsa; 1999. p. 36-252.

[39] Robers RA, Roberts SO. *Exercise physiology.* WCB McGrow-Hill; 2000. p. 318-336.

[40] Knight KL. Strength imbalance and knee injury. *Phys Sports Med* 1980;8:140.

[41] Lermen J, Bruce RA, Sivarajan E, Pettet GE, Trimble S. Low-level dynamic exercises for earlier cardiac rehabilitation: Aerobic and hemodynamic responses. *Arch Phys Med Rehabil 1976;*57:335-360.

[42] Lesmes GR, Costill DL, Coyle EF, Fink WJ. Muscle strength and power changes during maximal isokinetic training. *Med Sci Sports 1978;*10:266-269.

[43] Mersky H. Classification of chronic pain: Description of chronic pain syndromes and definition of pain terms. Pain Suppl 1986;3:S1-226.

[44] Morris A, Lussier L, Bell G, Dooley J. Hamstring/quadriceps strength ratios in collegiate middle-distance and distance runner. Phys Sportsmed *1983;11:*71-77.

[45] Morrissey MC. The relationship between peak torque and work of the quadriceps and hamstrings after meniscectomy. *J Orthop Sports Phys Ther* 1987;8:405-408.

[46] Myers JN. Perception of chest pain during exercise testing in patients with coronary artery disease. *Med Sci Sports Exerc 1994;*26:1082-1086.

[47] Negus RA, Rippe JM, Freedson P, Michaels J. Heart rate, blood pressure, and oxygen consumption during orthopaedic rehabilitation exercise. *J Orthop Sports Phys Ther 1987;*8:346-350.

[48] Ostering LR. Isokinetic dynamometry: implication for muscle testing and rehabilitation. Exerc Sport Sci Rev 1986;14:45-80.

[49] Perrin DH. *Isokinetic exercise and assessment.* Champaign, IL: Human Kinetics; 1993.

[50] Perrin DH. Reliability of isokinetic measures. *Athletic Training 1986;21:*319-321.

[51] Staublr WT. Eccentric action of muscles: physiology, injury, and adaptation. Exerc Sport Sci Rev 1989;17:157-185.

[52] Stratford PW, Bruulsema A, Maxwell B, Black T, Harding B. The effect of inter-trial rest interval on the assessment of isokinetic thigh muscle torque. *J Orthop Sports Phys Ther 1990;*11:362-366.

[53] Swain DP, Leutholtz BC. *Exercise prescription : A case study approach to the ACSM guidelines.* Champaign, IL: Human Kinetics Publishers; 2002.

[54] Taylor GB, Sallis JF, Needle R. The relation of physical activity and exercise to mental health. *Public Health Rep 1985;*100:195-202.

[55] Tomberlin JP, Basford JR, Schwen EE, Orte PA, Scott SG, Laughman RK, Ilstrup DM. Comparative study of isokinetic eccentric and concentric quadriceps training. *J Orthop Sports Phys Ther 1991;*14:31-36.

[56] Torg JS, Barton TM, Pavlov H, Stine R. Natural history of the posterior cruciate ligament-deficient knee. Clin Orthop Relat Res *1989;*246:208-216.

[57] Westing SH, Seger JY, Thorstensson A. Isoacceleration: A new concept of resistive exercise. Med Sci Sports Exerc *1991;*23:631-635.

[58] Dvir Z. Isokinetics: muscle testing, interpretation and clinical applications. 2nd Eds. Churchill Livingstone; 2004.

[59] Song JY, Park JW, Lee CB, Eun D, Jang JH, Lee HJ, Hyun GS, Park JM, Cha JY, Cho NH, Ko IG, Jin JJ, Jin YY, Ham DW, Jee YS. Analysis of ipsilateral and bilateral ratios in male amateur golfers. J Exerc Rehabil 2016;12:99-108.

[60] Kim SE, Hong J, Cha JY, Park JM, Eun D, Yoo J, Jee YS. Relative appendicular skeletal muscle mass is associated with isokinetic muscle strength and balance in healthy collegiate men. J Sports Sci 2016;34:2114-2120.

[61] Cha JY, Kim JH, Hong J, Choi YT, Kim MH, Cho JH, Ko IG, Jee YS. A 12-week rehabilitation program improves body composition, pain sensation, and internal/external torques of baseball pitchers with shoulder impingement symptom. J Exerc Rehabil 2014;10:35-44.

Chapter 4. Clinical Kinesiology

[1] American College of Sports Medicine. *ACSM's guidelines for exercise testing and prescription.* 9th ed. Philadelphia: Lippincott Williams & Wilkins; 2013.

[2] Bompa TO. *Periodization of Strength: The new wave in strength training.* Veritas Publishing Inc; 1996. p. 60-82.

[3] Franklin BA. *ACSM's guidelines for exercise testing and prescription.* 6th ed. Philadelphia: Lippincott Williams & Wilkins; 2000. p. 145-150.

[4] Lang PB, Latin RW, Berg KE, Mellion MB. The accuracy of the ACSM cycle ergometer equation. *Med Sci Sports Exerc* 1992;24:272-276.

[5] Latin RW, Berg KE. The accuracy of the ACSM and a new cycle ergometry equation for young women. *Med Sci Sports Exerc 1994;26*:642-646.

[6] Londeree BR, Moffitt-Gerstenberger J, Padfield JA, Lottmann D. Oxygen consumption of cycle ergometry is nonlinearly related to work rate and pedal rate. *Med Sci Sports Exerc 1997;29*:775-780.

[7] National Strength & Conditioning Association. NSCA's essentials of personal training. 2nd ed. Champaign, IL: Human Kinetics Publishers; 2011.

[8] Swain DP, Leutholtz BC, editors. *Exercise prescription : A case study approach to the ACSM guidelines.* Champaign, IL: Human Kinetics Publishers; 2002.

Chapter 5. Clinical Sports Medicine

[1] Adams HP Jr, Bendixen BH, Kappelle LJ, Biller J, Love BB, Gordon DL, Marsh EE 3rd. Classification of subtype of acute ischemic stroke. Definitions for use in a multicenter clinical trial. TOAST. Trial of Org 10172 in Acute Stroke Treatment. Stroke 1993;24:35-41.

[2] Ades PA, Waldmann ML, Poehlman ET, Gray P, Horton ED, Horton ES, LeWinter MM. Exercise conditioning in older coronary patients. Submaximal lactate response and endurance capacity. *Circulation 1993;*88:572-577.

[3] *American Association of Cardiovascular and Pulmonary Rehabilitation.* Guidelines for Cardiac Rehabilitation Programs. 2nd ed. Champaign, IL: Human Kinetics; 1991.

[4] Kim SE, Ko IG, Kim BK, Shin MS, Cho S, Kim CJ, Kim SH, Baek SS, Lee EK, Jee YS. Treadmill exercise prevents aging-induced failure of memory through an increase in neurogenesis and suppression of apoptosis in rat hippocampus. Experimental Gerontology 2010;45:357–365.

[5] American College of Sports Medicine. *ACSM's guidelines for exercise testing and prescription.* 8th ed. Champaign, IL: Human Kinetics; 2010.

[6] Appel LJ, Moore TJ, Obarzanek E, Vollmer WM, Svetkey LP, Sacks FM, Bray GA, Vogt TM, Cutler JA, Windhauser MM, Lin PH, Karanja N. A clinical trial of the effects of dietary patterns on blood pressure. DASH Collaborative Research Group. N Engl J Med 1997;336:1117-1124.

[7] Aro A, Soimakallio S, Voutilainen E, Ehnholm C, Wiljasalo M. Serum lipoprotein lipid and apoprotein levels as indicators of the severity of angiographically assessed coronary artery disease. Atherosclerosis 1986;62:219-225.

[8] Aronow WS, Ahn C, Kronzon L. Prognosis of congestive heart failure in elderly patients with normal versus abnormal left ventricular systolic function associated with coronary artery disease. *Am J Cardiol 1990;*66:1257-1259.

[9] Beeh KM, Kornmann O, Lill J, Buhl R. Induced sputum cell profiles in lung transplant recipients with or without chronic rejection: correlation with lung function. *Thorax 2001;*56:557-560.

[10] Bloomfield SA. *Osteoporosis. In:* American College of Sports Medicine. *ACSM's exercise managements for persons with chronic disease and disability.* Champaign, IL: Human Kinetics; 1991. p. 161-166.

[11] Braunwald E. Valvular heart disease. In: Braunwald E, editor. Heart disease: *A textbook of cardiovascular medicine.* 4th ed. Philadelphia: Saunders; 1992.

[12] Bray GA. Exercise and obesity. In: Bouchard C, Shepard R, Stephens T, Sutton JR, McPherson BD, editors. Exercise, fitness and health: *A consensus of current knowledge.* Champaign, IL: Human Kinetic; 1990.

[13] Buckley LM, Leib ES, Cartularo KS, Vacek PM, Cooper SM. Calcium and vitamin D3 supplementation prevents bone loss in the spine secondary to low-dose corticosteroids in patients with rheumatoid arthritis. *Ann Intern Med 1996;*125:961-968.

[14] Celli BR. Is pulmonary rehabilitation an effective treatment for Chronic Obstructive Lung Disease? *Am J Respir Critical Care Med 1997;*155:781-783.

[15] Chagnon YC, Rankinen T, Snyder EE, Weisnagel SJ, Perusse L, Bouchard C. The human obesity gene map: The 2002 update. *Obes Res 2003;*11:313-367.

[16] Chaitman BR. Exercise testing. In: Braunwald E, Zipes DP, Libby P, editors. Heart disease. 6th ed. Philadelphia: Saunders; 2001. p. 129.

[17] Cooper CB. *Pulmonary disease. In:* American College of Sports Medicine. *ACSM's Exercise managements for persons with chronic disease and disability.* Champaign, IL: Human Kinetic; 1991. p. 74-80.

[18] Corbin CB. *Concepts of physical fitness and wellness with laboratories.* Brown & Benchmark Publishers; 1994.

[19] Dougherty AH. Congestive heart failure with normal systolic function. *Am J Cardiol* 1984;54:778-782.

[20] Drinkwater BL. Physical activity, fitness, and osteoporosis. *In: Bouchard C, Shephard RJ, Stephens T, editors. Physical activity, fitness, and health.* Champaign, IL: Human Kinetic; 1994.

[21] Durstine JL. Exercise and optimization of the lipid profile. *In:* Torg JS, Shehard RJ, editors. *Current therapy in sports medicine.* 3rd ed. Mosby; 1995. p. 668-676.

[22] Fletcher GF, Froelicher VF, Hartley LH, Haskell WL, Pollock ML. Exercise standards: a statement for health professionals from the American Heart Association. *Circulation 1990;82:*2286-2322.

[23] Franklin BA, Bonzheim K, Wetherbee S, Gordon S, Timmis GC. Exercise and fitness. *Obstet Gynecol Clin North Am* 1990;17:817-835.

[24] Franklin BA. Coronary artery bypass grafting and angioplasty. *In:* American College of Sports Medicine. *ACSM's exercise managements for persons with chronic disease and disability.* Champaign, IL: Human Kinetics; 1991. p. 26-31.

[25] Franklin BA. Myocardial infarction. *In:* American College of Sports Medicine. *ACSM's exercise managements for persons with chronic disease and disability.* Champaign, IL: Human Kinetics; 1991. p. 19-25.

[26] Frayniarz K, Mahler DA. Writing an exercise prescription for patients with COPD. *J Respir Dis 1990;*11:638-644.

[27] Friedman D. Angina and silent ischemia: *In:* American College of Sports Medicine. *ACSM's exercise managements for persons with chronic disease and disability.* Champaign, IL: Human Kinetics; 1991. p. 32-36.

[28] Geltman EM. Mild heart failure: diagnosis and treatment, *Am Heart J 1989;*118:1277-1291.

[29] Goldberg AP. Aerobic and resistive exercise modify risk factors for coronary heart disease. *Med Sci Sports Exerc 1989;*21:669-674.

[30] Goldberg L, Elliot DL, editors. *Exercise for prevention and treatment of illness.* Philadelphia: FA Davis Company; 1994. p. 228-238.

[31] Gordon DJ, Rifkind BM. High-density lipoprotein--the clinical implications of recent studies. *N Engl J Med 1989;*321:1311-1316.

[32] Gordon NF. *Hypertension. In:* American College of Sports Medicine. *ACSM's exercise managements for persons with chronic disease and disability.* Champaign, IL: Human Kinetics; 1991. p. 59-63.

[33] Gordon T, Castelli WP, Hjortland MC, Kannel WB, Dawber TR. High density lipoprotein as a protective factor against coronary heart disease. The Framingham Study. *Am J Med 1977;62*:707-714.

[34] Hagberg JM. *Exercise, fitness and hypertension.* In: Bouchard C, Shepard R, Stephens T, Sutton JR, McPherson BD, editors. Exercise, fitness and health: *A consensus of current knowledge.* Champaign, IL: Human Kinetic; 1990.

[35] Hanrath P, Schlüter M, Sonntag F, Diemert J, Bleifeld W. Influence of verapamil therapy on left ventricular performance at rest and during exercise in hypertrophic cardiomyopathy. *Am J Cardiol 1983;*52:544-548.

[36] Harris KA, Holly RG. Physiological response to circuit weight training in borderline hypertensive subjects. *Med Sci Sports Exerc 1987;*19:246-252.

[37] Hartard M, Haber P, Ilieva D, Preisinger E, Seidl G, Huber J. Systematic strength training as a model of therapeutic intervention. A controlled trial in postmenopausal with osteopenia. *Am J Phys Med Rehabil 1996;75*:21-28.

[38] Higuchi MT, Tamai T, Kobayashi S, Nakai T. Plasma lipoprotein and apolipoprotein profiles in aged Japanese athletes. Med Sports Sci *1992;37:*126-136.

[39] Hurley BF, Hagberg JM, Goldberg AP, Seals DR, Ehsani AA, Brennan RE, Holloszy JO. Resistive training can reduce coronary risk factors without altering VO_2max or percent body fat. *Med Sci Sports Exerc 1988;*20:150-154.

[40] Jee YS, Yoon JH, Im JH. Establishment of rehabilitative object through the differences of lumbar extension strength and subjective pain degrees between chronic low back pain patients and normal group. Exercise Science 2003;12:319-330.

[41] Jee YS, Yu BK, Lee WH. Comparison Study on Lumbar Strength and Lumbar Flexor/Extensor Ratio of Spondylolisthesis Patients and Herniated Disc Patients. Journal of Korean Physical Therapy 2002;14:133-141.

[42] Jee YS. Analysis of bone mineral density among the elderly participated in the exercise programs weekly for 1 year. Journal of Korean Geriatrics Society 2001;5:185-195.

[43] Jee YS. The effects on rehabilitative exercise on pain degree, bone mineral density, and muscular functions in patients with knee osteoarthritis. Korean Journal of Sports Medicine 2005;23:152-160.

[44] Joint National Committee (JNC) on Detection, Evaluation and Treatment of High Blood Pressure. The fifth report of the joint national committee. *Arch Intern Med 1993;*153:154-183.

[45] Kannel WB, Neaton JD, Wentworth D, Thomas HE, Stamler J, Hulley SB, Kjelsberg MO. Overall and coronary heart disease mortality rates in relation to major risk factors in 325,348 men screened for the MRFIT. Multiple Risk Factor Intervention Trial. Am Heart J 1986;112:825-836.

[46] Kappagoda CT, Haennel RG, Serrano-Fiz S, Davies DH, English TA. The hemodynamic responses to upright exercise after orthotopic cardiac transplant. *Arch Phy Med Rehabi 1993;*74:484-489.

[47] Kelemen MH. Resistance training safety and assesment guidelines for cardiac and coronary prone patients. *Med Sci Sports Exerc 1989;21*:675-677.

[48] Kelley GA, Kelley KS. Progressive resistance exercise and resting blood pressure: A meta-analysis of randomized controlled trials. Hypertension 2000;35:838-843.

[49] Kennedy HL, Whitlock JA, Sprague MK, Kennedy LJ, Buckingham TA, Goldberg RJ. Long-term follow-up of asymptomatic healthy subjects with frequent and complex ventricular ectopy. N Engl J Med 1985;312:193-197.

[50] Keteyian S, Ehrman M, Fedel F, Rhoads K. Heart rate-perceived exertion relationship during exercise in orthotopic heart transplantation patients. J Cardiopulm Rehabil Prev *1990;*10:287-293.

[51] Keteyian SJ, Levine AB, Brawner CA, Kataoka T, Rogers FJ, Schairer JR, Stein PD, Levine TB, Goldstein S. Exercise training in patients with heart failure: a randomized, controlled trial. *Ann Intern Med 1996;124*:1051-1057.

[52] Kim KJ, Shin YJ. Review of association of $Trp^{64}Arg$ polymorphism of β3-adrenergic receptor gene with obesity development. Journal of Coaching Development 2004;6:65-75.

[53] Jee YS, Ko IG, Sung YH, Lee JW, Kim YS, Kim SE, Kim BK, Seo JH, Shin MS, Lee HH, Cho HJ, Kim CJ. Effects of treadmill exercise on memory and c-Fos expression in the hippocampus of the rats with intracerebroventricular injection of streptozotocin. Neurosci Lett 2008;443:188-192.

[54] Lampman RM, Schteingart DE. Moderate and exercise obesity. *In:* Franklin BA, Gordon S, Timmis GC, editors. *Exercise and modern medicine.* Philadelphia: Williams & Wilkins; 1989.

[55] Lauer MS, Levy D, Anderson KM, Plehn JF. Is there a relationship between exercise systolic blood pressure response and left ventricular mass? The Framingham Heart Study. *Ann Intern Med 1992;*116:203-210.

[56] Lele SS, Scalia G, Thomson H, Macfarlane D, Wilkinson D, Stafford W, Khafagi F, Frenneaux M. Mechanism of exercise hypotension in patients with ischemic heart disease. *Circulation 1994;*90:2701-2709.

[57] Leutholtz BC, Ripoll I. *Exercise and disease management.* Boca Raton, Florida: CRC Press; 1999.

[58] Manninen V, Elo MO, Frick MH, Haapa K, Heinonen OP, Heinsalmi P, Helo P, Huttunen

JK, Kaitaniemi P, Koskinen P, Maenpaa H, Malkonen M, Manttari M, Norola S, Pasternack A, Pikkarainen J, Romo M, Sjoblom T, Nikkila EA. Lipid alterations and decline in the incidence of coronary heart disease in the Helsinki Heart Study. *JAMA* 1988;260:641-651.

[59] Martel GF, Hurlbut DE, Lott ME, Lemmer JT, Ivey FM, Roth SM, Rogers MA, Fleg JL, Hurley BF. Strength training normalizes resting blood pressure in 65- to 73-year-old men and women with high normal blood pressure. J Am Geriatr Soc 1999;47:1215-1221.

[60] McKelvie RS, Teo KK, McCartney N, Humen D, Montague T, Yusuf S. Effects of exercise training in patients with congestive heart failure: a critical review. *J Am Coll Cardiol 1995;*25:789-796.

[61] Meyer K, Samek L, Schwaibold M, Westbrook S, Hajric R, Lehmann M, Essfeld D, Roskamm H. Physical responses to different modes of interval exercise in patients with chronic heart failure-application to exercise training. Eur Heart J 1996;17:1040-1047.

[62] Moorcroft AJ, Dodd ME, Webb AK. Long-term change in exercise capacity, body mass, and pulmonary function in adults with cystic fibrosis. *Chest 1997;*111:338-343.

[63] Morris JN, Heady JA, Raffle PAB, Roberts CG, Parks JW. Coronary heart-disease and physical activity of work. *Lancet 1953;265*:1111-1120.

[64] National Asthma Education Program Expert Panel Report. *Guidelines for the diagnosis and management of asthma.* U.S. Department of Health and Human Services. Public Health Service. National Institutes of Health Publication; 1992.

[65] National Heart, Lung, and Blood Institute Consensus Development Panel. Treatment of Hypertriglyceridemia. *JAMA 1984;*251:1196-1200.

[66] Nickerson BG. *Asthmatic patients and those with exercise-induced bronchospasm. In:* Franklin BA, Gordon S, Timmis GC, editors. *Exercise in Modern Medicine. Philadelphia:* Williams & Wilkins; 1989.

[67] Packer M, Bristow MR, Cohn JN, Colucci WS, Fowler MB, Gilbert EM, Shusterman NH. The effect of carvedilol on morbidity and mortality in patients with chronic heart failure. U.S. Carvedilol Heart Failure Study Group. N Engl J Med 1996;334:1349-1355.

[68] Packer M, O'Connor CM, Ghali JK, Pressler ML, Carson PE, Belkin RN, Miller AB, Neuberg GW, Frid D, Wertheimer JH, Cropp AB, DeMets DL. Effect of amlodipine on morbidity and mortality in severe chronic heart failure. Prospective Randomized Amlodipine Survival Evaluation Study Group. N Engl J Med 1996;335:1107-1114.

[69] Palatini P, Graniero GR, Mormino P, Nicolosi L, Mos L, Visentin P, Pessina AC. Relation between physical training and ambulatory blood pressure in Stage I hypertensive subjects. Results of the HARVEST trial. Hypertension and Ambulatory Recording Venetia Study. *Circulation 1994;*90:2870-2876.

[70] Palmer-Mclean K, Harbst KB. Stroke and brain injury. In: American College of Sports Medicine, Durstine JL, Moore G, Painter P, Roberts S, editors. *ACSM's exercise management for persons with chronic diseases and disabilities. 3rd ed.* Champaign, IL: Human Kinetics; 2009.

[71] Palmer-McLean K. *Stroke and head injury. In: American College of Sports Medicine. ACSM's exercise managements for persons with chronic disease and disability.* Champaign, IL: Human Kinetics; 1991:169-174.

[72] Perticone F, Ceravolo R, Pujia A, Ventura G, Iacopino S, Scozzafava A, Ferraro A, Chello M, Mastroroberto P, Verdecchia P, Schillaci G. Prognostic significance of endothelial

dysfunction in hypertensive patients. *Circulation 2001;*104:191-196.

[73] Redwood DR, Goldstein RE, Hirshfeld J, Borer JS, Morganroth J, Morrow AG, Epstein SE. Exercise performance after septal myotomy and myectomy in patients with obstructive hypertrophic cardiomyopathy. *Am J Cardiol 1979;*44:215-220.

[74] Rose G. Physical activity and coronary heart disease. *Proc R Soc Med 1969;*62:1183-1187.

[75] Seo TB, Kim BK, Ko IG, Kim DH, Shin MS, Kim CJ, Yoon JH, Kim H. Effect of treadmill exercise on Purkinje cell loss and astrocytic reaction in the cerebellum after traumatic brain injury. *Neurosci Lett 2010;*13;481:178-182.

[76] Shephard RJ. Aging respiratory function and exercise. J Aging Phys Act *1993;1*:59-83.

[77] Smith EL, Reddan W, Smith, PE. Physical activity and calcium modalities for bone mineral increase in aged women. *Med Sci Sports Exerc 1981;*13:60-64.

[78] Squires RW. Cardiac rehabilitation issues for heart transplantation patients. J Cardiopulm Rehabil Prev *1990;*10:159-168.

[79] Stenstrom CH. Therapeutic exercise in rheumatoid arthritis. *Arthritis Care Res 1994;7*:190-197.

[80] Grundy SM, Bilheimer D, Chait A, Clark LT, Denke M, Havel RJ, KrisEtherton P. Summary of the second report of the National Cholesterol Education Program (NCEP) Expert Panel on Detection, Evaluation, and Treatment of High Blood Cholesterol in Adults (Adult Treatment Panel II). *JAMA 1993;*269:3015-3023.

[81] Szlachcic J, Massie BM, Kramer BL, Topic N, Tubau J. Correlates and prognostic implications of exercise capacity in chronic congestive heart failure. *Am J Cardiol 1985;*55:1037-1042.

[82] Thompson CE, Thompson TR, Albers JJ, Decedue CJ. Response of HDL cholesterol, apoprotein A-I, and LCAT to exercise withdrawal. Atherosclerosis 1985;54:65-73.

[83] Wallace JP. Obesity. *In:* American College of Sports Medicine. *ACSM's exercise managements for persons with chronic disease and disability.* Champaign, IL: Human Kinetics; 1991. p. 106-111.

[84] Williams RS. Exercise training of patients with ventricular dysfunction and heart failure. In: Wenger NK, editor. Exercise and the heart. 2nd ed. Philadelphia: FA Davis Company; 1985. p. 219-231.

[85] Wood PD, Haskell WL, Blair SN, Williams PT, Krauss RM, Lindgren FT, Albers JJ, Ho PH, Farquhar JW. Increased exercise level and plasma lipoprotein concentrations: a one-year, randomized, controlled study in sedentary, middle-aged men. Metabolism 1983;32:31-39.

[86] Wynne J, Braunwald E. The cardiomyopathies and myocardiotides: toxic, chemical, and physical damage to the heart. In: Braunwald E, editor. Heart disease: *A textbook of cardiovascular medicine.* 4th ed. Philadelphia: Saunders; 1992.

[87] Zhang X, Zhao SP, Li XP, Gao M, Zhou QC. Endothelium dependent and independent functions are impaired in patients with coronary heart disease. *Atherosclerosis 2000;*149:19-24.

[88] American College of Sports Medicine. *ACSM's guidelines for exercise testing and prescription.* 9th ed. Wolters Kluwer: Lippincott Williams & Wilkins; 2014.

[89] Dvir Z, Keating JL. Trunk extension effort in patients with chronic low back dysfunction. Spine 2003;28:685-692.

[90] Rivera-Casas C, Gonzalez-Romero R, Garduño RA, Cheema MS, Ausio J, Eirin-Lopez JM. Molecular and Biochemical Methods Useful for the Epigenetic Characterization of Chromatin-Associated Proteins in Bivalve Molluscs. Front Physiol 2017;8:490.

[91] Anuurad E, Yamasaki M, Shachter N, Pearson TA, Berglund L. ApoE and ApoC-I polymorphisms: association of genotype with cardiovascular disease phenotype in African Americans. J Lipid Res 2009;50:1472-1478.

[92] Ko IG, Park EM, Choi HJ, Yoo J, Lee JK, Jee YS. Proper exercise decreases plasma carcinoembryonic antigen levels with the improvement of body condition in elderly women. Tohoku J Exp Med 2014;233:17-23.

Appendix

[1] Garrick JG, Radersky P, editors. *Peak Condition.* New York: Harper & Row; 1988.

[2] Horowitz MB, Littenberg B, Mahler DA. Dyspnea ratings for prescribing exercise intensity in patients with COPD. *Chest 1996;109*:1169-1175.

[3] McRae R, editor. *Clinical orthopaedic examination.* London: Churchill Livingstone; 1983.

[4] Novich MM, Taylor B, editors. *Training and conditioning of athletes.* Philadelphia: Leg & Febiger; 1983.

[5] American College of Sports Medicine. *ACSM's guidelines for exercise testing and prescription.* 9th ed. Wolters Kluwer: Lippincott Williams & Wilkins; 2014.

Appendices

Appendix A. Exercise prescription formula

[Appendix A] lists the 'prescription formulas' necessary for the clinic worker who is working in the clinic to make exercise prescriptions and provide patients with more detailed exercise programs. The exercise formula should be prescribed taking the target heart rate zone of each patient into consideration. However, attention should be paid to patients who should not be prescribed at the target heart rate zone (such as those who are taking medications that can change their heart rate, or peripheral vascular disease due to diabetic complications). The exercise intensity calculated as the target heart rate is generally 40/50 to 85% of the $\dot{V}O_2max$. For patients with poor physical condition, the initial exercise intensity is set at 40% or lower. In the case of the general public, it is preferable to prescribe 50%. Of course, the goal of ultimate exercise intensity for patients and the general public is to raise the intensity to 85%.

The patient must be trained to check the heart rate on his / her wrist in order to proceed with the exercise program in the target heart rate zone. The carotid or temporal arteries can also promote heart rate, but it can be measured below the heart rate measured on a common radial artery because the baroreceptor reflex can be activated.

The heart rate is measured by palpating the pulse for 10 seconds, counting from zero at the same time as the 'start', and after 10 seconds, multiplying the pulse by 6 to convert to heart rate per minute. For example, suppose that a patient with heart failure is trying to measure a pulse at rest, 0 times at the second hand alignment, and 12 times at 10 seconds. At this time, the patient's pulse rate for 10 seconds is 12 times/10seconds, and the pulse rate for 1 minute is 72 bpm. Of course, checking the heart rate for 10 seconds may miss irregular arrhythmia. Therefore, it is desirable to measure the heart rate for 1 minute or to present exercise program using RPE for this arrhythmia patient. On the other hand, the fingers that should be used to palpate the pulse must be index and middle finger, and care should be taken not to use the thumb. This is because the thumb itself has minute pulsations, which makes it difficult to accurately measure heart rate.

[Formula 1] Maximum heart rate formula by age prediction

The method of predicting with age to calculate target heart rate is one of the simplest methods. This method is widely used in aerobic exercise and found in the walls of most health clubs. The principle is to regard the maximum predicted heart rate as 220 bpm and regard the figure as the 'maximum heart rate' by subtracting the age of the person from 220. The predicted maximum heart rate is decremented once per minute for every year. The physiological cause of decreasing the maximum heart rate one beat per minute is presumed to be functional decline of the heart and decrease of elasticity, but it is reported that there is a deviation of ± 10 bpm according to the individual. On the other hand, this method is simple but it is less used because it provides a target heart rate zone during a somewhat lower exercise than other formulas. The following 'heart rate reserve formula (Karvonen formula)' is recognized as a better exercise prescription formula. An example of maximum heart rate calculation by age is shown below.

Example 1] When a patient 58 years old is trying to exercise at 60% of his/her maximum heart rate, what is the target heart rate?

Answer] 97 bpm

Explanation] Target heart rate = (0.60) * (220 - Age)

= (0.60) * (220 - 58)

= (0.60) * (162)

= 97.2

If the patient is taking a drug that can change the heart rate (such as a beta blocker) or has a pheripheral neuropathy or chronotropic incompetence, the exercise regimen using this method is inaccurate It is considered. If the patient is taking cardiologic medications, the patient is encouraged to participate in the exercise after directly measuring the graded exercise test given in [Appendix B].

[Formula 2] Heart Rate Reserve or Karvonen method

The Heart Rate Reserve or the Karvonen method is made by taking into account the patient's resting heart rate and the maximum heart rate directly measured in the graded exercise test or the age prediction (220 - age) presented in [Formula 1]. The resting heart rate is measured with the patient taking a comfortable rest for several minutes. If the temperature is too hot or if the patient is taking caffeine, smoking, or taking other medications, it is not considered as an accurate resting heart rate. An example using a heart rate reserve or Karvonen method is as follows.

Example 2] When applying walking exercise with 40% of exercise intensity to the elderly (aged 82 years old, resting heart rate = 81bpm), what is the target heart rate?

Answer] 103 bpm

Explanation] Target heart rate = (0.40) * {(220 - Age) - resting heart rate} + resting heart rate

= (0.40) * [(220 - 82) - 81] + 81
= (0.40) * (138 - 81) + 81
= (0.40) * (57) + 81
= 22 + 81
= 103

Example 3] The heart rate was 121 times / minute when the elderly who were 79 years old and had a resting heart rate 77 times / minute walked five times in the playground. How many percent of the exercise intensity did the elderly do?

Answer] 85%

Explanation] Heart rate immediately after exercise = (Intensity) * {(220 - Age) - resting heart rate} + resting heart rate

121 = (Intensity) * {(220 - 79) - 77} + 77
121 = (Intensity) * (141 - 77) + 77
121 = (Intensity) * (64) + 77
121 = (Intensity) * 141
(Intensity) = 121÷141
(Intensity) = 0.85 * 100
(Intensity) = 85%

This formula should not be recommended for patients with pheripheral neuropathy, chronotropic incompetence, or patients taking medications that can alter resting heart rate.

[Formula 3] Rate Pressure Product Formula

The method of calculating the target heart rate by the rate pressure product (RPP) is a very unique and recommended formula. Specifically, rate refers to the rate of heart rate, pressure refers to the pressure of blood pressure, and product refers to multiplication. In other words, the heart produces electrical impulses at regular intervals, causing heart rate, and then the ventricles are opened and the blood is delivered to the whole body along the aorta at a constant blood pressure. This process is referred to as 'myocardial oxygen consumption' because its ability to deliver depends on how much oxygen the myocardium consumed. The unit of RPP has not been considered until recently, but apparently it is calculated by heart rate × blood pressure, so the unit may be expressed as bpm·mmHg. Although this formula is highly desirable for patients with ischemic thresholds, it is not recommended for patients with peripheral neuropathy or heart failure. And this method should calculate the maximum SBP, so it should be combined after GXT is done.

Example 4] The following data were reported after the graded exercise test.

SBPmax : 155 mmHg
HRmax : 128 bpm
SBPrest : 110 mmHg
HRrest : 65 bpm
RPPmax = SBPmax × HRmax/100
RPPrest = SBPrest × HRrest/100

RPPmax) = (155×128)/100 = 198 bpm*mmHg
RPPrest) = (110×65)/100 = 71 bpm*mmHg

The use of RPP can be done by substituting RPP for the Karvonen formula and dividing by 100 to simplify the calculation. From the data presented above, the target heart rate at 50% intensity can be calculated as follows.

Answer] Target RPP : 135 bpm*mmHg
Answer] Target HR : 87bpm
Explanation] Target RPP = (0.50) (RPPmax − RPPrest) + RPPrest
= (0.50) (198 − 71) + 71
= (0.50) (127) + 71
= 63.5 + 71
≒ 135

Below is a formula to determine the target heart rate corresponding to 135 bpm·mmHg, calculated as the target RPP of 50%.

$$\text{Target HR} = \frac{\text{RPPmax} = 198}{\text{TargetRPP} = 135} \qquad \frac{\text{HRmax} = 128}{\text{Target HR} = X}$$

The result of the diagonal multiplied target heart rate is about 87 bpm. This value is calculated to be 22 bpm higher than 64 bpm (128 bpm × 0.50) which is the result of calculation of the target heart rate using [Formula 1], and it can be mistaken as a somewhat high exercise intensity. However, it should be noted that 64 bpm was calculated to be lower than the resting heart rate of 65 bpm.

[Formula 4] SBP Formula

SBP can be used to suggest exercise intensity similar to heart rate. This formula is a very useful way to prescribe exercise for hypertensive patients, heart transplant patients with potential hypertension, or peripheral vascular disease. A graded exercise test is required to calculate maximum SBP, and the maximum SBP and the resting SBP calculated from the test are substituted into the Karvonen formula given in [Formula 2]. On the other hand, the age-based prediction formula presented in [Formula 1] is not recommended because it produces a lower target SBP than the patient's resting SBP. An example of SBP formulas is follows.

Example 5] A GXT was performed on patients with hypertension. The maximum SBP was 185 ㎜Hg and the resting SBP was 140 ㎜Hg. What is the corresponding target SBP when prescribing cycling with 50% exercise intensity for this patient?

Answer] 163 ㎜Hg

Explanation] Target SBP

$$\begin{aligned} &= (0.50) * (\text{SBPmax} - \text{SBPrest}) + \text{SBPrest} \\ &= \{(0.50) * (185 - 140)\} + 140 \\ &= \{(0.50) * (45)\} + 140 \\ &= 22.5 + 140 \\ &\fallingdotseq 163 \text{ mmHg} \end{aligned}$$

[Formula 5] Ratings of Perceived Exertion Formula

RPE is an easy way to record and prescribe exercise intensity and can be easily applied to patients who do not record their heart rate during exercise or are reluctant to record. Ratings of perceived exertion can be found in the RPE / Borg scale, the Dyspnea Scale, and the Angina Scale. These scales should be determined after a period of 3~5 minutes, during which the body can adapt to aerobic exercise or weight-bearing exercise. It is necessary to focus on what the body feels over the entire workout period and to educate the patient not to think of only a part of the body. For example, when walking or riding a bicycle, consider how the whole body feels, and do not think fatigue in a local part such as a leg. On the other hand, in the case of a worried person or type A person, the actual exercise intensity can be calculated to be low, and about 10% of these people can not use each scale accurately.

[Formula 6] Maximum Oxygen Uptake Formula

The $\dot{V}O_2max$ is a good standard way of describing an individual's fitness level. $\dot{V}O_2max$ is calculated by measuring the exhalation gas during the GXT and is directly proportional to the heart rate. This suggests that exercise should be prescribed at the target heart rate zone where the ratio of the target heart rate to the patient's functional capacity is equal. For example, the range of exercise intensity recommended by the ACSM is typically between 40/50 and 85% of the functional capacity. It is important to use an initial exercise intensity of 40% for patients with poor physical condition and 50% for the general people, but to provide an exercise program with an aim of 85% after improvement. On the other hand, the formula based on the $\dot{V}O_2max$ can also be calculated by multiplying the exercise intensity with the Karvonen formula. An example of this is shown below.

Example 6] GXT was performed on diabetic patients. The $\dot{V}O_2max$ was calculated as 36 ㎖/㎏/min. What is the target oxygen uptake and target heart rate when prescribing walking with 60% exercise intensity for this patient?

Answer] Target oxygen uptake : 23 ㎖/kg/min

Explanation] Target oxygen uptake = $(0.60) * (\dot{V}O_2max - \dot{V}O_2rest) + \dot{V}O_2rest$

$$= \{(0.60) * (36 - 3.5)\} + 3.5$$
$$= \{(0.60) * (32.5)\} + 3.5$$
$$= 19.5 + 3.5$$
$$= 23 \text{ ㎖/kg/min}$$

[Formula 7] Anaerobic Threshold Formula

The anaerobic threshold (AT) is defined as the point at which ventilation increases rapidly during an graded exercise test. It is hypothesized that this point occurs when exercise intensity increases lactic acid abruptly. Lactic acid has a buffering effect and is released into the body in the form of CO_2, resulting in an increase in the amount of ventilation. It is desirable to prescribe the exercise slightly below the AT or AT point, since the intensity above AT will cause fatigue and prevent the exercise from continuing. Many studies have shown that exercise in this zone can be performed by most patients without difficulty. In order to calculate the AT point, expiratory gas measurement by GXT is inevitable. On the other hand, the point indicated by hyperventilation may not be the actual AT point, and it is a professional technique of the clinical exercise prescriber to distinguish it.

[Formula 8] Ventilation Formula

Exercise prescription by the amount of ventilation is useful for patients with chronic lung disease. Specifically, the analytical process that sets 70~80% of the maximum voluntary ventilation (MVV) derived from the graded exercise test or the target heart rate zone that matches the AT is a necessary process for clinical exercise prescribers.

Appendix B. Graded Exercise Test

[Appendix B] explained the reasons why clinician exercise prescribers should conduct GXT directly in the clinic and how to interpret the variables in the derived data. In fact, a GXT can be equally named when proceeding with either a cardiac stress test or a cardiopulmonary stress test. Specifically, it is called 'cardiac stress test' when only ECG test is performed, and 'cardiopulmonary stress test' when ECG and respiratory gas test are combined.

[Test 1] Medical Screening Prior to Exercise

Medical screening prior to exercise is widely recommended for everyone to prevent disease and promote health, but there is a widespread belief that it is not necessary to do it for economic problems, temporal conditions, or younger age groups. However, men aged 40 or older and women aged 50 or older need to consult with a professional or clinician before taking part in an exercise program, even if they think they are healthy. In particular, people who start their first workouts, who have smoking, family history of heart disease or other diseases, hypertension, hyperlipemia, and long-term sedentary lifestyle are at risk for injury or sudden death during sudden exercise. Therefore, the above people must go through 'medical screening prior to exercise'. For medical screening prior to exercise, as described in the text, physical examination and blood tests may be sufficient if there is no symptoms or is below the over-age. However, for those who are over-age (male 40 years old, female 50 years old) or who are determined to require specialist observation on the symptom factor or risk factor presented in the screening test, It is desirable to perform comprehensive screening including blood test and radiography. On the other hand, the physical examination includes tests to find heart rate and blood pressure measurements and signs of musculoskeletal diseases. Blood tests help detect potential diseases through blood count, blood glucose, cholesterol, and creatinine levels.

[Test 2] Cardiac Stress Test

There was much controversy concerning the fact that cardiac stress tests should be carried out on healthy people. In particular, cardiac stress tests were performed on 3,617 patients aged 35 to 59 years. As a result, the sensitivity to detect a true positive was only 18%. This means low reliability in cardiac stress testing. However, since sudden death is a variable that can not be predicted by anyone, it is recommended to perform tests and exercise in order to minimize it. In particular, the ACSM recently recommended that all over-aged people should undergo cardiac stress testing before they begin intense exercise. In addition, ACMS suggests that patients with high cholesterol levels without symptoms are more likely to have higher exercise-related injuries and therefore have to undergo cardiac stress testing. The specific algorithm for cardiac stress testing is shown in [Fig. A.1].

In spite of the algorithms presented above, the GXT or the cardiac stress test should not be performed in the case of the following diseases or symptoms, or the symptom-limited test should be carried out based on clinical experience and knowledge. The former is called 'absolute contraindications', and the latter is called 'relative contraindications'.[5]

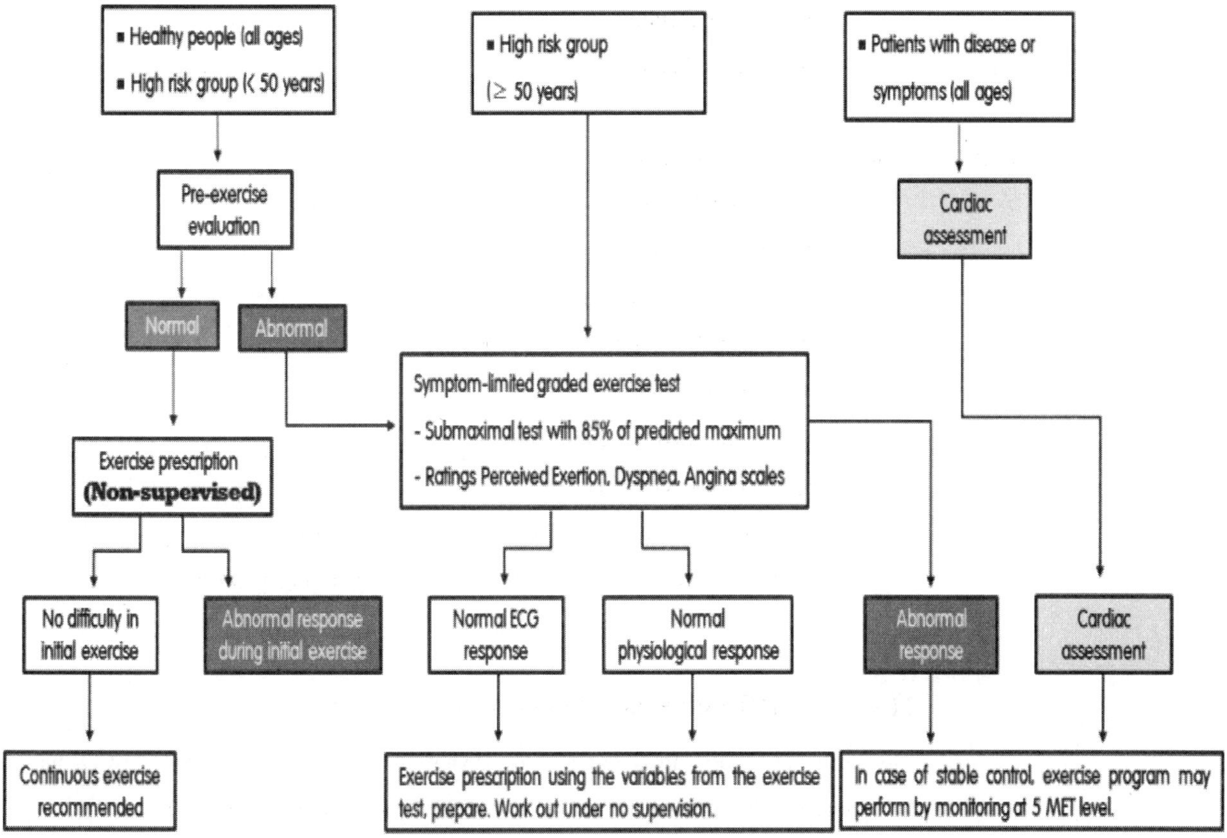

Fig. A.1 *Algorithm for cardiac stress test for each group*[5]

❖ Absolute contraindications :

- Recent changes in myocardial infarction[77)]
- Unstable CAD
- Uncontrolled arrhythmia[78)]
- 3° atrioventricular block
- Acute congestive heart failure[79)]
- Severe aortic stenosis[80)]
- Dissecting aneurysm[81)]

---

77) Myocardial infarction: Necrosis of the myocardial layer as a result of blood flow disorders, such as coronary artery thrombosis.
78) Arrhythmia: Fluctuations in normal heart rhythm (sinus arrhythmia, atrial flutter, atrial fibrillation).
79) Congestive heart failure: Clinical syndrome due to heart failure, characterized by poor breathing, swelling, and abnormal sodium and water retention.
80) Stenosis: Diseases caused by narrowed blood vessels.

- Thrombus[82] or Embolus[83]
- Acute infection
- Mental illness

❖ Relative contraindications :

- Resting blood pressure of 200/115 mmHg or more
- Moderate valve disease
- Electrolyte abnormality
- Patients with fixed rate pacemaker[84] insertion
- Ventricular aneurysm[85]
- Uncontrolled metabolic disease
- A chronic epidemic
- Musculoarticular disorder increased by exercise
- Progressive or complex disease occurring during pregnancy

[Test 3] Cardiopulmonary Stress Test

The cardiopulmonary stress test has the advantage of being able to assess ECG, lung function and metabolic changes. In this test, ECG can assess the likelihood of CAD. The pulmonary function part can assess respiratory (R), respiration rate (RR) and tidal volume (VT). The metabolic portion assesses changes in MET or calories (kcal) and the energy requirements of the work being performed. This allows for seeing at a glance how the heart, lungs and muscles are being controlled. In fact, the 'dyspnea' that occurs during intense exercise is not caused solely by the deterioration of pulmonary function, but is a symptom expressed by a specific disease such as muscle and heart. A cardiopulmonary stress test allows the examiner to determine what causes the symptoms for a patient with one or more diseases and to identify the differences between the components.

Cardiopulmonary tests can be used to diagnose functional impairment of the human

---

81) Dissecting aneurysm: Disease in which the arterial wall separates in the direction of travel due to bleeding caused by rupture of the arterial lining.

82) Thrombus: It refers to the aggregation of blood components composed of platelets and fibrin surrounding the cellular components.

83) Embolus: A blood clot carried by blood from other blood vessels. When it enters a small blood vessel, it blocks blood vessels and closes the circulation.

84) Fixed rate pacemaker: An implanted pacemaker that stimulates the heart with a predefined rhythm.

85) Ventricular aneurysm: Aneurysmal enlargement of the left ventricular wall, or a small overhang through the left ventricle.

body, to measure the degree of damage, to provide treatment, to prescribe appropriate exercise for the recovery of people with diseases, or to provide special training instructions for athletes. A stationary cycle or a treadmill can be used as a load device using the lower body, and an arm ergometer or a rowing machine can be used as an upper body device. In the following, we will learn the principles related to cardiopulmonary stress testing and how these data can be used in exercise prescriptions.

Aerobic fitness

The most demanding for aerobic endurance exercise is aerobic capacity. This is also called aerobic fitness, which refers to the ability of the heart, lungs, and circulatory system to supply oxygen to muscles and remove waste products. It is academia's opinion that an aerobic exercise program that is appropriate for individuals, whether general or athletic, heart disease, lung disease or healthy person, is very effective and safe. Cardiopulmonary stress testing provides basic information to prescribe an aerobic exercise program. For example, in healthy people, information is usually provided to exercise comfortably in a range of 50~85% of their $\dot{V}O_2max$ for 20~60 minutes. On the other hand, in the case of heart disease, information can be given to exercise within the range of $\dot{V}O_2max$ 40~70% for 15~30 minutes.

Aerobic exercise

During exercise, our skeletal muscles use carbohydrates and fats (free fatty acids) as the primary source of energy. The term 'aerobic' means that only when there is oxygen, energy can be mobilized and utilized. When exercise intensity is high, carbohydrate plays a role as energy source, and when exercise intensity becomes low, free fatty acid acts as main energy source. In fact, aerobic exercise is a long-lasting exercise that allows you to continue exercising for a long time, depending on fat stored in large quantities in many parts of the body rather than relying on carbohydrates stored in small amounts in liver and muscle.

Maximal oxygen uptake

Individual aerobic capacity means how much oxygen can be used during maximal or exhaustive exercise, which can be determined by the $\dot{V}O_2max$. In other words, the $\dot{V}O_2max$ is an individual's functional ability and is an important variable that enables the lungs to carry oxygen to the blood and the blood pump action of the heart and the process of feeding the pumped blood to the muscles . In other words, $\dot{V}O_2max$ accounts for lung, heart, and blood vessel function during maximal exercise. Ultimately, $\dot{V}O_2max$ is the "most important criterion" for evaluating fitness.

Efficiency of oxygen utilization

The efficiency of oxygen utilization is also known as the oxygen economy, which is how much muscle activity can be maximized with a relatively small amount of oxygen. In other words, it means 'maximum exercise effect of minimum oxygen use'. Strength, flexibility, appropriate weight and technical ability are important variables to support the oxygen economy. For example, a trained runner who has a good muscle strength, a flexible and light body weight can run faster, even if he uses the same amount of oxygen compared to a poor runner who has a weak muscle strength, a stiff and heavy body weight. In order to improve oxygen economy, it is necessary to improve muscular strength and flexibility with decreasing body fat, and training time for perfect technique is also important. Mathematically, oxygen economy is expressed as $\dot{V}O_2 \times work$, which is called the 'economic curve of oxygen'. Ultimately, if this slope is flat, the oxygen economy means high.

Anaerobic exercise

An anaerobic exercise is a form of exercise performed by obtaining an energy source without the use of oxygen. For example, during low intensity exercise below 50% of the maximum oxygen uptake, the energy source is produced through an aerobic biochemical pathway. However, when the work rate is increased to reach a certain point, the aerobic mechanism alone does not produce all necessary energy sources and an anaerobic mechanism is activated. However, anaerobic energy sources are 18 times more inefficient than energy sources produced aerobically. The energy source used during anaerobic exercise is derived from energy stored in the muscle or from stored glycogen in the liver, and substances such as lactic acid are produced that prevent exercise for a long time. The amount of lactic acid accumulated by anaerobic exercise is proportional to the size of excessive post-exercise oxygen consumption (formerly oxygen debt).

Oxygen debt and Excessive post-exercise oxygen consumption

Muscles also have an energy charge like a battery. The muscle maintains a charged state of the energy source in the form of chemical energy, a phosphate bond of a molecule such as ATP. If you perform a high intensity exercise (lifting, jumping, running 100-m) in a short time, the muscle will use the charged energy source to perform this exercise. Afterwards, the energy source used combusts glucose or fat with oxygen to compensate for deficiencies. In the past, the amount of oxygen used to fully supplement this shortage of energy source was called 'oxygen debt'. But now the idea of borrowing the oxygen already stored in the body and replenishing the energy source to compensate for the deficit has disappeared. Instead, the term "excessive post-exercise oxygen consumption (EPOC)" refers to the concept that the body recharges the energy source with more oxygen to compensate for the energy source shortly after exercise. It is considered to be a correct concept.

On the other hand, short-term high-intensity anaerobic exercise reduces the amount of energy in muscle and forms EPOC, but lactic acid does not necessarily accumulate in large quantities. For example, a 100-m run for 15 seconds does not produce lactic acid, but if you exercise at the same speed for a long time, the production and accumulation of lactic acid becomes excessive and the EPOC level becomes high. On the other hand, runners who are playing high-intensity, high-speed marathons are adjusting their pace with speed just before lactic acid is produced. Thus, most of the energy sources used by these runners are aerobic, and if they remain at this pace in the second half of the game, very low amounts of lactic acid accumulate or lactic acid is not produced and low EPOC is formed.

Anaerobic threshold

An AT is defined as the point at which serum lactate concentration begins to increase as exercise intensity increases. Here, serum lactate is defined as the amount of oxygen consumption that increases in proportion to exercise intensity. At this time, the slope of the ventilation curve in a straight line state is increased. Exercise intensity below AT does not produce large amounts of lactic acid to cause fatigue, but exercise intensity above anaerobic threshold gradually increases lactate and lowers serum bicarbonate concentration and increases ventilation and heart rate. In other words, the exercise above AT can not last without causing fatigue. In general, AT is formed between 50 and 85% of the maximum oxygen uptake, which is formed at a higher level of maximum oxygen uptake for a player who has continued regular training. On the other hand, in patients with long-term disease, AT is formed at a lower level of $\dot{V}O_2max$. On the other hand, if the AT level is low, anemia, heart disease, abnormalities of the systemic circulation and the pulmonary circulation due to damage of the oxygen delivery system can be . suspected. There is also a report that rarely, low levels of AT may cause musculoskeletal disorders.

Heart rate and exercise

Heart rate during exercise is an indicator of the severity of the myocardium. The heart rate does not indicate the amount of exercise performed in the peripheral muscles, but rather the intensity of the exercise. For athletes who have been trained, the resting heart rate is low and the stroke volume is high, while for the general population, the resting heart rate is high and the stroke volume is low. That is, even when two subjects are stable under the same conditions, the resistance of the athletes to the load on the atmospheric pressure is more dominant. On the other hand, it is the most accurate way to measure and record your heart rate as soon as you open your eyes in the morning in order to measure your condition or fatigue status. If you have a lot of training or disease, your heart rate measured in the morning will be high. Generally, if the heart rate measured in the morning is higher than the average by 5 bpm, it is evaluated as a disease or excessive training. If the heart rate after exercise is higher than the average by 5 bpm even though the exercise is performed at the same exercise intensity, it can be interpreted as the degree of the effect of the above-described symptoms or training.

Heart Rate, AT and RPE

Since the heart rate increases proportionally with exercise intensity, those who check their heart rate frequently during exercise may be able to guess the relationship between heart rate and exercise level. Heart rate is closely related to the level of anaerobic threshold and RPE during exercise. Let's look at an example. First, exercise below AT is perceived as easy or moderate exercise. At this time, you can talk with the other person or pronounce the long sentence clearly. When the exercise is over, the heart rate and respiration are easily returned to normal. Second, exercise in accord with AT or slightly higher than AT is self-perceived as difficult or very difficult, in which case it is not possible to communicate during exercise or it is pronounced as a short sentence. At this time, when the exercise is stopped, the short EP is continued by the high EPOC, and the heart rate is kept high. Third, exercise intensity above AT seems to be severely difficult, and exercise can not be sustained, and it maintains extreme fatigue and very high heart rate state within a short time.

[Test 4] Graded Exercise Test for Cardiopulmonary Patients

Heart Failure Patients

Cardiac output of patients with heart failure is mostly dependent on heart rate, and maximum heart rate is relatively high even at low exercise intensity. In particular, in patients with severe heart failure, exercise increases pressure (carbon dioxide partial pressure) by increasing pulmonary circulation, but this change does not necessarily cause dyspnea. Patients with heart failure have low levels of anaerobic threshold and maximum oxygen uptake. In general, AT levels in patients with heart failure are reported to be less than 40% of the predicted $\dot{V}O_2max$. Severity of patients with heart failure is somewhat related to AT and $\dot{V}O_2max$.

- In mild or absence of heart failure, $\dot{V}O_2max$ is 20 mℓ/kg/min.
- In mild to moderate heart failure, $\dot{V}O_2max$ is 16 to 20 mℓ/kg/min.
- In moderate to severe heart failure, $\dot{V}O_2max$ is 10 to 15 mℓ/kg/min.
- In severe heart failure, $\dot{V}O_2max$ is 6~9 mℓ/kg/min.
- In extremely severe heart failure, $\dot{V}O_2max$ is 6 mℓ/kg/min.

On the other hand, when patients with heart failure receive a detailed clinical exercise prescription and carry out a continuing management program, the level of AT and $\dot{V}O_2max$ can be improved. Conversely, if no intervention measures are taken, the AT and $\dot{V}O_2max$ level will continue to fall. That is, AT and $\dot{V}O_2max$ can be used as an objective evaluation index for patients with heart failure.

Pulmonary Vascular Impairment

Patients with pulmonary vascular impairment (pulmonary hypertension[86]), pulmonary embolism[87]), scleroderma[88])) exhibit similar responses to patients with heart failure during exercise and have low levels of $\dot{V}O_2max$ and AT levels during cardiopulmonary stress testing. However, there is a way to distinguish patients with pulmonary vascular

---

86) Pulmonary hypertenstion: Increased pressure in the pulmonary circulation (SBP/DBP 30/12 mmHg or higher).

87) Pulmonary embolism: Closed state due to embolization of the pulmonary artery.

88) Scleroderma: Chronic hardening and atrophy of connective tissue in all parts of the body, including the lungs.

impairment from patients with heart failure. In patients with pulmonary vascular impairment, high ventilation equivalents ($\dot{V}E/\dot{V}O_2$ and $\dot{V}E/\dot{V}CO_2$) are measured at AT and high dead space ventilation ($\dot{V}D/\dot{V}T$) is measured at maximal exercise. Other abnormalities observed in patients with pulmonary artery disease include increased oxygen partial pressure difference in the alveolar artery and increased partial pressure of CO_2 at the aortic end. On the other hand, as with patients with heart failure, the severity of pulmonary vascular disease is somewhat related to AT levels and $\dot{V}O_2max$.

Using AT level in Patients with Heart Failure or Pulmonary Vascular Impairment

Patients whose disease is managed to a certain degree of stability are able to perform low-intensity exercise with their heart rate below their AT level. However, you should refrain from exercise that belongs to the exercise intensity equal to or higher than the AT level. If you continue exercising beyond the AT level, you may endanger life.

Restrictive Pulmonary Diseases

Patients with restrictive pulmonary diseases have lower lung volumes than normal people. Patients with restrictive pulmonary disease in both lungs and limited pulmonary disease in patients with local pulmonary disease or outside the lung (e.g, pleura or chest) can be classified as diffusing capacity. During exercise, the tidal volume (TV: breathing air volume per breath) increases until it reaches half of lung capacity (the amount of air taken from the maximal inspiration to the maximal expiration), and this increase is achieved by increasing respiratory rate. Patients with restrictive pulmonary disease are characterized by a respiration rate of more than 40 reps per minute and may exhibit abnormal responses to oxygen transport from the lung to arterial blood. There is, of course, a high correlation between the degree of diffusing capacity impairment and the observed abnormalities during exercise, but the degree of abnormal oxygen transport can not be predicted solely by the pulmonary function test data obtained from the clinic.

Obstructive Impairment

Patients with obstructive impairment are characterized by reduced air volume. These patients are generally divided into two groups. Type A is called "Pink Puffers," which are patients with emphysema[89)] who have lost the elasticity of the lungs, with a high number of broken alveoli, a reduced alveolar surface area, and poor gas carrying capacity. Also, arterial oxygen and carbon dioxide partial pressures are usually normal or low. On the other hand, Type B is called "Blue Bloaters", which are suffering from chronic bronchitis. Type B patients did not have larger lung volume than normal Type A patients, and the alveolar surface area was normal. However, it is characterized by the fact that the lungs are insufficiently ventilated and thus cause problems in gas transportation. Their arterial oxygen partial pressure is normal or low, and arterial carbon dioxide partial pressure is normal or high. Exercise reverses arterial oxygen partial pressure.

Patients with emphysema have a tendency to lower arterial oxygen partial pressure, but patients with bronchitis tend to have increased arterial oxygen partial pressure. The changes in arterial oxygen partial pressure during exercise can not be predicted from the resting data, but can be confirmed by the forced expiratory volume-one second (FEV_1). Patients with FEV_1 less than 1.0 tend to have decreased arterial oxygen partial pressure during exercise. The tidal volume increases during exercise, but unlike patients with restrictive pulmonary disease, the tidal volume does not reach half of the lung capacity. In spite of the increased respiratory quotient, the respiratory rate does not exceed 40 per minute.

Patients with mixed pulmonary disease and impairment often have low fitness levels. If the muscles become weak, they cause dyspnea during exercise, and when the respiratory damage worsens, the dyspnea becomes even worse. Walking, stair climbing, shopping, and other daily activities also have many difficulties to perform. Furthermore, in patients with sedentary lifestyle due to illness, muscle weakness is exacerbated, making dyspnea worse. On the other hand, exercise programs are not appropriate for patients with lung problems, but can increase their athletic performance. If there is cardiopulmonary stress testing and metabolic control data, exercise prescriptions for patients with pulmonary disease can be prescribed by one of the methods in [Table A.1].

89) Emphysema: A state of morbid air accumulation in lung tissues or organs.

Table A.1 ***Exercise prescription and basis for patients with lung disease***

① Exercise at the same target heart rate as AT and exercise at 70~80% or less of MVV
Some patients may not be able to reach the AT because the condition of the lungs is too damaged, but if the patient can reach the AT, set the heart rate to be slightly below that level. On the other hand, it is reasonable to prescribe exercise at a heart rate consistent with 70~80% of MVV for patients who can not exercise to AT or who use a respiration volume close to 100% at AT.
② Exercise at AT level
A significant effect can be expected if the patients with mild lung disease perform the exercise at a point that matches the AT level. In a study of patients with mild chronic obstructive pulmonary disease (COPD) admitted to the hospital, the variables including the decrease in the ventilation rate per minute were significantly improved compared with the patients who exercised at the AT level or below the AT level.
③ Exercise at MVV 95%
Patients with moderate to severe COPD were able to maintain ventilation at high MVV levels. According to one study, 52 patients exercised at their MVV 95% intensity and the majority of patients did not continue to exercise for a few minutes, but their endurance was significantly increased. In addition, it was observed that the exercise time of the patients was increased and dyspnea and fatigue were decreased.
④ Exercise with Dyspnea scale
It is desirable to use the Dyspnea scale when patients with moderate to severe respiratory disease have limited exercise due to dyspnea. The Dyspnea scale is similar to the RPE, ranging from 0.5 (rarely seen) to 10 (no longer patronized). On the Dyspnea scale, 3 corresponds to 50% of VO_2max and 6~7 corresponds to 85%. Horowitz, Littenberg, and Mahler (1996) analyzed the cardiopulmonary stress test and the Dyspnea scale for COPD patients, which proved to be highly accurate and reliable. Therefore, it is desirable to educate these patients in advance to observe their condition by checking the Dyspnea scale themselves when performing routine tasks.

Ultimately, the exercise prescription chart for patients with pulmonary disease is shown in [Fig. A.2], the test results for general clinical exercise prescription in [Fig. A.3], the exercise program record chart in [Fig. A.4], and the management chart in [Fig. A.5].[1,2,5]

EXERCISE PRESCRIPTION
(Pulmonary Dx)

Name :
I.D. # :
Date :
M.D. :
Referring physician :

Age :
Sex :
Height :
Weight :

History :

	BEFORE :	AFTER :	% CHG
PFTS	FVC =	FVC =	% =
(liters)	FEV_1 =	FEV_1 =	% =
	MVV =	MVV =	% =
	FEV_1/FVC =	FEV_1/FVC =	% =

AEROBIC :	Measured	Measured
$\dot{V}O_2max$ (liters)		
$\dot{V}O_2max$/pred.	85%	
HRmax (220-age)		
HR @ 60% HRR		
HR @ 70% $\dot{V}Emax$		
HR @ AT	*	
O_2/HR (mℓ/beat)	*	
AT as % of $\dot{V}O_2max$	>40%	
$\dot{V}O_2$ @ AT	*	

Reason for stopping the test :

BREATHING RESERVE :	NORNAL	Measured
	1 - ($\dot{V}Emax$/MVV) > 30%	
	MVV - $\dot{V}Emax$ > 15L	

RESPIRATORY :	Predicted	Measured
$\dot{V}E$ (liters)		
$\dot{V}D/\dot{V}T$: Rest/Max	0.35/0.25	
$\dot{V}E/\dot{V}O_2$: $\dot{V}E/\dot{V}CO_2$	24~26	
Pulse oximetry :	Rest/Max > 85%	

CARDIAC : BP : Rest : ____________ Max : ___________
ECG :

IMPRESSION :

(AT = Anaerobic Threshold), HRR = Heart Rate Reserve)

Fig. A.2 *Exercise prescription chart for patients with pulmonary disease*[2]

EXERCISE TEST RESULTS

ID: - - Name: F / M years Test date : YY-MM-DD

Cardiopulmonary Function

$\dot{V}O_2$peak	Max HR	Intensity	Test time	VT(or AT)
mℓ/kg/min	bpm	MET	min sec	mℓ/kg/min

Results

$\dot{V}O_2$peak level : Low Fair Average Good High

Target Heart Rate :

Respiratory Quotient Ranges :

ECG opinion :

GXT opinion :

Body Composition

Height	Weight	WHR	Fat Mass	% Fat	Lean Mass
cm	kg		kg	%	kg

Results

Lipid profiles

TC : mg/dℓ

TG : mg/dℓ

HDL: mg/dℓ

LDL: mg/dℓ

CDRR :

BMD(T-score) :

Musculoarticular Function

Total Opinions

Fig. A.3 *Test results for general clinical exercise prescription*

Exercise Session Programs

Prescribed Date : YY-MM-DD

ID	Name	Gender / Age	Exercise Objects
			* *

Comment & Attention

	Retest	①	YY-MM-DD	③	YY-MM-DD
		②	YY-MM-DD	④	YY-MM-DD

Exercise Prescription

Warm Up	Standing Stretch & Calisthenic Exercise × 5min

		Items	THR	Speed	Intensity	Time	other
Work Out	Aerobic Exercise	Leg-Ergometer	bpm	rpm	watt	min	
		Arm-Ergometer	bpm	rpm	watt	min	
		Treadmill	bpm	kph		min	

		Items	1RM	TRM		Rep			Sets			Setting		
				%	Kg							L	A	T
Work Out	Weight Training	① Leg press		40		10	12	15	1	2	3			
		② Leg extension		45		10	12	15	1	2	3			
		③ Leg curl		50		10	12	15	1	2	3			
		④ Back extension		55		10	12	15	1	2	3			
		⑤ Abdomen curl		60		10	12	15	1	2	3			
		⑥ Torso		65		10	12	15	1	2	3			
		⑦ Chest press		70		10	12	15	1	2	3			
		⑧ Butter fly		75		10	12	15	1	2	3			
		⑨ Pull down		80		10	12	15	1	2	3			
		⑩ Rowing		85		10	12	15	1	2	3			
		⑪ Biceps		90		10	12	15	1	2	3			
		⑫ Triceps		95		10	12	15	1	2	3			

Work Out	Rehab Protocol	Joint : Lumbar/ Cervical/ Hip/ Knee/ Ankle/ Shoulder/ Elbow/ Wrist Manual intervention : ( ) part × ( ) min TENS intervention : ( ) part × ( ) min Cybex exercise (CPM/ Isokinetics/ Isometrics) : [ ] Others : [ ]
Warm Down		① Basic Stretch / ② Stretch for LBP / ③ Specific Stretch c̄ PNF [sign]

Fig. A.4 *Exercise program record chart*

EXERCISE TEST RESULTS

ID		Name		Gender		Birth		Test Date	

Items	Variables		Result	Reference
Body Composition	Height(㎝)			
	Weight(㎏)			
	Muscle Mass(㎏)			
	Fat Mass(㎏)			
	Percent Fat(%)			
	WHR			
	BMI(㎏/㎡)			
	BMR(㎉)			
	Ideal Weight(㎏)			
	Ideal Fat(㎏)			
	Ideal Muscle(㎏)			
	Posture			
Graded Exercise Test	GAS	VO_2 max		
		Exercise Time		
		VE BTPS		
		RR/min		
		VT BTPS		
		VCO_2 STPD		
		VO_2 STPD		
		R		
		VEO_2		
		$VECO_2$		
		METS		
		㎉/min		
		Work Watt		
		O_2 Pulse		
	VT	VO_2/㎏		
		R		
		VE BTPS		
		RR/min		
		Work Watt		
		METS		
		㎉/min		
	ECG	RHR(bpm)		
		MHR(bpm)		
		RSBP(㎜Hg)		
		MSBP(㎜Hg)		
		RDBP(㎜Hg)		
		MDBP(㎜Hg)		
		RPP		
		MPP		
		RSTlevelII(㎜)		
		MSTlevelII(㎜)		
		RSTlevelV2(㎜)		
		RSTlevelV2(㎜)		
		RSTlevelV5(㎜)		
		RSTlevelV5(㎜)		

Items	Variables		Result	Reference
Isokinetic Muscular Function Test	KNEE 60d/s	RF		-
		RE		-
		R HQR		50%
		LF		-
		LE		-
		L HQR		50%
		F DR		±10%
		E DR		±10%
	KNEE 180d/s	RF		-
		RE		-
		R HQR		55%
		LF		-
		LE		-
		L HQR		55%
		F DR		±10%
		E DR		±10%
	KNEE 240d/s	RF		-
		RE		-
		R HQR		60%
		LF		-
		LE		-
		L HQR		60%
		F DR		±10%
		E DR		±10%
	TRUNK 30d/s	E		-
		F		-
		TEF		≥100%
	TRUNK 60d/s	E		-
		F		-
		TEF		≥100%
	TRUNK 120d/s	E		-
		F		-
		TEF		≥100%
Bone Scan	Total BMD(g/㎠)			
	Total T-score2			-1.0≤
	Calcium (g)			
	Region BMD (g/㎠)	HEAD		
		ARMS		
		LEGS		
		TRUNK		
		RIBS		
		PELVIS		
		SPINE		
Evaluation				

Fig. A.5 *Exercise program management chart*

Appendix C. Exercise and Injury

As with both sides of the coin, exercise is fun, but also dangerous. However, exercise injuries are not common. On the other hand, the most common athletic injuries can be trauma or overuse, but it should not be overlooked as all organs of the human body may be injured by exercise. Therefore, this chapter divided the human body by the organ system and examined what kind of injury may occur during exercise.

[Injury 1] Cardiovascular system

Exercise increases the size of the heart and may also indicate changes in the ECG accompanied by disease-free arrhythmia. This is called "athlete's heart" and its function is considered to be superior to "normal heart". However, these heart changes can also lead to misleading diagnoses in the case of unskilled examiners. On the other hand, intense exercise can cause myocardial infarction in patients with CAD. This is one reason why exercise testing is recommended for patients suspected of having CAD, and it is helpful for subjects who want to participate in intense exercise even if the sensitivity is low. CAD and cardiac arrhythmia are the most serious diseases of sudden death associated with exercise. Symptoms of the aforementioned diseases include palpitations[90)], dizziness, light-headedness, pain or discomfort in the chest and upper abdomen, the jaw and left arm.[3,4]

[Injury 2] Endocrine system

Abnormal menstrual cycles are common in female athletes with low body fat (< 20%). However, the menstrual cycle returns to normal with weight gain. In abnormal cases, estrogen[91)] production is presumably decreased. An important problem associated with reduced estrogen levels is not the irregularity of the menstrual cycle, but the demineralization[92)] of the bones due to low estrogen levels, and the resulting osteoporosis

90) Palpitation: Excessive heartbeat that the patient can feel. It may be regular or irregular.

91) Estrogen: Female hormone. In humans, estrogen is produced in the ovaries, adrenal cortex, testes, and fetal placenta. It has various functions in the development. It manifests the second characterization of women and creates an environment suitable for menstrual cycle interval, exercise of female genitalia, fertilization, implantation, and nutrition of the early embryo. Estrogen is also used as an oral contraceptive pill, postmenopausal breast and prostate cancer progress inhibitors. Other uses include reduction of post-menopausal discomfort, inhibition of lactation, osteoporosis, ovarian disease, and severe menstrual hyperactivity.

92) Demineralization: Mineral loss in bone. It is present in pulmonary tuberculosis, cancer, and osteomalacia.

is considered a serious problem. On the other hand, other endocrine diseases can be summarized as hypoglycemia which can occur in diabetic patients.[3,4]

[Injury 3] Ophthalmology

The injuries associated with exercise-induced ophthalmologic injuries are not except for direct eye trauma. Only patients with diabetic retinopathy may have visual disturbances due to capillary rupture during intense exercise. However, there is a conflicting opinion that it may not be.

[Injury 4] Gastrointestinal system

Exercise often causes heartburn93) symptoms due to acid reflux from the stomach to the esophagus. On the other hand, exercise is good for relieving constipation because it increases the fluidity of the gastrointestinal system, but it can cause abdominal cramps and sometimes diarrhea. Gastrointestinal hemorrhage is observed in marathon runners and athletes experiencing ulcerative colitis94) when these conditions worsen.

[Injury 5] Hematologic system

The problem of exercise-related hematologic systems is abated by iron deficiency, regardless of anemia. Patients with chronic gastrointestinal blood loss experience iron-deficiency anemia, and athletes are reported to experience iron-deficiency reactions without anemia. The so-called "sports anemia" is not actually anemia. This is due to a dramatic increase in training intensity in the early stages of the sport program. Sports anemia is caused by an increase in plasma volume that can contribute to cardiac output, resulting in diluted hemoglobin concentration in the blood. Whether iron-deficiency without anemia is beneficial to an athlete or not is unknown.[3,4]

[Injury 6] Muscle pain/injury

Vigorous exercise results in a proportional muscular injury depending on the strength, time, or type of exercise. Muscle pain caused by exercise is related to the regulation of

---

93) Heartburn: Burning sensation in the posterior part of the sternum.

94) Ulcerative colitis: It is a recurrent ulcer. It occurs in the mucous membrane and in the lower part of the mucous membrane and the cause is unclear. Clinically, it is characterized by abdominal pain, rectal hemorrhage, blood, pus, and diarrhea with a very small division of mucus. Symptoms include hemorrhoids, abscesses, colon perforations, pseudopolyps, and cancer.

muscle fibers and collagen. The best way to prevent muscle pain is to continue low intensity exercise until the pain disappears. Exercise in an extremely vigorous situation can cause life-threatening muscular injuries.[3,4]

[Injury 7] Pulmonary vascular system

Injury caused by exercise associated with the pulmonary vascular system is asthma, which accounts for about 5~12% of the population. See the text.

[Injury 8] Integumentary system

Skin-related diseases are usually mild and are easy to prevent. The disease includes Papillitis and the like, which are usually found in people who are jogging. Although the clothes rub against the nipple, it can be prevented by attaching a bandage to the nipple. Inflammation of the inside of the femur and axilla is caused by friction between skin and skin, which can be prevented by Vaseline. Tinea pedis95) and tinea cruris96) are also common skin diseases. This can be treated with tolnaftade cream. The hemorrhage under the toenail (often seen on the toes of the runners, tennis players) can be prevented by wearing half-size-large shoes. Eventually, exercise can cause itching and skin rash diagnosed by sweat allergies. This is called "exercise-related urticaria" and is caused by histamine release.[3,4]

[Injury 9] Urinary system

Exercise-induced hemodynamics and hormonal changes cause renal vasoconstriction and markedly decrease glomerular filtration rate. Drugs that cause renal vasoconstriction cause exercise-induced kidney failure in athletes, but this is rarely reported. Typical exercise-related urticaria, including proteinuria and microscopic hematuria, is a mild disease. One danger is that these mild illnesses are likely to worsen into serious diseases such as nephritis97). Exercise-induced renal failure can be caused by the complications of rhabdomyolysis98) and secondary dehydration associated with heat, vigorous exercise, and the use of renal arteriovenous fistulas such as non-steroidal anti-inflammatory agents.

---

95) Tinea pedis: It is a chronic superficial mycosis between the toes and the soles of the feet. It is caused by trichophyton species or dermatophytes. Symptoms are skin maceration, cracking, desquamation and severe itching.

96) Tinea cruris: It appears well in the groin, perineum and adjacent areas, and is acute or chronic. It is often accompanied by tinea pedis. The causative organism is the same and it is characterized by severe pruritus.

97) Nephritis: Diffuse, proliferative, destructive inflammation that invades the tubules, neonatal vaginal tissue.

98) Rhabdomyolysis : Collapse or dissolution of muscle accompanied by urinary excretion of myoglobin.

[Injury 10] Musculoskeletal system

Injuries occur as a result of accidents and trauma. Pain and disability occur suddenly when an injury occurs, and accurate assessment, diagnosis, and treatment are required. Pain is not caused by an accident or trauma but by overuse of the body part or abnormal structure. Such pain usually starts slowly, it is difficult to recognize the cause, and a case of misdiagnosis or improper treatment occurs. It is not possible to cause injury or pain with only the wrong attitude, and most of the problems are caused by flexibility. Specifically, injuries do not occur even if there is a problem with the posture when the flexibility of the joint is good. However, in spite of maintaining a good posture, lack of flexibility can not endure the stimulation of the exercise and eventually causes injury. The ligaments and tissues surrounding the less flexible joints are torn apart as a result of the activity. These mild ruptures proceed through inflammation, swelling and pain for a long time. Pain is caused by compensatory changes to minimize disability. Appropriate flexibility, posture, and strength measurements should be avoided if the subject has pain. After the pain has subsided, a policy for correcting the problem should be established. Exercise programs to increase endurance, strength, and flexibility are not enough, and the program should include proper balance training and posture correction.[3,4]

Exercise therapy needed to correct erroneous biomechanical problems is presented in the 'back pain' section of this book. For reference, a reinforcement program is recommended because the abdominal muscles will fall when low back pain occurs. However, inaccurate sit-ups to strengthen the abdominal muscles can aggravate low back pain. If it is difficult to perform sit-ups, it may be desirable to strengthen the abdominal muscles through hip flexion exercises.

[Injury 11] Overuse injuries

Overuse injuries can be divided into acute and chronic. In the case of acute injury, it is mainly a result of trauma. Pain, swelling and functional incompetence occur during acute injury. If the pain worsens, continuous care and treatment are needed. There are other types of sports injuries that progress slowly due to frequent trauma to bones or guns. Early pain is negligible and can be tolerated easily. This is often considered simply annoying to the players. For an athlete, pain is easily overlooked in daily life as well as during exercise, but should not be neglected.

Other injuries are chronic. Overuse injuries occur frequently, accounting for 30~50%

of all sports injuries. Unlike acute injuries, chronic injuries are often misdiagnosed and misdiagnosed. Chronic overuse injuries are most often caused by biomechanical problems, lack of training, or problems associated with the facility. Rest and anti-inflammatory drugs can treat these injuries, but injury is likely to recur if the biomechanical condition is abnormal but not corrected. Examples of biomechanical abnormal conditions include 'shin splint[99]' and bowleg. Wrong training usually means "too much too soon", and if you run too many distances too quickly, you may experience fatigue fractures in your tibia. On the other hand, a tennis elbow is an overuse injury caused by a lack of skill in which an elbow is excessively moved forward or a wrist is opened during a backhand stroke.[3,4]

Overuse injuries caused by improper equipment or tools include running on a hard surface, using too much racket, or using inappropriate shoes. Overuse injury can affect tendons, bones, bursae, ligaments, muscles and even nerves involved in movement. Ironically, there are also a number of studies showing that physical activity is not harmful to joints and that overuse does not cause arthritis, and exercise plays an important role in rehabilitation and treatment for patients with joint problems.

[Injury 12] Tendinitis

The tendon is a connective tissue that connects muscles and bones. Tendon is reported to be at high risk of injury due to insufficient blood circulation. Tendinitis, on the other hand, occurs easily when a bad posture is caused by excessive friction between the tendon and bone, when it is too much stimulation, or when the tendon is weak. Treatment of tendinitis includes physical therapy such as 3 days rest after heat treatment (hot pack) and cold treatment (ice pack), and anti-inflammatory medicine is also helpful. Steroid[100] injections can only be injected once. Two times are dangerous, and three times are absolutely prohibited. Steroids can only be injected around the tendon, not the tendon itself. Ultrasound[101] is used to inject drugs into infected areas. A massage that causes intense friction improves blood circulation and helps stretch tendons. If the inflammation subsides, rehabilitate with muscle strength and stretching exercises and strengthen the wound area with progressive principle to prevent recurrence.

---

99) Shin splint: It is characterized by pain along the tibia as a contusion of the long flexor muscle of toes that occurs to the athlete.

100) Steroid: Name for a group of lipids containing hydrogenated cyclopentophenanthrene rings. These include progesterone, corticosteroids, sex hormones, bile acids, sterols [cholesterol], saponins and some carcinogenic hydrocarbons.

101) Ultrasound: Mechanical radiant energy with a frequency of at least 20,000 cycles per second.

[Injury 13] Bursitis

Bursitis[102)] refers to a state of inflammation in the bursa. The bursa is a small pouch that is filled with oily fluid, and the tendon or ligament is located in the area where the bone rubs. Overuse occurs due to excessive friction of tendons or ligaments and bones, resulting in tendonitis or bursitis, and both. Occasionally, bursitis may also be caused by direct trauma to the bursa. When the bursa is infected, the area becomes thick, and the oily fluid is mixed and filled with calcium. If inflammation persists, the bursa turns into a hard scar filled with calcium. Bursitis is treated with rest and anti-inflammatory drugs. Calcium-precipitated furuncle bursa rapidly progresses. Fluid and steroid aspiration[103)] improves bursitis, after which the calcium deposits disappear. If the treatment process is too late and there is no response to treatment, surgery is the only type of treatment available.

[Injury 14] Fatigue fracture

Bones have the ability to grow and recover by themselves. When starting training or increasing the intensity of training, the bones are adapted by muscle activity. This creates a new part of the bone, and is directed to the cell to remove the old bone. In other words, better bones are created to accommodate new demands. However, if the training is too excessive, it will cause problems. That is, when new bone formation fails to keep up with the rate at which bone is removed, fatigue fractures occur. Fatigue fractures occur frequently in areas such as bones of foot, tibia, and femoral neck that are in contact with the hip joint, which must endure weight bearing. Renal disease, malnutrition, secondary amenorrhea, or prolonged joint fixation can make the bones weaker and double the risk of fatigue fractures.[3,4]

Fatigue fractures are accompanied by pain at the same time as activity, and the degree of pain can be confirmed by palpation. If the fracture has progressed for the first 3 weeks, it may not appear on the X-ray, but most can be identified. The average duration of treatment for fatigue fractures is 7~8 weeks, and medications that reduce pain include magnesium, calcium, or vitamin B and hormone replacement therapy. It is better to modify the type of exercise than to stop exercising. At least once a week for stability, alternating low-intensity and high-intensity training, and cross-training through sport of other sporting events help prevent fatigue fractures.

---

102) Bursitis: It is an inflammation of the bursa. This may be accompanied by calcification in the underlying Supraspinatus tendon. The most common is Deltoid Bursitis.

103) Aspiration: A treatment technique that sucks out liquid or gas from the hole.

[Injury 15] Nerve entrapment

The human body has several nerves flowing through the muscles and into the special course between the bone pathways and the ligaments, where nerve entrapment can occur. Weightlifting and rowing athletes can compress the median nerve[104)] and radial nerve[105)] near the elbow because the brachial muscles are overdeveloped. Athletes with frequent wrists, such as cyclists, can constrain the median nerve (carpal tunnel syndrome) or ulnar nerve[106)] (handlebar paralysis) of the wrist. In case of runners, running on a road can also cause compression of the posterior tibial nerve or fibula of the foot. The result is weakness accompanied by pain, paralysis or tingling. This is similar to a patient with a spinal disease. If you have any of these symptoms, you should consult your doctor.

Sometimes the opposite happens. Patients with nerve compression may think that the spine is abnormal. The sciatic nerve[107)] is very close to piriformis (a small muscle located under the gluteus maximus muscle in the buttocks). About 20% of the population has sciatic nerve penetrating piriformis. Eventually, the nerve is pressed by these muscles, causing pain in the buttocks, and the pain on the back of the legs and feet. Therefore, most patients with this type of pain suffer from lumbar spine, which is likely to be mistaken for back pain. The more confusing it is that the "Straight-Leg Raising Test" shows the same positive response in patients with piriformis and sciatica. It should be diagnosed by examiner to see if it is pain caused by lifting the leg while bending the knee or pain caused by piriformis stretching method. Treatment of nerve compression includes anti-inflammatory, steroid injections, surgery, and rehabilitation.

[Injury 16] Thermal injuries

Energy produced during exercise is converted to work energy (25%) and thermal energy (75%). The heat produced is removed by radiation[108)], convection[109)], and

104) Median nerve: It is distributed in all flexor muscles of the forearm including lumbricals and flexes the forearm.

105) Radial nerve: It is distributed in triceps brachii and spirally surrounds the back of the upper arm. It is distributed in all muscles of the back of the forearm and receives perception from the skin of the forearm and hand. Because it is close to the upper arm, fracture of humerus can cause serious injury.

106) Ulnar nerve: It is mainly distributed in the ulnar flexor of wrist and deep flexor muscle of fingers, and the sensory nerve also plays a role in this area. If you are hit by the nerve, you will feel stabbing pain.

107) Sciatic nerve: It is the largest and longest nerve in the human body. It is divided into the common peroneal nerve and tibial nerve, which are two end points, descending from the pelvis to the buttocks and coming down the back of the thigh.

108) Radiation: Direct heat transfer to surrounding objects. Regardless of the air temperature around the body, the lower the object temperature, the greater the amount of heat transferred.

109) Convection: The movement of heat by the movement of air. The warmer air rises and the colder air falls.

evaporation. Evaporation of sweat is very important. Dehydration, older age, drugs (diuretics and anticholinergics) that interfere with body temperature control make it prone for people to get heat-related diseases. This is called thermal injuries. Symptoms of thermal injuries in the body include heat cramps, heat stroke, and heat exhaustion. Heat cramps refer to muscle cramps due to dehydration associated with exercise. Patients with heatstroke complain of fever (usually higher than 39.44°C), nausea, convulsions, headaches and dizziness, but sweat naturally spills. On the other hand, the symptoms of heat exhaustion patients are similar to those of heat stroke patients, but they are different from heat cramps in that the mind is confused, the skin becomes dry, and hypotension occurs. Preventing thermal injuries is to take moderate water and avoid exercise in hot, humid weather. It is necessary to drink plenty of water before and during exercise, and drinking salt or electrolytes is not very helpful.[3,4]

On the other hand, cold-related diseases have hypothermia and frostbite. Exposure to cold weather or entering cold water can lower the core temperature and cause hypothermia (core temperature falling below 35℃). Symptoms include confusion, tremor, and chills, which can lead to muscle stiffness, lethargy, coma, metabolic acidosis, and arrhythmia. Frostbite cases are common in the toes, fingers, ears, nose, and penis. The symptoms start with pain and are accompanied by paralysis and paleness of the infected site. The treatment of the frostbite is to warm the body slowly in warm water (42℃). At this time, the infected area may be reddened and painful. Patients with hypothermia should be covered with a blanket and moved to a warm place. Covering an electric blanket too quickly or bathing too quickly in warm water should be avoided as deep temperature and redistribution of blood to the skin may not occur.

Appendix D. Flowchart of clinical exercise prescription and rehabilitation exercise

Exercise for the general public or for the patient offers several advantages as described in the text. However, if the subject does not exercise well, it can cause "adverse effects". For example, if a person performs an erroneous exercise, his or her physical structure and function may be impaired, psychologically unstable or depressed, and socially lost or shrinked. Therefore, exercise should be scientifically and precisely prescribed to prevent such injuries. As shown in [Fig. A.6], it is most desirable to prescribe exercise by combining with health screening at the clinic. Depending on the outcome of the prescription, patients with independent gait or cerebrovascular disease (CVD) should be treated with a treatment program in the motor function care unit. Patients with an abnormality in the muscles of the joints should have a treatment program in the relaxation room. Patients with an joint problem and uncomfortable gait need to be treated in a rehabilitation room. After a certain improvement in health, it is advisable to carry out exercise programs in the aquatic and healthcare facilities.

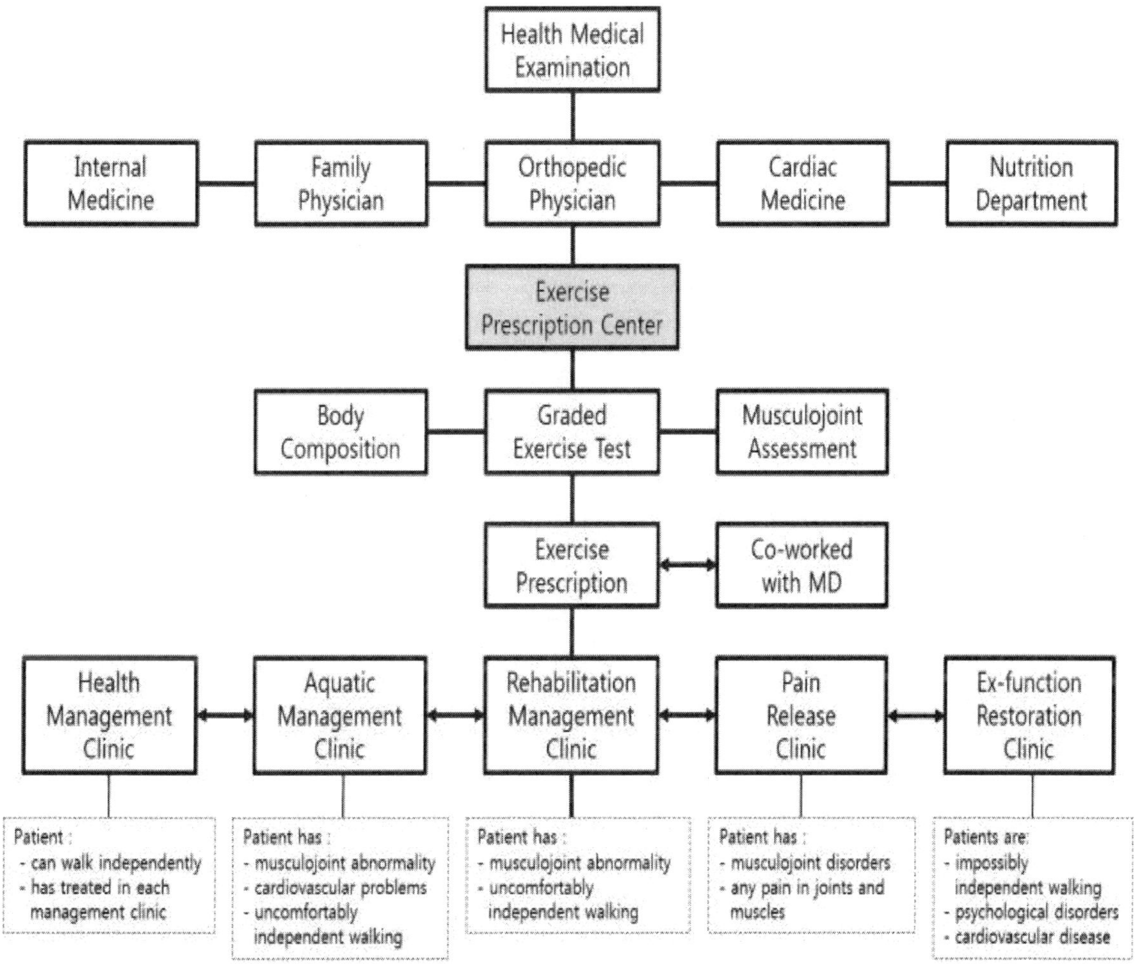

Fig. A.6 *Flowchart of clinical exercise prescription and rehabilitation movement in the clinic*

Index

(B)

(C)

(D)

(E)

(N)

(O)

(P)

(Q)

(R)

(S)

(T)

Mechanisms of Clinical Exercise Prescription

Author Yong-Seok Jee · Kang-Ho Kim
Publisher Kyoung-Hwa Lee
Publishing company 21st Publishing

Address (3F, Wonjin Plaza, Ssangnim-dong) 293-1, Toegye-ro, Jung-gu, Seoul, Republic of Korea, 04560
TEL 82-2-2269-6561
FAX 82-2-2269-6568
E-mail 21publish@naver.com

Registration 12 February 1991.(1-1128)

First printing 2 January 2018
First published 5 January 2018

₩ 25,000

ISBN 978-89-6131-052-9 93600